Vol. 29. **The Analytical Chemistry of Sulfur and Its Compounds** (*in three parts*). By J. H. Karchmer

Vol. 30. **Ultramicro Elemental Analysis.** By Günther Tölg

Vol. 31. **Photometric Organic Analysis** (*in two parts*). By Eugene Sawicki

Vol. 32. **Determination of Organic Compounds: Methods and Procedures.** By Frederick T. Weiss

Vol. 33. **Masking and Demasking of Chemical Reactions.** By D. D. Perrin

Vol. 34. **Neutron Activation Analysis.** By D. De Soete, R. Gijbels, and J. Hoste

Vol. 35. **Laser Raman Spectroscopy.** By Marvin C. Tobin

Vol. 36. **Emission Spectrochemical Analysis.** By Morris Slavin

Vol. 37. **Analytical Chemistry of Phosphorus Compounds.** Edited by M. Halmann

Vol. 38. **Luminescence Spectrometry in Analytical Chemistry.** By J. D. Winefordner, S. G. Schulman and T. C. O'Haver

Vol. 39. **Activation Analysis with Neutron Generators.** By Sam S. Nargolwalla and Edwin P. Przybylowicz

Vol. 40. **Determination of Gaseous Elements in Metals.** Edited by Lynn L. Lewis, Laben M. Melnick, and Ben D. Holt

Vol. 41. **Analysis of Silicones.** Edited by A. Lee Smith

Vol. 42. **Foundations of Ultracentrifugal Analysis.** By H. Fujita

Vol. 43. **Chemical Infrared Fourier Transform Spectroscopy.** By Peter R. Griffiths

Vol. 44. **Microscale Manipulations in Chemistry.** By T. S. Ma and V. Horak

Vol. 45. **Thermometric Titrations.** By J. Barthel

Vol. 46. **Trace Analysis: Spectroscopic Methods for Elements.** Edited by J. D. Winefordner

Vol. 47. **Contamination Control in Trace Element Analysis.** By Morris Zief and James W. Mitchell

Vol. 48. **Analytical Applications of NMR.** By D. E. Leyden and R. H. Cox

Vol. 49. **Measurement of Dissolved Oxygen.** By Michael L. Hitchman

Vol. 50. **Analytical Laser Spectroscopy.** Edited by Nicolo Omenetto

Vol. 51. **Trace Element Analysis of Geological Materials.** By Roger D. Reeves and Robert R. Brooks

Vol. 52. **Chemical Analysis by Microwave Rotational Spectroscopy.** By Ravi Varma and Lawrence W. Hrubesh

Vol. 53. **Information Theory As Applied to Chemical Analysis.** By Karel Eckschlager and Vladimir Štěpánek

Vol. 54. **Applied Infrared Spectroscopy: Fundamentals, Techniques, and Analytical Problem-solving.** By A. Lee Smith

Vol. 55. **Archaeological Chemistry.** By Zvi Goffer

Vol. 56. **Immobilized Enzymes in Analytical and Clinical Chemistry.** By P. W. Carr and L. D. Bowers

Vol. 57. **Photoacoustics and Photoacoustic Spectroscopy.** By Allan Rosencwaig

Vol. 58. **Analysis of Pesticide Residues.** Edited by H. Anson Moye

Vol. 59. **Affinity Chromatography.** By William H. Scouten

Vol. 60. **Quality Control in Analytical Chemistry.** By G. Kateman and F. W. Pijpers

Vol. 61. **Direct Characterization of Fineparticles.** By Brian H. Kaye

Vol. 62. **Flow Injection Analysis.** By J. Ruzicka and E. H. Hansen

(*continued on back*)

Applications of Fluorescence in Immunoassays

CHEMICAL ANALYSIS

A SERIES OF MONOGRAPHS ON ANALYTICAL CHEMISTRY AND ITS APPLICATIONS

VOLUME 117

A WILEY-INTERSCIENCE PUBLICATION

JOHN WILEY & SONS, INC.

New York / Chichester / Brisbane / Toronto / Singapore

Applications of Fluorescence in Immunoassays

ILKKA A. HEMMILÄ

Department of Biochemistry
University of Turku
Turku, Finland

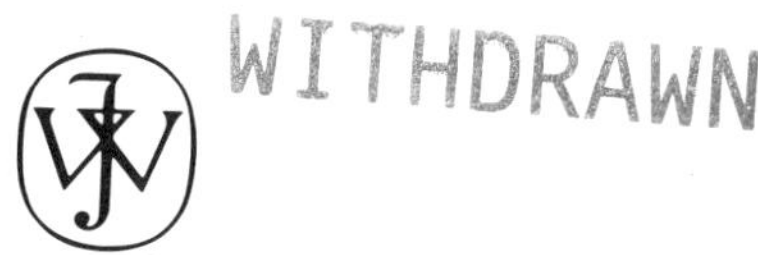

A WILEY-INTERSCIENCE PUBLICATION

JOHN WILEY & SONS, INC.

New York / Chichester / Brisbane / Toronto / Singapore

Library of Congress Cataloging in Publication Data:

Hemmilä, Ilkka A..

Applications of fluorescence in immunoassays / Ilkka A. Hemmilä.

p. cm. – (Chemical analysis, ISSN 0069-2883 ; v. 117)

"A Wiley-Interscience publication."

Includes bibliographical references and index.

ISBN 0-471-51091-2

1. Immunofluorescence. 2. Fluorescent antibody technique. 3. Fluorescent antigen technique. I. Title. II. Series.

QR187.I48H46 1991

616.07′56–dc20 90-27188

CIP

Printed in the United States of America

10 9 8 7 6 5 4 3 2 1

PREFACE

Fluorescence provides a diversified and sensitive detection system applied in the versatile field of immunological techniques. The application of antibodies labeled with fluorescent probes dates back to the 1940s, when Coons et al. introduced the microscopic immunofluorescence staining technique. During the 1970s fluorescence was considered as a promising and potentially very sensitive detection system in the search for alternative labels to replace radioisotopic tracers in immunoassays. Regardless of the number of assays developed and also successfully applied in certain areas, the inherent vulnerability of fluorescence detection to background interferences hindered its application in assays requiring high sensitivity. The recent development of fluorescence instruments, assay technologies and fluorescent probes has, however, resulted in assay techniques producing one of the highest available sensitivities, and fluorometric immunoassays also offer real alternatives to the sensitive radioisotopic immunoassays. The ability of fluorometric detection to combine spectral, temporal and spacial resolution offers a powerful tool for future immunoassay development, too.

The present monograph describes the basic prerequisites for a fluorometric immunoassay; the antibody, the immunological technology, the fluorescent probe and the instrument, as well as gives a profile of the clinical applications of the various assay technologies.

The author would like to express his gratitude to Mrs. Airi Toivonen for recording the fluorescence spectra included in the monograph, Mr. Raimo Harju, M.Sc., for updating the authors knowledge about lasers and detectors, and to Mr. Pertti Hurskainen, M.Sc., for proofreading the chapter discussing DNA-based assays.

ILKKA A. HEMMILÄ

CONTENTS

Applications of Fluorescence in Immunoassays

CHAPTER

1

INTRODUCTION

Immunoassays can be characterized as quantitative analytical methods applied for measuring biologically important compounds, methods employing antibodies as specific analytical reagents (Chapter 2). The methods rely, to a great extent, on the unique specificity of the recognition reaction between an antibody and the respective determinant site on an antigen—i.e., the chemical structure against which the antibody is formed. The high affinity and specificity of that reaction enable the use of immunological techniques for the detection and quantitation of millions of compounds of interest from various biological sources, where the constituents of the sample and the chemical similarity of the compounds makes routine chemical analysis impossible and respective biological assays too complicated and laborious to be adopted for routine clinical practice.

The introduction of reporter groups attached to one of the components of immunologic reaction has made the monitoring of the binding reaction easier and more sensitive. During the evolution of immunoassays the advent of radioactive isotopic labels, with the potent sensitivity they achieve, has had an enormous impact on biomedical research and clinical practice. In that sense the evolution of immunoassays coincides to a great extent with the evolution of radioimmunoassays (Chapter 3), and most of the basic technologies and performance characteristics of today's immunoassays were originally defined with use of radioisotopic tracers.

Even though radioimmunoassays have been the method of choice as sensitive and robust techniques, there has been a growing interest for non-isotopic alternatives since the late 1970s and early 1980s. Some of the drawbacks related to the use of radioisotopic labels have formed the driving forces towards non-radioisotopic challengers. Other reasons which have directed the efforts towards non-radioisotopic alternative labels are, for example, the desire to develop easy and rapid homogeneous assays, or ultimately to find even more sensitive assays (Chapter 4).

The group of techniques characterized as photon-emission techniques is the most rapidly growing non-isotopic technique and has the potential to offer a real alternative to radioisotopic labels, also in terms of sensitivity. Fluorometric determinations—determinations based on photon excitation of a fluorescent probe and the measurement of the resulting emission (Chapter

5)—can in principle be ultimately sensitive, reaching in well-defined pure conditions sensitivity of a single molecule detection. Although much less sensitive in routine practice, fluorometry provides a versatile, simple, and rapid detection system also able to reach high sensitivities.

However, the measurement of minute amounts of substances of interest from biological samples containing a huge amount of interfering compounds is a demanding task. The various background sources make fluorometric detection prone to background interferences, and the detection is generally limited. Therefore the fluorescent properties of the label, the fluorescent probe, are of utmost importance. The quantitation of a fluorescent compound with high sensitivity in routine conditions requires a very high fluorescence level (high absorptivity and quantum efficiency), and an especially important feature is the resolution of the specific signal from background noise (Chapter 7).

Fluorometers are becoming an integrated part of respective immunoassays. Relatively few of today's fluorometric immunoassays are measured with research fluorometers; rather, fluorometers developed for that particular type of assay and label are used. The most profound trend of immunoassay development during the late 1980s and early 1990s is the mechanization and automation of immunoassays. In automated instruments the fluorescence detector is an integral part of the whole system (Chapter 6). The sensitivity of the instrument is not generally a decisive factor unless all background noise interferences can be eliminated before detecting the specific signal.

Fluorescent labels were used in immunological staining systems before the advent of radioimmunoassays, and semiquantitative immunofluorescence is still routinely used as microscopic technology. Development of quantitative fluorometric immunological technologies has proceeded two ways: the quantitation and standardization of immunofluorescence and the development of simple homogeneous methods. The desire to replace radioisotopes with non-isotopic labels has put in an additional requirement for fluorometric techniques—sensitivity. Two of the current fluorometric techniques, time-resolved fluoroimmunoassays and enzyme immunoassays with fluorometric detection, have resulted in sensitivities adequate to make them real alternatives to radioimmunoassays.

Fluorescence is a versatile and potentially very sensitive detection technique which will certainly have extensive future applications, not only in future immunoassays but also with DNA-based specific binding assays (Chapter 10), in fluorescence immunosensors (Chapter 8), and in multiparameter analyzing systems (Chapter 11).

CHAPTER

2

ANTIBODIES AS ANALYTICAL REAGENTS

Antibodies are specific binding proteins functioning in the natural defense mechanism of animals against foreign intruders. Immunoassays are based on the unique recognition reaction between antibodies and the antigens which elicit their production. The great variability of antibody production and the ability of antibodies to bind to antigenic determinants on antigens with high affinity and specificity enables their use for the analytical determination of a tremendous number of analytes of biological, biochemical, and medical interest from samples containing an enormous assortment of chemically related compounds.

Antibodies are able to recognize and bind to a defined epitopic site on an antigen, which forms the basis for their specificity. Accordingly, immunoassays are defined as being structurally specific assays, in contrast to biological assays, bioassays, which are functionally specific methods; they measure the functional activity of the compound, such as the effect of a hormone on a certain tissue of the test animal. Regardless of the fact that certain discrepancies may occur between biological and immunological responses, in numerous cases there are no bioassays available, and in general biological techniques are too laborious, expensive, and time-consuming to be widely adopted for routine analysis.

Understanding antibody structure and its functional properties is of crucial importance when developing any immunoassays. Therefore, some of the major features of antibodies—their production, purification, fractionation, and also some of the interesting future aspects—are briefly discussed here, despite the availability of numerous reviews and textbooks dealing with immunological responses and antibodies (see, for example, references 1 and 2).

Production and properties of antibodies were known long before their exploitation in immunoassays started. The first reporter groups attached to antibodies without destroying their ability to react specifically with the respective antigens were colored dyes. As early as 1930 Reiner (3) suggested the use of labeled antibodies in the study of quantitative aspects of antigen-antibody reaction. In 1932 Heidelberger and Kendall (4) used antibodies as precipitating reagents in a study of pneumococcus polysaccharides by using the inherent nitrogen as a marker. The use of fluorescent compounds as sensitive marker substances coupled to antibodies was invented by Albert Coons and his colleagues in the early '40s, when they developed immunofluorescence staining techniques for microbes (5, 6).

The study of antibody production in diabetic patients treated with insulin led to the development of the radioimmunoassay in the late '50s by Berson and Yalow (7, 8); this method has had a major impact on the acceptance of immunological techniques in the field of routine clinical diagnosis.

In their early days radioimmunoassays were exclusively applied for determinations of peptide hormones. Since the pioneering work of Landsteiner in 1946 (9), antibodies have also been produced for small (molecular weight under 10,000) compounds called haptens, for compounds which as such are unable to elicit antibody production but must be bound to larger carrier molècules to form immunogenic conjugate. The production of antisera against haptenic molecules, such as steroids (10) or thyroid hormones (11), opened a new dimension for immunoassays. Since then antibodies have been produced against an enormous number of antigens and biological and synthetic compounds, and these have been applied in a variety of ways for analyzing those compounds. Modern biotechnology has revolutionized antibody production, and genetic engineering opens totally new perspectives for their future applications.

2.1. IMMUNOGENIC RESPONSE

An antigen is an immunogenic compound which can elicit a strong immune response in an immunized animal. An immunogenic antigen can be a peptide, protein, polysaccharide, polynucleotide, or almost any polymeric compound containing functional groups on its surface recognized by antibody producing B-lymphocytes. The primary recognition by the membrane bound receptor proteins of lymphocytes triggers the complex process of maturation of antibody producing B-cells and the subsequent production of large quantities of antibodies.

The production of antisera of high titer, affinity, and specificity requires substantial amounts of chemically pure antigens. A large amount is needed for repeated immunizations of test animals. High purity is an absolute necessity in order to obviate cross-reactivities with unrelated compounds. The purification and stability problems with some biological compounds can be a limiting factor in antiserum production, but these have been partly overcome with the development of methods for producing monoclonal antibodies (Chapter 2.2).

2.1.1. Haptenic Antigens

Haptenic antigens are compounds which because of their small size cannot elicit immunoresponse. Generally the molecular weight limit for immunogenic response is around 10,000. Because of the difficulties in producing anti-hapten antibodies, the first real immunoassays were developed for peptides or proteins, and actually the first "specific protein binding assays" of haptenic molecules, developed by Roger Ekins et al. in the early '60s, used naturally occurring specific binding proteins, thyroxine binding globulin for labeled thyroxine (12) and intrinsic factor for labeled B_{12}-vitamin (13).

The production of anti-hapten antibodies was invented in the late '40s (9), and anti-steroid antibodies were produced in 1957 (10). It was several years, however, before these were applied for making radioimmunoassays. For eliciting immunoresponse the haptenic molecules need first to be coupled to a suitable carrier. Bovine serum albumin is the most often used carrier protein for immunizations, mainly because of its solubility and availability. Other proteins, like keyhole limpet hemocyanin, have been preferred later on because of their high immunogenicity and coincident contribution of the production of anti-hapten antibodies with high titer and affinity (14).

The production of anti-hapten antibodies of predetermined specificity is often problematic, partly because the coupling of the compound to a carrier can block important epitopic sites needed for specificity and partly because of recognition of the linking arm between the hapten and carrier by the produced antibodies. Since the antibodies are able to bind structures equal to about 7 amino acid residues (15), an anti-hapten antibody most often recognizes simultaneously part of the linking group and spacer arm used in conjugation reaction for immunization (bridge recognition).

Bridge recognition is especially problematic for steroid immunoassays (16, 17) and is encountered when labeled steroids (tracer) or immobilized steroids (e.g., solid-phase reagent) are prepared using the same position of the steroid (site homology) or same linking arm (bridge homology) as used for preparing the immunogenic conjugate. With such conjugates the competitive binding between the limited amount of antibody, labeled antigen, and the unknown amount of sample antigen (or standard) favors the reaction between tracer and antibody with poor replacement; the rate constant k_1 is much higher than k_2 (Eq. 2.1). The poor replacement results in insufficient slope to the standard curve and low assay sensitivity because the sample antigen is unable to compete with the tracer in binding to antibodies.

Accordingly, the production of immunogenic conjugates for steroid immunization is better performed after selecting different spacer arms or sometimes even different positions for attachment on the steroid structure (Fig. 2.1).

$$\text{Ab}\begin{cases} + \text{Ag} - \text{F} & \overset{k_1}{\underset{\dashleftarrow}{\longrightarrow}} \quad \text{Ab} - \text{Ag} - \text{F} \\ \\ + \text{Ag} & \overset{k_2}{\underset{\dashleftarrow}{\longrightarrow}} \quad \text{Ab} - \text{Ag} \end{cases} \tag{2.1}$$

For example, considerably higher sensitivity was obtained in an assay of 17-hydroxyprogesterone when using a bridge heterologous tracer as compared to a respective homologous system (18). Similarly, the equilibrium time required for ligand displacement in an assay of estradiol shortened from 10 h to 1 min when changing from a homologous system to heterologous (19). The requirement of site homology depends greatly on the analyte and antibodies used. In EIA of cortisol Arakawa et al. (20) used cortisol-6α-hemisuccinate for producing the antigen conjugate for solid-phase immobilization and 3-carboxymethyloxime conjugate for producing the marker-enzyme tracer. On the other hand, in the experiments of Kobayashi et al. (21) and Mikola and Miettinen (22), cortisol could be assayed only with a site homologous system. Tiefenauer and Andres (23) tested spacer arms between estradiol and biotin for use in EIA. They found that a reasonably long spacer was an absolute necessity and that the chemical structure of the spacer may also have a major effect on bridge recognition.

2.2. MONOCLONAL ANTIBODIES

In 1975 Köhler and Milstein (24) made the first monoclonal antibodies of predetermined specificity by fusing a spleen cell line producing the specific antibodies with a myeloma cell line capable of continuous growth in cell culture. Since then the advent of monoclonal antibodies has had an enormous impact on many fields of biomedical research (25, 26). It was soon realized that the technique would revolutionize the immunoassay field as well, and it has raised great expectations also in immunotherapy, imaging, and biotechnology.

Monoclonal antibodies are rapidly gaining a dominant position in immunoassays, especially from a commercial point of view, because of their unlimited supply, molecular homogeneity, and defined, unchanged properties. The production and use of monoclonal antibodies has also become a

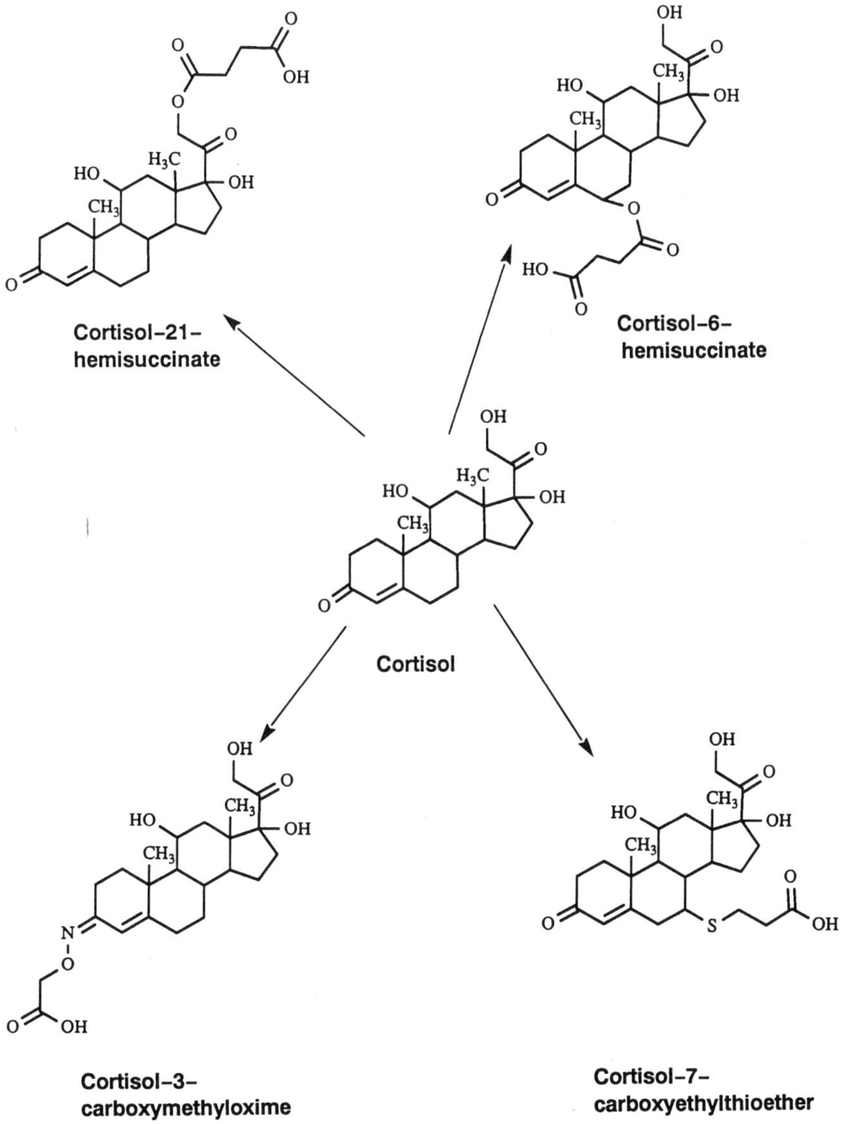

Cortisol-21-hemisucinate

Cortisol-6-hemisuccinate

Cortisol

Cortisol-3-carboxymethyloxime

Cortisol-7-carboxyethylthioether

Fig. 2.1. Site heterologous routes to prepare cortisol derivatives for immunization and for labeling.

matter of extensive litigation and restrictions due to numerous patents issued about their use in immunoassays, regardless of the rather questionable inventiveness of such patents (27).

2.2.1. Production of Monoclonal Antibodies

Monoclonal antibodies are uniform homogeneous proteins produced by a single cell line, clone. The clones are produced by immunizing a mouse (or rat) and fusing the mouse spleen cells with a nonsecretory myeloma cell line using polyethylene glycol. The myeloma cell line used is not able to survive in the specified growth medium ("HAT" medium), which makes it easy to select the formed hybridoma clones. From the mixture of cell lines, antibody producing clones are selected, and clones producing monoclonal antibodies with desired properties are screened and chosen for further production.

The selected antibody producing clones are subsequently grown either *in vivo,* in ascites fluid of the host animal, or *in vitro,* in cell cultures. For small-scale production the growth of intraperitoneal tumors in mice (ascites) is most convenient. Several different fermentor-like mass culture technologies have been applied for *in vitro* production. Techniques like "cell factories" with free suspension cultures or reactors, where cells are entrapped on permeable beads or into microcapsules, ceramic cartridges, or hollow fiber cartridges, allow large-scale production of pure monoclonal antibodies (28). For example, production of antibodies with scales up to 500 mg per day can be achieved with hollow fiber systems (29). *In vitro* production has the advantages of avoiding the use of animals and producing antibodies free from extraneous antibodies and other rodent proteins; it also allows for production in economic scales in ratio of labor and capital cost and for a reproducible production process.

In addition to *in vitro* production, immunization also can be made *in vitro* (30). *In vitro* immunization obviates possible problems related to immunological tolerance and the danger of antigen breakdown in the test animal.

2.2.2. Polyclonal or Monoclonal?

Monoclonal antibodies are beginning to displace their antiquated progenitors, polyclonal antibodies, in the field of immunoassays. Their superior advantages have not been always acknowledged, and they still have certain shortages. Table 2.1 summarizes some of their advantages and weak points. The most profound advantage is the unlimited supply of well-defined, homogeneous antibodies, which makes them perfect analytical reagents. The low affinities somewhat inherent with monoclonal antibodies can be

Table 2.1. Properties of Monoclonal Antibodies

Advantages	Disadvantages
Constant, well-defined characteristics	Often lower affinity
Can be produced against small amount of impure antigen	Does not form precipitation
Specificity can be selected	Does not always react with protein A
Indefinite supply	Can express individual unwelcome properties
Easy purification	May be too specific (polymorphism of antigens)
Low nonspecific bindings in immunoassays	Special techniques required for production

overcome by the careful selection of high affinity antibody producers, and currently many monoclonal antibodies have affinities in the range of 10^{-10}–10^{-12} L/mol.

The production and application of monoclonal antibodies have created new dimensions for immunoassays. Large amounts of unchanged reagent raise the possibility of the standardization of assays. By selecting the epitopes —and respective monoclonal antibodies—specificities can be stipulated according to clinical situations. The availability of antibodies against many different epitopes on a protein enables epitope mapping of the antigen for elucidation of its three-dimensional structure.

2.3. CHEMICAL STRUCTURE OF ANTIBODIES

Antibodies belong to the globular fraction of serum proteins and consist of five main types of glycoproteins: IgG, IgM, IgE, IgA, and IgD. IgG is the most common class of antibodies comprising the major component of molecular immunity, and in most animals the immunological memory resides primarily in the IgG response. IgG antibodies are also the most important class of antibodies for immunological techniques.

2.3.1. Immunoglobulin G

IgG consists of two identical pairs of heavy (H,γ) and light (L) polypeptide chains (mw. 50,000 and 25,000 respectively) linked together by disulfide bridges (Fig. 2.2). Disulfide bridges create the intra-chain linkages forming domains.

The IgG structure can be divided into three fractions: two immunologically active, antigen combining sites, Fab-fragments, and into one constant, non-

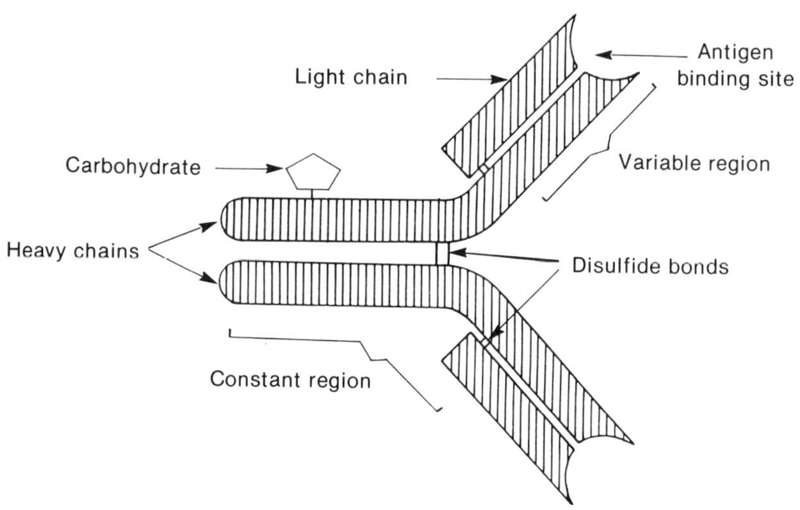

Fig. 2.2. Structure of immunoglobulin G (IgG).

binding fraction Fc-fragment (crystallizable part) (Fig. 2.2). The antibody binding site of Fab consists of two variable region domains; the other parts of the molecule consist of constant regions and a carbohydrate moiety linked to the Fc part.

The immunoglobulin molecule is biologically bifunctional. It brings together a specific antigen and a nonspecific mechanism that inactivate and degrade antigens. The binding sites are located in different domains of the molecule, which can even be separated by proteolytic cleavage with retention of their activities. Fab forms the basis for the specific recognition reaction, and the Fc is important for linking the primary immunologic binding to secondary reactions, including complement binding.

When using antibodies as analytical reagents, one can sometimes take advantage of the bifunctionality of antibodies. For example, the binding of the complement to complex-forming antibodies can be utilized as a universal labeling system for complexed IgG (31), or it can be used to make precipitation more complete in traditional precipitation-based competitive binding assays. The activation of the complement by antibody binding is also used in complement mediated lysis of erythrocytes or sensitized liposomes (Chapter 8.3.5). The binding of protein A to the Fc part of most of the subtypes of IgG is frequently applied in IgG purifications and also as an universal reagent for IgG measurement. The Fc-fraction functions also as a bulk of available amino acid residues for conjugation reactions.

On the other hand, the bifunctional nature of antibodies can lead to artifacts and incorrect interpretations of results. The Fc-fraction is responsible for most cross-reactivities between anti-species antibodies, and it may cause nonspecific signals in two-site assays due to the existence of rheumatoid factors. For these reasons the Fc-fraction is sometimes cleaved off in preparing labeled reagents of low nonspecific binding (Chapter 2.5.3).

IgG can further be divided into several subclasses. The main subclass-related differences are in the hinge region (Fig. 2.2) and in the number of cross-linking disulfide bridges. Chemically IgG subtypes are rather similar, but they differ in many biological functions, including their ability to activate complement, to cross the placental barrier, and to bind to Fc-receptors (32), occasionally encountered in the purification of monoclonal antibodies with protein A. Also the expression of IgG subtypes is different; for example, IgG_1 and IgG_3 subclasses are mainly expressed against protein antigens (33) and IgG_2 subclass is mainly produced in the T-cell independent way against carbohydrate antigens (34).

2.3.2. Other Immunoglobulins

From the other four immunoglobulin classes, only IgM is frequently applied as an immunological reagent. Clinically IgM is responsible for the first immunoresponse after exposure to a immunogenic substance, and it is also the major class of antibodies with neonates. It is a multivalent antibody containing ten antigen-combining sites. Because of its multivalent nature it has high avidity, and it is an efficient activator for antibody mediated phagocytosis.

Secretory IgM is a pentameric molecule with five L and H (μ) chains in addition to one joining J-chain, with a total molecular weight of 950,000. Because of its early response after immunogenic exposure, it is measured in studies of recent infections. Its use as an immunological reagent is more or less restricted to hybrid clones producing IgM antibodies.

IgA is the predominant antibody in secretions. It has an analogous structure with IgG (α-chain as H) but occurs mostly as polymeric forms. IgE is related to allergic reactions and is an important analyte in allergy research. IgD appears mainly on the surface of lymphocytes as antigen receptors. The function of IgD is not fully elucidated (35).

2.4. IMMUNOCHEMICAL PROPERTIES OF ANTIBODIES

Titer. The antisera produced for immunoassays were traditionally "titrated" with an appropriate amount of labeled antigen to determine the antiserum titer. The binding capacity is determined from the serial dilution of serum.

The titer reflects both the amount of produced antibodies and their average avidity. Normally it corresponds to the dilution needed for the actual immunoassay.

Affinity. Antibody affinity is a measure of the strength of the bond between a single antigen-combining site and an antigen determinant. From a simple binding reaction in equilibrium, affinity can be calculated from reactant concentrations (Eq. 2.2) or from respective reaction rate constants (Eq. 2.3).

$$[Ab] + [Ag] \underset{k_d}{\overset{k_a}{\rightleftharpoons}} [Ab - Ag] \tag{2.2}$$

$$K\ (L/mol) = [Ab - Ag]/[Ab][Ag] = k_a/k_d \tag{2.3}$$

The affinity is traditionally determined using the Scatchard equation (Eq. 2.4) (36) and so-called Scatchard plotting, where r is the number of occupied sites on the antibody, [Ag] is the free antigen concentration, and n is the antibody valency.

$$r/[Ag] = -Kr + nK \tag{2.4}$$

With polyclonal antibodies the affinity does not have any well-defined value but reflects the average affinities of different antibodies present in the serum, and the blotting does not form a straight line. It is more relevant with monoclonal antibodies. Affinity of the antibodies is a very important factor in determining the assay performance. The optimal sensitivity obtainable with an immunoassay is inversely related to the antibody affinity (37).

Avidity. This is a measure of antigen-antibody binding strength and is a direct function of the affinity and the number of antigen-combining sites. The binding strength is enhanced when multiple epitopes are present for binding.

Kinetics. The kinetics of immunoreaction depends on the association rate constant, k_a (Eq. 2.2). Generally high-affinity antibodies have high binding kinetics (Eq. 2.3). High kinetics is required to make immunoassays rapid, a feature which is especially important for the automation of immunoassays. On the other hand, simple single-reagent assays based on ligand displacement (LIDIA) presuppose that the dissociation rate constant, k_d, is high. The kinetics of immunoreaction can be enhanced by manipulation of the assay buffer (e.g., with detergents) or by choosing suitable bridge or site heterology (see Chapter 2.1.1).

Specificity. Specificity is a crucial feature of antibodies. For each antibody used it is obligatory to determine its cross-reactivities to antigen-related compounds. High specificity is very critical in assays of peptide hormones having identical subunits in their structure and in assays of steroid hormones. The presence of several related steroid structures in serum and especially their metabolites in urine set a high demand for antibody specificity. In many cases those samples need to be pretreated (e.g., with extraction) to assess the overall assay specificity.

The use of two specific antibodies in two-site assays is frequent for peptide hormones, where the obtained response is a result of two simultaneous recognition reactions; it will also enhance the total assay specificity (Fig. 2.3).

On the other hand, high specificity is not needed for assays where the existence of a group of related compounds is measured. For example, screening for illicit drugs in urine, with their numerous metabolites, requires antibodies with rather wide cross-reactive properties.

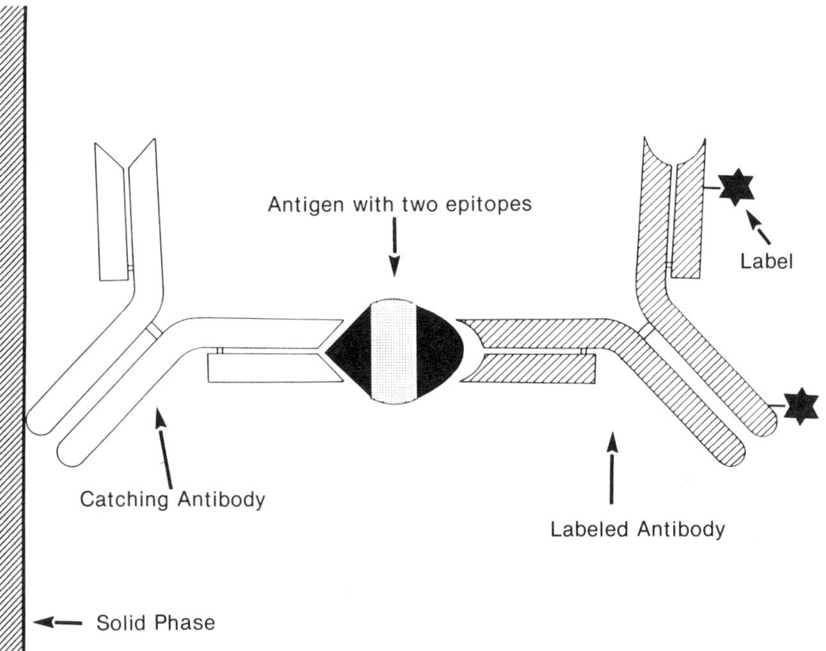

Fig. 2.3. Two-site sandwich immunoassay on a solid surface.

2.5. PROCESSING OF ANTIBODIES

For use in immunoassays, antibodies are almost invariably processed to some extent. Their use as an analytical reagent may require purification, precipitations within assay, conjugations with reporter groups or insolubilizations to various matrixes, or fractionation into fragments. As the antibodies are biologically active proteins, their processing has to preserve all their natural characteristics needed for immunoassays.

2.5.1. Purification

The purity of the labeled antibodies depends greatly on the assay system used, on the nonspecific binding characteristics of labeled antibodies, and on the required sensitivity of the assay. Traditionally, in the competitive immunoassays (e.g., RIA) the antiserum is used without any further purification. Actually, the precipitation employed requires the existence of nonspecific globulins to facilitate complete precipitation of the antigen-antibody complex. The "sandwich" type noncompetitive assays with labeled antibodies —assays which are functioning in a wide range of analyte concentrations and with a large excess of labeled antibodies—require very low nonspecific binding properties for the labeled antibodies. Accordingly, the purity and purification methods of antibodies have become more important factors in developing those assays. The various methods commonly used to purify IgG fractions, or to prepare pure antibodies, are described in numerous reviews (1, 2, 28, 38).

Fractionation of the total globulin fraction from serum is most often accomplished by simple salt precipitation with, for instance, half-saturated ammonium sulfate. Chemically pure IgG, the most important class of antibodies in antiserum, can be purified with ion-exchange chromatography or may be fractionated with various precipitation methods. Recently IgG purifications have been commonly accomplished with affinity chromatography using insolubilized protein A or protein G. The highest purity of polyclonal antibodies is achieved with affinity purification with immunosorbents (immobilized antigens), by eluting with acid, chaotropic agents, or with the antigen. However, the highest purity is not always any advantage if the purification process causes losses of immunoreactivity or affinity.

The rapidly increasing use of monoclonal antibodies in immunoassays has reduced the need for elaborate purification processes obligatory with polyclonal antibodies. When the cell line produces only one type of specific antibodies, the purification of that type of globulin is enough to produce pure reagent. The most often used method with monoclonal antibodies is affinity purification with protein A (1).

2.5.2. Chemical Modification

The insolubilization of antibodies on solid matrixes has become a standard practice for a convenient separation of bound immunoreagents from unbound reagents (Chapter 3.4). For immobilization antibodies are either "coated" to solid surfaces by physical absorption or coupled to derivatized surfaces by covalent reactions. The coated surfaces have to preserve the immunological properties of antibodies and such orientation that they are still capable of specific recognition. The leakage of antibodies from the surface must be minimized to guarantee extended stability of coated surfaces, stored either wet or dried. Antibodies on the coated surfaces can be stabilized by treatment with suitable carrier proteins (albumin) or sugars.

Quite many immunoassays (e.g., all noncompetitive assays) are based on labeled antibodies, which are chemically coupled with one or several marker groups. Different amino-acid residues of antibodies (lysine, cysteine, tyrosine, tryptophan, aspartate, or glutamate) have reactive groups which can be utilized for conjugations, but the carbohydrate moiety of the Fc part also has been used for conjugation reaction—for instance, after periodate oxidation. Periodate coupling is commonly used for labeling antibodies with enzymes (HRP) and also has been used for labeling antibodies with fluorescein through a thiosemicarbazide derivative (39). Free amines of lysine provide the most convenient side chains for conjugations, and mild coupling of markers with lysine (ε-amino groups) does not cause such losses in immunoreactivities that are encountered with modifications of, for instance, histidine or tyrosine residues (40).

2.5.3. Fractionation

Antibodies are occasionally fractionated into smaller fragments in order to obviate unwanted binding reactions related to the Fc-fragment (rheumatoid factors, complement binding, or binding with protein A when it is used as a universal reagent) or to produce Fab′-fragments containing a suitable SH-group for covalent coupling with enzymes.

Antibody fragments are prepared by combining enzymatic hydrolysis, selective reduction of disulfide bridges, and gel-chromatographic purification of resulting fragments (41).

Fab-fragment contains only one antigen-combining site (Fig. 2.4). It is prepared by papain digestion of IgG. The respective Fab′-fragment, which contains an additional SH-group, is prepared by pepsin digestion and partial reduction. $F(ab')_2$ has two antigen-combining sites and differs from natural IgG only by lack of the Fc part (Fig. 2.4). It is prepared by pepsin digestion.

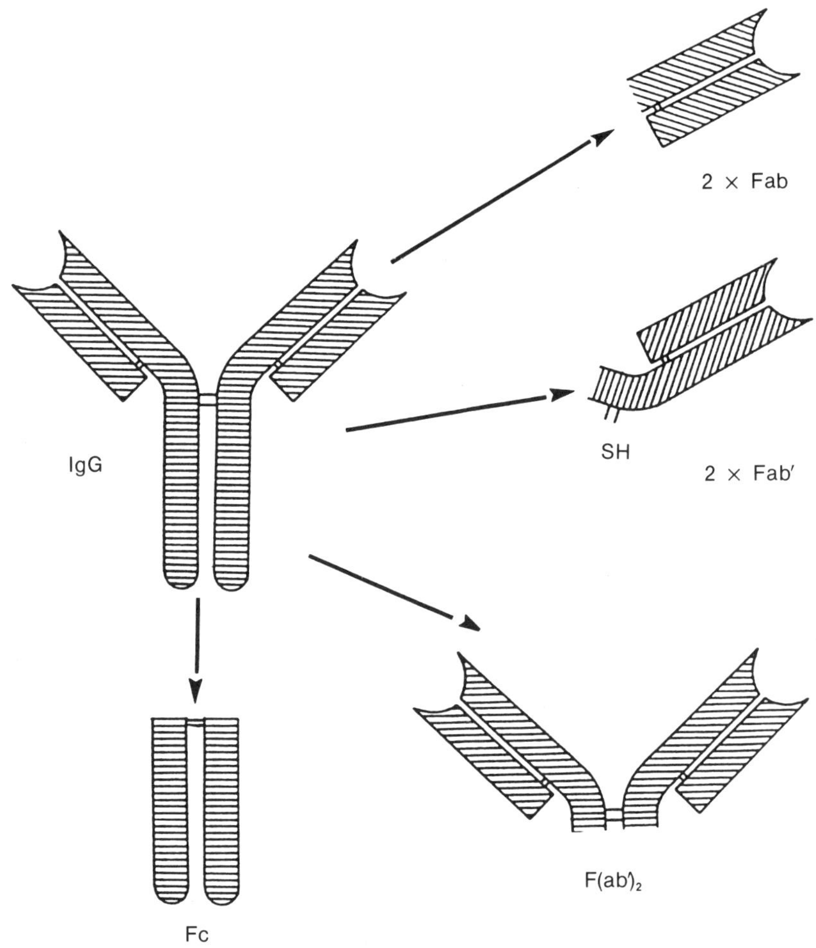

Fig. 2.4. Fractionation of IgG.

2.6. IMMUNOREACTION CONDITIONS

2.6.1. Assay Buffer

Antibodies are biological compounds which require physiological conditions for their optimal function. The optimal pH for most immunoassays is near neutral; a higher pH, up to 8.5, is occasionally used, and a lower pH can be applied as a blocking system (Chapter 2.6.2). The ionic strength of the buffer is generally kept at physiological range with 0.9% sodium chloride. Physiologic saline is needed for antibody stability and for restricting nonspecific bindings.

Assay buffers developed for immunoassays contain almost invariably high concentrations of proteins, most often bovine albumin (BSA). Proteins act as a stabilizer of antibodies; they mask the matrix differences related to variations in protein concentrations in samples and are needed to prevent nonspecific bindings of labeled reagents to solid surfaces. The addition of globulins can eliminate the potential interference in two-site assays which arises from the presence of anti-immunoglobulin antibodies in serum samples. These may be produced initially as a response to bovine immunoglobulins in milk, but can cross-react with IgG of various sources—with mouse IgG, for example. The incidence of such antibodies may be as high as 7% (42), and problems arising from anti-mouse antibodies are frequently reported in assays using monoclonal antibodies. Addition of bovine globulins can saturate the majority of these antibodies, but mouse IgG in the form of nonimmune serum, ascites, or globulins is needed to eliminate problems derived from specific mouse-allergic antibodies (43–45). The problem of human anti-mouse antibodies (HAMA) has had a minor importance so far, but the increasing use of monoclonal antibodies in diagnosis, particularly in therapy, may increase the occurrence of high titers of HAMA.

Detergents are frequently added to assay buffer primarily to restrict nonspecific bindings. In addition to albumin, detergents are an efficient means to saturate binding sites on plastic surfaces used as solid-phase (46). The use of high concentrations of detergents is restricted by the sensitivity of some antibodies to detergents and the releasing effect of detergents on surface-coated antibodies.

2.6.2. Blocking of Carrier Proteins

Many hormones circulate in blood as complexes with their binding proteins. These hormones need to be released from those proteins to measure their total concentrations in serum. Also, the binding of antigen-analog, a tracer, to those proteins must be prohibited.

Anilinonaphthalene sulfonic acid (ANS) is a blocking agent often applied (47, 48), especially in assays of thyroid hormones. Others, like merthiolate and sodium salicylate, are used with, for example, thyroxine (49) and cortisol (50). Steroid analogs, like danazol, or related non-cross reactive steroids can be used in steroid assays, as can a low pH in the assay buffer (51, 52) or chaotropic ions, such as trichloroacetate (53). Triton X-100, at a relatively high concentration (1%), is used to remove luteinizing hormone-releasing hormone from its binding protein (54).

Another way to obviate the interference of binding proteins is to use sample pretreatment—extraction with an organic solvent such as ethanol (55), heat denaturation (56) or denaturation with sodium dodecyl sulfate (SDS), or enzymatic degradation (57).

2.6.3. Physical Conditions of Assays

The general tendency in immunoassays is to allow reaction to reach equilibrium before its termination. When the reaction has proceeded to completion, the response range is maximal, and miscalculations caused by different kinetics of standard and samples due to matrix effects are thus obviated.

Raising the incubation temperature to +37 °C, or sometimes even higher, can accelerate reaction kinetics. With solid-phase reaction, where the reaction rate is diffusion limited, the kinetics can be enhanced either by shaking or by decreasing the diffusion distances (e.g., by using microparticle suspensions as solid-phase). Microwaves have also been used to speed up immunologic binding reaction.

2.7. OTHER SPECIFIC BINDING PROTEINS

Some of the very first published specific binding assays were actually performed with other binding proteins than antibodies (12, 13). Those nonimmunological binding proteins are frequently used in immunological techniques either as alternatives to antibodies, complements to antibodies, or as amplifiers in antibody-based immunoassays. Some of the proteins applied and their respective ligands are listed in Table 2.2.

2.7.1. Avidin-Biotin Complex

Due to its unique high affinity, easy coupling of biotin derivatives to various macromolecules, and the multivalent binding characteristics of avidin, the avidin-biotin binding pair has found wide application in various biotechnological methods (58, 59). Table 2.3 summarizes the properties of egg-white avidin and bacterial streptavidin. Both are tetrameric structures having four binding sites for biotin, with an affinity of 10^{-15} M^{-1}. Avidin is a basic glycoprotein with an isoelectric point (pI) at pH > 10. Streptavidin, purified from *Streptomyces avidii,* has about the same molecular weight and affinity to biotin as avidin. The fact that streptavidin is neither basic nor glycosylated implies that many of the problems frequently encountered with avidin, like occasionally high nonspecific interactions, can be circumvented by replacing avidin with streptavidin.

Table 2.2. Specific Binding Proteins Applied in Binding Assays

Protein	Ligand
Avidin	Biotin
Streptavidin	Biotin
Thyroxine binding globulin	Thyroxine
Intrinsic factor	B_{12}-vitamin
Protein A	Fc of IgG
Protein G	Fc of IgG
Concanavalin A	D-mannosyl or D-glycosyl groups
Complement components	Immunocomplexes

Because only the intact ureido ring of biotin is required for its strong interaction with avidin, it can be easily coupled to proteins from its side chain carboxylic acid without interfering in the binding reaction. Many activated biotin derivatives have been synthesized for covalent conjugations, and many of them are also commercially available.

Avidin-biotin linkages are routinely used for amplification of signal in immunohistochemistry and flow cytometry. Avidin-biotin augmented complexes (ABC) are frequently applied with different variations of peroxidase staining (60, 61), FITC-labeled avidin is used both in microscopic immunofluorescence (62) and in flow-cytometric methods. Avidin or streptavidin also has been used as a carrier for phycoerythrin (63)—for example, in double label flow-cytometric experiments (64, 65)—and as a universal labeled reagent after coupling to fluorochromes—via loaded liposomes, for instance (66).

Like the ABC-immunofluorescence system, avidin-biotin complex also is used in some enzyme immunoassays (EIA) developed, for example, for bacterial antigens (67) and thyrotropin (68). Streptavidin-β-galactosidase has been used as an amplifier in fluorometric enzyme immunoassays (ELFIA) in the detection of hepatitis B surface antigen (69) and interleukin-2 receptors (70).

Table 2.3. Properties of Avidins

	Avidin	Streptavidin
Molecular weight	67,000	60,000
Subunit	15,600	14,600
Affinity to biotin (M)	10^{-15}	10^{-15}
Absorptivity, 280 (mL/mg)	1.54	3.4
pI	> 10	< 7
Lysines	9	4

Avidin labeled with Texas red was used as a fluorescence energy donor for phycoerythrin-labeled antigen in a fluorescence energy transfer immunoassay of phenytoin performed with an immunosensor (71). Bador et al. (72) tested the use of europium (Eu^{3+})-labeled streptavidin for a time-resolved fluoroimmunoassay (TR-FIA), but they did not achieve the expected increase in sensitivity. On the other hand, in two-site TR-IFMA of thyrotropin both Eu-labeled avidin and Eu-labeled streptavidin were able to improve both the signal level and also, slightly, the sensitivity of the assay as compared to directly labeled primary antibodies (73). Eu-chelator labeled streptavidin is applied in all of the commercial TR-FIAs of CyberFluor (Chapter 8.4.2), both as a signal amplifier and as a means to avoid the direct contact of the chelator with the sample (74).

Although in the majority of the published articles the use of avidin-biotin improved the signal obtained and the assay sensitivity, its actual effect on assay performance depends on how the antibody is biotinylated and on the nonspecific interactions caused by labeled avidin. An example of the unsuccessful use of avidin is an ELFIA of nerve growth factor (75), in which the directly labeled antibody gave a hundredfold higher sensitivity than the assay with labeled streptavidin.

2.7.2. Fc-Reactive Proteins

Protein A is the most often used Fc-reactive protein, both in biotechnology for purification of IgG and in immunoassays. It is purified from *Staphylococcus aureus* and binds specifically to the Fc part of most subtypes of IgG from a majority of mammalian species (40). Protein G, a cell surface protein of group G streptococci, is a Type III Fc receptor. Protein G has slightly different IgG-binding specificity. It has a molecular weight of about 17,000 and an isoelectric point at pH 4.1.

Protein A is widely used as a universal reagent for IgG determinations (e.g., for measuring of circulating antibodies) in RIA (76), in fluorescence microscopic studies (77), and in immunofluorometric assays (78–80).

Complement component, C1q, can recognize formed immunocomplexes, and it also can be applied as a universal labeled reagent for bound IgG (31). A wide patent application of its use in energy-transfer-based homogeneous binding assays has also been issued (81).

Lectins are proteins of nonimmune origin characterized by their affinity to carbohydrates in glycoproteins. Lectins are purified from different sources, including plants, microorganisms, invertebrates, etc. Because the Fc-fragment of IgG contains carbohydrate moiety, some lectins will also recognize IgG. Concanavalin A is used analogously to antibodies in immunosensors, for example, to detect glucose by competitive binding assay using FITC-labeled dextran as a tracer (82). Fluorescein-labeled *Helix pomatia* lectin is used in lieu of antibodies in immunofluorescence tests of *herpes simplex* virus types (83) and *Triticum vulgaris* lectin for detection of molds in food (84). Lectins can be applied also as specific catching proteins for sandwich-type "lectin immunometric assays." Nagata and Komoda (85) measured CEA concentrations with lectin-based IRMA using nine different lectins coupled to agarose beads and labeled monoclonal antibodies for detection. Concanavalin A is used for assay of interleukin (86) and agglutinins from *Bandeiraea simplicifolia* and *Ricinus communis* to measure abnormal glycosylation levels of glycoproteins in rheumatic patients (87, 88). *Lens culinaris* agglutinin is used for determination of the fucosylation level on AFP (89).

2.7.3. Universal Catching Proteins

In addition to the use of some labeled proteins as universal labels, some proteins are also applied as universal catching proteins immobilized on solid surfaces. Anti-species antibodies (e.g., anti-mouse IgG) are the most commonly used universal reagents, used both as labeled reagent and as catching proteins on solid-phase.

Streptavidin (or anti-biotin antibodies in some applications) are commonly utilized in affinity-based-collection (ABC) types of hybridization assays (Chapter 10.3). It has also, although less frequently, been applied in immunoassays (90, 91)—for example, in a commercial automated immunoassay system, VISTA™ of DuPont.

Protein A (92) and protein G (93) are also used as common catchers for polyclonal and monoclonal antibodies (similarly to complement component C1q attached to Stiq-samplers) for autoimmune disease screening (94). They are attached to microbeads for detecting circulating immunocomplexes by flow cytometry (95) or in enzyme immunoassay (96).

2.8. FUTURE ASPECTS

The production of large quantities of monoclonal antibodies has offered the possibility of using those well-defined antibodies in human immunotherapy. In immunotherapy, however, human monoclonal antibodies would be better tolerated by humans. The development of human hybridoma lines has generally not been successful, and the hybridomas formed with human-lymphocyte–mouse-myeloma cell lines proved to be unstable (25). Hybrid hybridomas and genetically engineered antibodies may overcome these problems.

Anti-idiotypic antibodies, originally discovered by Oudin and Michel

(97), are antibodies formed against the variable region of IgG. These antibodies complement the antigenic binding sites of the primary antibodies (''internal images'' of antigens) and can be used as surrogates for antigens (98)—for instance, in competitive solid-phase EIA of cotidine (99). The development of anti-idiotypic antibodies has also created a challenge to develop noncompetitive sandwich-type assays for haptenic molecules. By using two anti-idiotypic antibodies, recognizing different epitopes within the hypervariable region of the primary antibody, Barnard and Kohen (100) were able to construct a noncompetitive immunoassay for a small molecular weight antigen, estradiol. The assay was based on a back-titration of unoccupied sites of solid-phase antibodies with beta-type anti-idiotype antibody and the steric hindrance it caused to the binding of a second, Eu-labeled anti-idiotype (alpha-type).

Bispecific or heterodimeric antibodies were originally produced by chemical aggregation and reconstitution methods; later on, hybrid-hybridoma techniques and also genetic engineering using chimeric genes were used as well. Bispecific antibodies have been developed to produce simple staining methods for histochemistry, uniform reagents for immunoassays, and bifunctional antibodies for immunotherapy.

Chemical chimers are produced by the reduction of $F(ab')_2$, protection of SH-groups, dissociation into half molecules in acid, and random reassociation of the fragments with the re-formation of single disulfide bond (101, 102). An example of such a chimeric antibody is an antibody against both ferritin and IgG (103).

Hybrid-hybridomas, sometimes also called second generation hybridomas, are produced by fusing two hybridoma cell lines (104, 105). A tetradoma antibody, anti-FITC & HRP, is used in fluorometric cell sorting (106) and anti-human lymphotoxin & HRP in a one-step EIA for human lymphotoxin (107).

Modern biotechnology and genetic engineering is revolutionizing antibody production (108, 109). The ability to genetically manipulate antibody genes and express these altered genes with transection techniques make possible the production of monoclonal antibodies with desirable properties, the addition of artificial properties to antibodies, and the combination of antibodies with enzymatic activities, toxins or hormones, and so on (110–113). Genetically produced mouse-human chimers have already been developed with the use of plasmid vectors to overcome problems related to immunotherapy with pure mouse antibodies (114).

Another approach offered by biotechnology is the development of synthetic antisens-peptides which could replace antibodies (115) and which could be genetically or chemically coupled to suitable markers.

CHAPTER

3

EVOLUTION OF IMMUNOASSAYS

Even though the components required for quantitative immunoassays were known long before the renowned publications of Berson and Yalow (7, 8, 116–118), early immunoassay techniques did not gain such the wide acceptance that radioimmunoassay achieved rapidly after its introduction in early '60s. The reason for the enormous attention the work received may relate to the fact that it introduced for the first time a competitive assay design suitable for haptenic molecules and a radioactive tracer which provided robust and highly sensitive detection not achieved earlier. The fact that at that time there was a definite need for such sensitive technique also may have been a factor.

Radioimmunoassays rapidly revolutionized the routines in many areas of clinical and scientific investigation, especially endocrinology, where the previous methods for measuring hormones often had insufficient sensitivity and dubious specificity.

Thus 1960 proved to be an important milestone in the development of quantitative sensitive immunoassays. During the next two decades radioimmunoassays had a dominating position, and the main developments in immunoassay technology took place via RIA. Therefore the evolution of immunoassays coincides to a great extent with the evolution of RIA. Not until the late '70s and '80s were alternative, non-isotopic methodologies developed; they since have opened totally new perspectives in technological research.

3.1. HISTORY OF IMMUNOASSAYS

Antibodies have been produced, purified, and used in the research of immunological reactions since the beginning of the twentieth century (119). Labeled antibodies were already in use in 1930, when Reiner (3) suggested the use of labeled antibodies for quantitative measurements of an immunoreaction.

Heidelberger and Kendall (4) made quantitative immunoassays in 1932 using unlabeled antibodies as reagents for measuring either antibodies, antigens, or haptens. They measured polysaccharides of pneumococcus by antibody-augmented precipitation reaction, using the nitrogen content of antibodies as internal tracer, determined with the micro Kjeldahl method.

The same authors used also azo-dye labeled antibodies for quantitative colorimetric determinations of immunoreaction (120).

Coons et al. (5, 6) were the first to introduce fluorescent compounds as labels for immunological techniques. They used labeled antibodies as reagents for detecting bacterial strains with fluorescence microscopes. It is surprising that the use of antibodies in competitive immunoassays did not appear until 18 years later with the introduction of RIA. The basic technology using labeled antibodies or labeled secondary antibodies (indirect staining) was not applied in quantitative immunoassays until much later with the advent of immunoradiometric assays in 1967, introduced by Wide et al. (121).

The immunofluorescence staining technique has remained unchanged since then and is still a widely applied technique in histology, pathology, virology, and microbiology. The same basic staining technique is also applied in flow-cytometric studies. The attempts to quantitate immunofluorescence resulted in "quantitative immunofluorescence" tests and later on led to its part in the development of immunofluorometric assays (IFMA).

The first homogeneous, quantitative immunoassay employing labeled antigen was based on hemagglutination reaction (HA) and was invented by Stavitsky and Arquilla in 1953 (122). They used tannic-acid-treated erythrocytes activated with insulin to detect anti-insulin antibodies by detecting the complement mediated lysis of erythrocytes by photometry. It is noteworthy that the occurrence of anti-insulin antibodies with insulin-treated diabetic patients has played a very important role in the development of radioimmunoassays (7, 8, 116–118). Stavitsky and Arquilla were able to detect microgram amounts of insulin and nanogram amounts of anti-tetanus, -albumin, and -diphtheria toxin antibodies with their homogeneous HA-assay (123, 124).

Radioisotopically labeled antigens were introduced in late '50s also for the determination of circulating antibodies. During 1957 and 1958 Farr (125, 126) reported the use of ^{131}I-labeled bovine albumin (BSA) for measuring antigen binding capacity by using polyethyleneglycol (PEG) augmented precipitation of formed immunocomplexes. The technique is still widely applied as a "Farr-assay" for determination of, for instance, anti-DNA antibodies using tritium-labeled DNA and precipitating the formed immunocomplexes with half-saturated ammonium sulfate (127). The Farr-assay differs from RIA, which was invented a few years later, only in that it measures antibodies, not antigens, and does not involve competition.

3.2. ADVENT OF RADIOIMMUNOASSAY

Quantitative immunological determination of antigen with RIA in the beginning of the 1960s was the origin of modern immunoassay technology. In the early '60s it was soon recognized that the general simplicity, potential sensitivity, and wide applicability of this type of assay made it the undoubted method of choice for most hormones. It offered a robust, sensitive, and easy method for the clinical chemist. The method rapidly replaced laborious bioassays.

In 1956 Berson and Yalow (7) demonstrated the presence of insulin antibodies in insulin-treated patients with the use of ^{131}I-labeled insulin. They showed that in the reversible binding of labeled insulin to a given amount of anti-insulin antibodies the ratio bound tracer/free tracer is an inverse function of the concentration of free insulin. In 1959 they constructed different theoretical models for the assay and were able to detect 1 ng amounts of anti-insulin antibodies (117) and finally constructed a competitive assay for insulin (116–118). At the same time those findings were confirmed by Grodsky et al. (128, 129) who were able to measure insulin with a detection limit of 20 μU/ml, which was not, however, enough for serum samples.

Soon after these studies Ekins et al. developed similar competitive binding assays using other specific binding proteins. The assay of blood vitamin B_{12} was based on ^{57}Co-labeled B_{12} and a circulating carrier protein (12), and the assay of thyroxine used thyroxine binding globulin as a binding protein for labeled thyroxine (13). Ekins also further developed the mathematic models and the theory behind the "limited reagent" or "saturation" assay as he named those competitive protein binding assays.

In the same year Weiler et al. (130) developed a similar assay based on inhibition of the precipitation of ^{131}I-labeled human globulin by globulins of samples in the presence of a limited amount of anti-globulin antibodies.

In spite of the work of an immunologist, Landsteiner, who produced anti-hapten antibodies as early as 1946 (9) and the studies of Erlanger et al. (10, 131), who synthesized steroid conjugates for immunization in 1957, a decade elapsed between the introduction of protein and steroid immunoassays (132).

All the early radioimmunoassays were competitive assays (RIA), which relied on competitive binding between an accurate, small amount of labeled antigen and an unknown amount of sample antigen for a limited amount of antibodies.

3.3. LABELING OF IMMUNOREAGENTS

Labeling antigens with dye molecules was introduced in the early study of the immunogenicity of those protein antigens (119). Labeling in immunoreagents with marker molecules, which facilitates the sensitive monitoring of immunological binding reactions, was introduced by Coons et al. (5, 6). Since then various marker substances have been applied, and almost any compound which can be detected with reasonable sensitivity has been used also as a label in immunoassays (Chapter 4.2). In addition to detectability, the marker used needs to be coupled to an immunoreagent without interfering with the primary recognition reaction.

The first radioimmunoassays all relied on antigens labeled with a radioisotopic nuclei. In the simplest cases suitable atoms of antigens were replaced with respective radioisotopic nucleus, like iodine of thyroxine for ^{131}I or later on for ^{125}I, or cobalt of vitamin B_{12} for ^{57}Co.

Different labeling procedures have been developed especially for protein antigens and antibodies, which after iodination need to preserve their binding activity. The chloramine T-method is one of the most often applied techniques, but it may include oxidative changes to the target molecule (133). Lactoperoxidase is used for enzymatic iodination with H_2O_2 and $Na^{125}I$ (134, 135). Other systems applied include electrolytic iodination (136) and iodination with iodine monochloride (137). In the Bolton-Hunter method, a free aminogroup of a suitable amino acid side chain is acylated with N-succinimidyl-3-(4-hydroxy-5-^{125}I-iodophenyl)-propionate (138).

Gamma emitting isotopes are the most often used labels in RIA techniques, but lately also β emitters, like tritium or the Auger electrons of ^{125}I, are applied for solid-scintillator based assays. The short distance penetration of β particles (4 μm with ^3H β particles or 35 μm for ^{125}I Auger electrons) can be exploited to construct homogeneous "proximity" assays (139, 140), commercialized by Amersham International (Bucks, UK). The homogeneous assays were long considered impossible with radioactive isotopes.

3.4. SEPARATION SYSTEMS

The early immunoassays almost invariably required the separation of bound labeled reagent from unbound reagent before measurement of either of the fractions took place. The precipitated or surface bound antibody-reacted fraction of labeled antigen is the fraction most often measured in those assays, which because of the separation of reaction components into two phases are generally termed heterogeneous assays (Eq. 3.1).

$$\begin{array}{c} Ab + Ag^* + Ag_x \leftrightarrow AbAg^* + AbAg_x + Ag^* + Ag_x \\ \downarrow \text{Separation} \\ \underset{\text{Counted}}{AbAg^* + AbAg_x} \qquad \qquad \underset{\text{Discarded}}{Ag^* + Ag_x} \end{array} \tag{3.1}$$

The measurement of bound fraction in competitive assays results in a typical inverse relationship between analyte concentration and the resulting response within the working range of the assay between zero-level binding (B_0) and nonspecific binding (response representing infinite analyte concentration) (Fig. 3.1a). As competitive assays generally have limited dynamic range, the dose-response curve is often drawn in a linear scale, the percentage of bound tracer (B/B_0) as a function of antigen (Ag_x) concentration (Fig. 3.1b).

An ideal separation system should perform complete separation without interfering with the primary equilibrium, be simple, rapid, and economic, and should not be prone to matrix differences of samples (e.g., variations in protein concentrations or lipid content).

Paper chromatoelectrophoresis was the separation system applied by Yalow and Berson in the early RIA (118), but later on a variety of precipitation techniques were employed in a majority of RIAs. Precipitation of the antigen-antibody complex, or all immunoglobulins present in an assay mixture, has been the most often used technique in competitive heterogeneous assays. Precipitation with half-saturated ammonium sulfate or concentrated PEG, used already in Farr-assays (125–127), are also frequently applied in competitive RIAs. Sometimes organic solvents—for example, ethanol—are used in addition to PEG (141) or simple extraction of organic solvent soluble tracers is performed (142, 143). Double-antibody precipitation with anti-species antibodies is also a relatively commonly used separation system (144). Another technique frequently applied in RIAs is the absorption either of the components with charcoal (145), dextran-coated charcoal, silicates, or ion exchange resins (146). The fraction separation has sometimes also been accomplished by gel filtration (147).

3.4.1. Coated Surfaces

One of the most important improvements in radioimmunoassay techniques was the use of antibody-coated tubes for solid-phase separation, introduced by Catt and Tregear in 1967 (148). They used antibodies noncovalently adsorbed onto polystyrene and polypropylene test tubes for radioimmunoassays of growth hormone and prolactin. Since then solid-phase separation has become one of the most applied separation systems in heterogeneous immunoassays.

The use of solid surfaces which can be washed easily greatly enhances the efficiency of separation and facilitates the use of noncompetitive, reagent excess, immunometric assays, where the complete and efficient separation of bound labeled antibodies from a large excess of unbound labeled antibodies is an absolute necessity. Solid-phase separation also frees the tech-

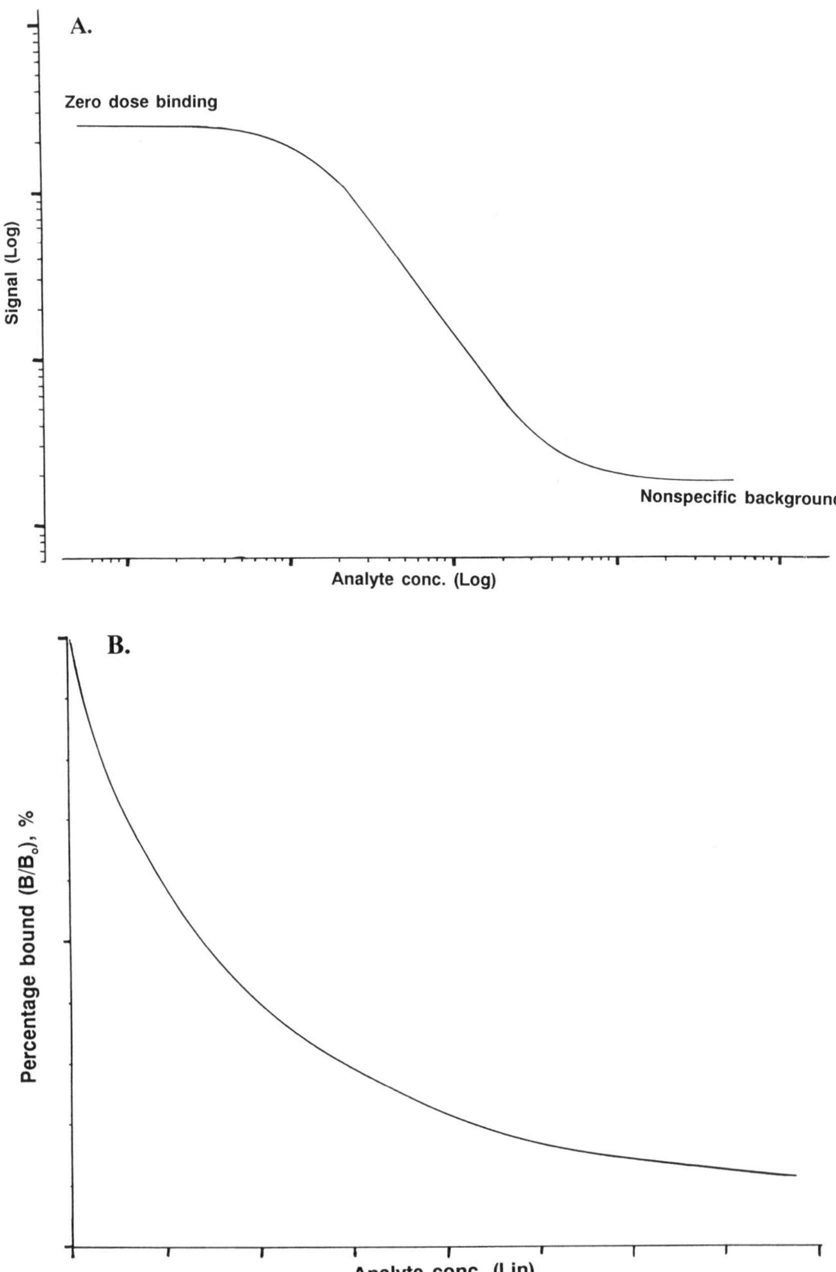

Fig. 3.1. Dose-response curves for a model competitive immunoassay, presented as logarithmic scales **(A)** and as a more conventional linear scale **(B)**.

nique from dependence on the centrifuge, thus opening possibilities for mechanized or more automated immunoassays.

Hydrophobic and Van der Waal forces are primarily responsible for the attachment of proteins to plastic surfaces. The absorbed proteins form a one-molecule-thick layer on plastic surfaces and the binding strength is directly proportional to the molecular size of the protein. For example, from the same amount of added IgM, IgG, or albumin the relative binding percentages of 85, 40, and 15% are recorded (149). The adsorptive coating is performed in a variety of buffers, pHs, and protein concentrations. The binding of proteins to surfaces is, however, extremely sensitive to the existence of detergents (46), which tends to detach coated proteins from the surfaces during the immunoassay. Reports about the detachment of bound proteins are, however, contradictory. The estimates of leaking vary between 0 and 50%.

The detachment of surface bound antibodies during the immunoassay is avoided by, for example, cross linking the proteins prior to coating in order to form larger molecules with stronger bindings (150). Partial acid denaturation of IgG prior to coating can produce more stable and active antibody-coated surfaces (151–153). Radiation with either UV light or X-rays is a method to produce "high-binding" surfaces with improved binding characteristics (154). DuPont de Nemours has developed a technique to increase the affinity of adsorption (155) by introducing fluorocarbon side chains on both the solid-phase and on the protein to create mutual high affinity between them.

Coating with haptenic antigens is generally performed after conjugation of the hapten to a suitable carrier protein, such as albumin (156), or better binding can be obtained by using larger proteins, such as thyroglobulin (157).

Very many materials have been tested as solid matrixes in immunoassays, the choice being partly dependent on the particular assay type, the detection system, the availability and price of the materials, and the convenience of use. Sedlacek et al. (158) evaluated several polymeric plastics and glass materials as solid-phases for IFMA with regard to specific binding, nonspecific background, and autofluorescence. In their study polymethylmethacrylate, polycarbonate, and polystyrene gave the best properties. Also, inorganic materials have been used as solid-phase, and glass fibers, for instance, are commonly applied in immunosensors (Chapter 8.5), generally after activation for covalent couplings. Wang et al. (159) used clear metal surfaces as a solid-phase for an IFMA of AFP.

In the development of nonisotopic immunoassays, microtitration plates (8 × 12 wells) or strips (8 or 12 wells in rows) made of polystyrene have become the most often used solid matrix. Because very few activation processes are useful for that kind of surface, the microtitration wells are generally coated with noncovalent adsorption. A problem frequently encountered with microtitration plates is the so-called "edge effect," an uneven coating giving higher signals to the edges of plates (160–163). The reason for the anomalous signal difference is unknown, but it can often be overcome by careful optimization of coating, washing, and stabilization of the surfaces. In the extreme cases the edges—the first and the last wells of the rows—are neglected in measurement (70).

Although the noncovalent, adsorptive coating method is frequently criticized, it is still the most frequently used and successful immobilizing technique for practical immunoassays.

3.4.2. Covalent Surfaces

In an attempt to improve the binding capacity and the stability of the coated surfaces, solid surfaces are chemically modified to make covalent linkages with proteins. The most frequently applied methods are direct activation of available plastics, grafting of surfaces with appropriate functional layers, precoating the surfaces with suitable polymers containing reactive groups, and preparation of reactive, molded plastic surfaces.

Nylon is used as an activated surface, because reactive aminogroups can easily be formed by partial surface hydrolysis of the amide-linkages. Hendry and Herrmann (164) used nylon balls, treated with HCl and activated with either water soluble carbodiimide (EDAC) of glutardialdehyde, for coupling with antibodies. The activation was claimed to increase the total capacity up to 74 $\mu g/cm^2$ (more than can be calculated from a monolayer) and to produce less desorption. Similarly surface hydrolyzed nylon balls were tested in EIA of antinuclear antibodies after activation with picryl sulfonic acid (165). Verschoor et al. used polystyrene microtitration plates crafted with a nylon layer and coated covalently with a hapten in a screening of hybridoma cultures producing anti-hapten antibodies (166).

The production of reactive aminogroups on polystyrene is more difficult. Neurath et al. used nitration of the polystyrene surface, reduction of the nitrogroups into amines, and activation with glutardialdehyde for coupling with antibodies (167) or coupling to aldehydes produced from glycoproteins via periodate oxidation (168) in their assays of hepatitis B antigens (HBsAg) and anti-HBsAg antibodies, respectively. Chu and Tarcha (169) prepared molded polystyrene balls for EIA via activation of the surfaces with chlorosulfonation to form sulfonamides subsequently coupled with antibodies after bromoacetyl activation (170). By roughening the surface with an abrasive wheel, the total binding capacity was increased tenfold.

Polymethylmethacrylate film was used as a solid-phase after reaction with hydrazine hydrate and activation with acid and nitrite to produce reactive diazogroups. The resultant covalent surface reportedly produced superior binding and nonspecific binding properties (158).

Glass fibers, applied to promote immunosensors (Chapter 8.4), are generally activated by silanization (171) to form stable reactive intermediates for covalent couplings. Plant et al. (172) used glass beads silanized with aminobutyldimethylethoxysilane and activated with succinimidyl-4(p-maleimidophenyl) butyrate for coupling with SH-groups of Fab ′- fragment and used them in a flow-injection fluoroimmunoassay technique. Alarie et al. (173) tested 7 μm diameter, 500 Å pore size silica beads (Synchron) for a fiberoptic fluoroimmunosensor after activation with different reagents—carbonyldiimidazole, glycidoxypropyltrimethoxysilane, fluoromethylpyridinium toluene sulfonate—and compared the results to those obtained with protein A coated beads in immobilizing antibodies. In their test, carbonyldiimidazole-activated beads and protein A coated beads gave the highest incorporation of active antibodies.

Grafting solid surfaces with a suitable polymeric layer, which can be subsequently activated, was done in 1966 to make covalently coated surfaces by Catt et al. (174). They used styrene-polytetrafluoroethylene as grafting material and activated the surface by nitrating, reducing, and converting the amines into isothiocyanates with thiophosgene. Larsson et al. (175) grafted polystyrene and polyvinylchloride surfaces with crotonic acid after radiation (forms free radicals) and coupled antibodies with EDAC. They were able to bind more proteins to the grafted surfaces than anticipated from a single monolayer, which might be a result of the aggregated clusters formed in the process.

One of the most frequently used covalent or "semicovalent" coating methods is precoating the surfaces with glutardialdehyde or polymerized glutardialdehyde (176, 177). Although the mechanism of glutardialdehyde reaction with aminogroups of proteins is not fully understood, glutardialdehyde is thought to form unsaturated condensation products with preserved aldehyde functions, which form relatively stable Schiff's bases with aminogroups. Other polymers used for precoating are polyimines and polypeptides. For example, phenylalanine-lysine copolymer is used as a source of amines activated after precoating with glutardialdehyde (178), and tyrosine-glutamate polyaminoacid as an acidic peptide for noncovalent ionic interaction with basic histone in assay of anti-histone antibodies (179).

Since the activation of most solid-phase materials is rather tedious, the availability of ready-to-use protein reactive molded plastic surfaces could find applications in immunoassays, especially in cases when noncovalent coating does not give satisfactory results. Various membranes attached to bottoms of microtitration plates or strips have recently found applications in immunoassays. Membranes of cellulose-acetate, nitrocellulose, nylon, or derivatized nylons, for example, are available from several commercial sources (Pall BioSupport, Portsmouth, England; Millipore, Bedford, MA;

Costar Co., Cambridge, MA; Micromembranes Inc., Newark, NJ). They can be used as supports for coating, covalent coupling, or particle capture assays (see, for instance, PCFIA by Pandex, Chapter 8.2.5). Derivatized polystyrene surfaces containing secondary amines in the form of microtitration strips were recently introduced by Nunc (CovaLink™, Nunc As Roskilde, Denmark).

3.4.3. Microbeads

Polymeric carbohydrates, dextranes, or celluloses, as microcrystals or porous beads, are extensively applied as solid carriers in affinity chromatography, biotechnology, and also immunoassays. Their activation is primarily performed with cyanogen bromide (180). Cyanogen bromide activated beads were applied, for instance, in the first published immunoradiometric assays (IRMA) (121, 181) and in early EIAs (182).

Cellulose was the matrix used in early attempts to standardize and quantitate the fluorescence microscopic test with the "soluble-antigen-fluorescent-antibody" (SAFA) technique (183–185) using cellulose discs coupled with antigens. Another approach to quantitative immunofluorometric assays was the use of "defined antigen substrate spheres" (DASS), composed of activated Sephadex (186), Sepharose, (187) or agarose beads (188, 189) coupled with antigens for microfluorometric determinations.

Polyacrylamide beads are used as solid-phases for various immunoassays (190). Also, commercial fluoroimmunoassay kits based on polyacrylamide beads, Immunobeads™, are marketed by Bio-Rad Laboratories (Richmond, CA, USA).

Monodisperse latex particles, plastic particles with accurately defined size, were first introduced as markers for antigens in scanning electron microscopy (191). Uniform latex particles are produced either by emulsion polymerization (size 0.04–3 μm), suspension polymerization (4–90 μm), or swollen emulsion polymerization (2–20 μm). Those beads with very accurate dimensions are used as standards for electron microscopy, flow cytometers, and particle counters. They are also used as carriers for fluors (fluorescent spheres, Chapter 7.5.3), gold, silver, or magnetite. Phillips et al. (192) used aminostyrene beads in their IFMA of virus diagnosis. Microspheres are also used in commercial immunoassay systems, such as PCFIA of Pandex, and in a microparticle capture enzyme immunoassay (MEIA), the IM_x system of Abbott (Chapter 9.2.2).

Magnetic or magnetizable particles are coupled with suitable carriers to facilitate precipitation of the particles to simplify separation with the aid of a magnetic field. Cellulose/iron oxide magnetizable particles, prepared according to Robinson and Dunnill (193), are frequently applied in immunoassays (194, 195) (see Chapter 8.2.5) after activation with cyanogen bromide.

Improvements in buoyancy properties and avoidance of activation with hazardous cyanogen bromide led to the development of polyacrolein-coated cellulose/iron oxide particles (196). The acrolein-coated cellulose/iron oxide particles do not require continuous mixing as do the heavier acrolein/iron oxide particles.

Chromium instead of iron is used in magnetic particles introduced by DuPont, Magni Sep™ (197), applied in the company's EIAs, such as the automated VISTA™ system (DuPont de Nemours & Co.). Reportedly those particles have the advantage of low remnant magnetism resulting in minimal magnetic aggregation, good wettability, stability in aqueous solution, and rapid separation in a magnetic field (197).

Magnetic separation is also applied in a commercial luminoimmunoassay system, Magic Lite™ of Ciba Corning. Various types of magnetizable microparticles are also commercially available from such sources as Technia Diagnostics (London), Scipac (Detling, Kent, UK) and Advanced Magnetic Inc. (Biomag™, Cambridge, MA, USA).

Other matrixes sometimes applied in immunoassays for solid-phase separation include the viable cell, used in hybridoma screening with a Pandex Screen Machine (198). Examples of the three-dimensional matrixes used as solid-phases are glass-fiber filters used in the Stratus system of Baxter and a water swellable, particle containing, protein binding gel, Collimune™ in the Track® system (Daryl Laboratories Inc., Santa Clara, CA), the matrix of which contains both scattering particles and light absorbing particles (199, 200).

Compared to plane surfaces, small beads have the benefits of a larger total area available when needed, easy activation processes which can be performed in bulk amounts, more rapid assay kinetics due to shorter diffusion distances, and the possibility of applying different separation systems, such as centrifugation, gradient separation, filtration, or magnetic separation. With beads, the analyte and the analyte-bound tracer can also be concentrated to a certain volume for measurement, used in the "Particle Concentration ImmunoAssay" PACIA of Pandex (a division of Baxter Health Care Co.).

Assays based on the use of microbeads, however, involve more steps than the assays applying simple surfaces due to the repeated incubations and washings of the beads. Avoiding the sedimentation of beads during immunoassays generally requires constant shaking, either mechanic or magnetic. Viscosity agents, like hydroxypropylmethylcellulose, sucrose, dextran, etc., are employed to avoid sedimentation of the dense particles during incubation.

3.4.4. Nonspecific Binding

Solid-phase separation systems provide not only a convenient but also a very efficient means of separating bound fraction from traces of unbound reagent, which is a very important factor in designing the assay performance—especially in noncompetitive assays. Efficient separation minimizes the error related to miscalculation of bound or free fraction. The sensitivity of noncompetitive, immunometric assays can be more dependent on the efficiency of separation than the ultimate detection sensitivity of the marker substance.

For easy, convenient, and efficient separation, the surface used needs to be easily washable. The nonspecific binding of labeled reagents to the surfaces might, however, have affinities that do not allow their removal by simple washing. Therefore both the labeling of the reagents (e.g., antibodies with a marker substance) and the properties of solid surfaces need to be optimized to give low nonspecific binding (NSB). Hydrophobic interaction chromatography with phenyl-sepharose has been found suitable for purification of labeled antibodies to get rid of hydrophobic fractions, which are responsible for high NSB in IFMA (201).

Bovine serum albumin has most often been used as a blocking agent for solid surfaces. It is used both to keep immobilized antibodies active and to restrict NSB. High concentrations of gelatin have on some occasions proven to be a more efficient blocker than albumin (202, 203). Because of their hydrophobicity, casein or hydrolyzed caseins are tested as surface blockers to avoid NSB (204). Unpurified, nonfatty, dried milk has also been used (205, 206), but its use is restricted by its interference of protein A binding (207) and biotin-avidin interaction (208). Addition of a salt concentration up to 0.4 M has restricted NSB in solid-phase assay (209). The effect of blocking proteins also depends on the label used. With BCPDA-ligand as the label (Chapter 7.4.4), thyroglobulin and casein were found to cause high nonspecific binding, whereas saturation with albumin, gelatin, ovalbumin, globulin, and polyvinylpyrrolidone gave acceptable results (210).

The nonspecific binding of labeled antibodies is charge dependent and almost directly proportional to the pI of the surface layer (211). Accordingly, the NSB has been decreased by co-coating antibodies with negatively charged polypeptides, such as α_1-acid glycoprotein (211) or polyglutaric acid (212). The acidic surface so produced actually mimics the surfaces of cells and membranes *in vivo*—in blood vessels, for instance.

NSB is particularly problematic when measuring small amounts of specific antibodies from samples (serum) containing milligram amounts of related IgG. Kohno and Ishikawa have introduced a technique they named immunocomplex transfer immunoassay to increase the assay sensitivities by means of NSB reduction (213–215). The technique is based on two sets of affinity reactions on solid surfaces, and a sensitivity increase up to 10,000-fold reportedly has been achieved.

3.5. IMMUNOMETRIC ASSAYS

Even though labeled antibodies have long been applied in direct and indirect immunofluorescence staining techniques for microscopic determinations of surface antigens, the introduction of radioactively labeled antibodies in noncompetitive, reagent excess assays has generally been credited to Miles and Hales in 1968 (216). They labeled anti-insulin antibodies with ^{125}I while bound to immobilized insulin (217). After releasing the labeled antibody, they used it for a noncompetitive, two-step IRMA-assay of insulin. After incubating sample insulin with an excess of labeled antibodies in the first step, the unbound antibodies were removed with solid-phase bound insulin (used in excess), and the analyte-bound labeled antibodies left were counted (Eq. 3.2). Miles and Hales termed their assay an immunometric assay (IRMA) because labeled antibodies were applied instead of labeled antigen.

$$
\begin{aligned}
&1.\quad Ab^* + Ag \leftrightarrow Ab^* + Ab^*-Ag \\
&2.\quad Ab^* + Ab^*-Ag + \blacksquare-Ag \leftrightarrow \blacksquare-Ag-Ab^* + Ab^*-Ag
\end{aligned}
\qquad (3.2)
$$

separation

$$\blacksquare-Ag-Ab^* \qquad\qquad Ab^*-Ag$$

counted

Later on the term *immunometric assay,* like IRMA, IFMA, etc., was more generally applied to describe assay design, which more precisely could be termed noncompetitive, sandwich-type or two-site assays. Since the pioneering work of Wide et al. in 1967 (121), who made a noncompetitive "RAST" assay of specific allergy-related antibodies, these types of immunoassays have proven to be the most suitable assays for most antigens having at least two epitopic sites. Noncompetitive sandwich-type assays are based on nonlabeled antibodies immobilized on solid surfaces for catching the antigens from samples, and the bound fraction is subsequently determined by additional immunoreaction with labeled antibodies forming a "sandwich" on the solid-phase (Eq. 3.3) (Figs. 2.3 and 3.2).

$$\begin{array}{llcl} 1. & \blacksquare - Ab + Ag & \leftrightarrow & \blacksquare - Ab - Ag \\ 2. & \blacksquare - Ab - Ag + Ab^* & \leftrightarrow & \blacksquare - Ab - Ag - Ab^* + Ab^* \\ & & & \quad \downarrow \text{ washing} \\ & & & \blacksquare - Ab - Ag - Ab^* \ / \text{ counted} \end{array} \tag{3.3}$$

Sandwich IRMA (later cited simply as IRMA) were rapidly gaining wide application in assays of peptide hormones, such as human growth hormone, HGH (218), and follitropin, FSH (219). Miles and Hales argued in 1968 on theoretical grounds that the IRMA technique should provide improvements in analytical sensitivity and specificity. They also proposed that further advantages could be gained by replacing the ^{125}I-label with a non-radioactive label, particularly if the signal detection could be amplified. Actually the very first sensitive enzyme immunoassays applied an immunometric assay design (182, 220, 221), and two-site assay technique has since then been applied for high sensitivity assays using different labels and detection principles.

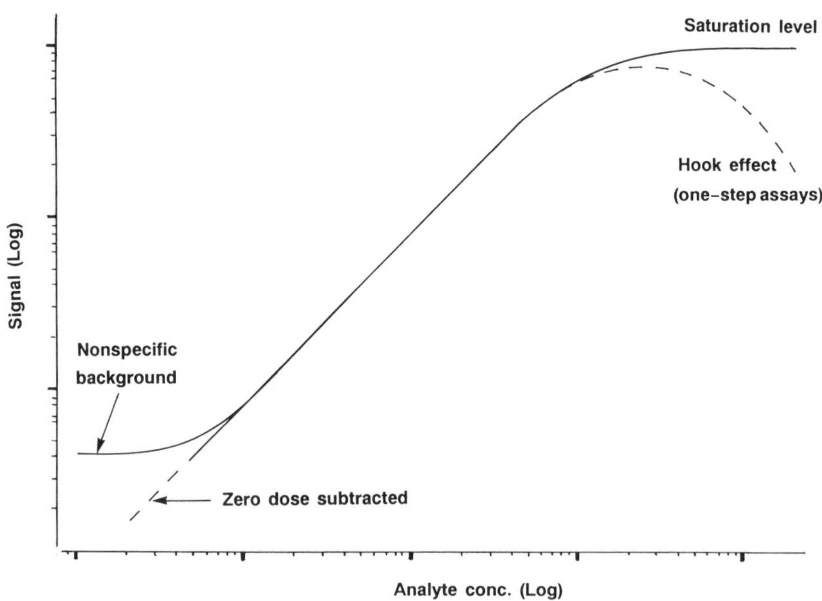

Fig. 3.2. Dose-response curve for a noncompetitive immunoassay.

3.6. SENSITIVITY OF IMMUNOASSAYS

Sensitivity of an assay system is one of the most important characteristics of analysis. Sensitivity, or the detection limit, has been defined in numerous ways, and discrepancies have prevailed about the most accurate and right definition of those terms. Unless common definitions are used it is difficult to evaluate different procedures from published articles.

Definitions of the terms *assay sensitivity* or *detection limit* have been made according to the slope of the dose-response curve, to the "midpoint" or midrange, ED_{50}, or 50% intercept, to a dose value giving $B/B_0 = 0.8$, etc. (222–225) . Different authors have also made different implicit assumptions in their theoretical calculations of optimal sensitivities; some workers have ignored the effect of errors in the estimation of response of zero dose; others have ignored uncertainty in the mean response for replicates, etc.

Most often the sensitivity of an assay has been defined from the precision of a zero dose (225–229), but even then different confidence limits have been applied. Sensitivities are presented as a dose giving the response of zero plus one, two, or three standard deviation of zero response (zero + $1-3 \times$ SD). If the measurement has been carried out using a zero calibrator, which can be even an artificial buffer, the definition does not take into consideration any matrix effects of sample nor biological variations (227, 230). The actual sensitivity of any immunoassay could be defined as the minimal dose of the analyte in samples which can be measured with reasonable confidence limits.

Similar discrepancies prevailed about the respective merits and disadvantages of noncompetitive immunometric assays as compared to original competitive assay design (231). It has been shown in theory and in practice that noncompetitive assays are potentially more robust and sensitive (232, 233). Rodbard and Weiss (234) stated that optimal sensitivity of competitive RIA is defined by the association constant of antibodies, $1/k_a$. Later on Ekins (235) demonstrated that the potential sensitivity of any competitive protein binding assay is strictly governed by factor E/K, where E is total error and K is the effective equilibrium constant.

On the other hand, the basic difference in optimizing noncompetitive assay is that optimal concentration of labeled antibodies is towards infinity, unless restricted by their nonspecific binding. Accordingly, the optimal sensitivity of immunometric assay is defined by factor E $\times$ NSB/K, where E is total error, NSB is the fractional nonspecific binding, and K is affinity. As a result, the noncompetitive assays can be several orders of magnitude more sensitive than competitive assays (232).

The sensitivity of immunoassays relying on radioisotopic labels permits the measurement of analyte concentrations above 10^7 molecules per ml. The limitation derives primarily from "manipulation" errors and the specific activity of labeled antibodies. In order to develop more sensitive assays, it is already generally recognized that noncompetitive assay design needs to be adopted with a high specific activity label and highly efficient discrimination between specifically bound fraction and nonspecific binding. Indeed, in two-site sandwich-type immunometric assays using nonradioactive labels, such as enzymes or fluorescent or luminescent probes, higher sensitivities have been achieved than those obtained with RIA or IRMA.

CHAPTER

4

NON-ISOTOPIC IMMUNOASSAYS

During the 1960s and '70s immunoassays relying on radioisotopic labels gained wide acceptance in various fields of clinical and medical science and practice. Since then a growing interest in alternative, non-radioisotopic techniques has evolved, and gradually those methods are replacing radioimmunoassays in several areas. Even though radioimmunoassays have their unquestionable advantages, certain of their limitations have created a strong demand to develop non-radioisotopic alternatives. Alternative labels and techniques have been adopted primarily in order to achieve simpler or more sensitive assays that do not involve radioisotopes.

4.1. LIMITATIONS OF RADIOISOTOPES

The disadvantages of radioisotopes and the problems related to their handling have been the strongest driving forces toward non-radioisotopic immunoassay techniques and labels. Some of the advantages of radioisotopic tracers together with the limitations and restrictions related to their use are listed in Table 4.1.

Table 4.1. Advantages and Disadvantages of Radioisotopic Labels

Advantages	Disadvantages
High sensitivity	**Limited shelf life**
low and stable background	short lifetimes of isotopic tracers
Robust detection	deterioration of reagents by decay catastrophe
not sensitive to sample interferences	**Specific activity limited to one ^{125}I per IgG**
insensitive to environmental factors	**Radiation hazard**
Small size of isotopes	handling, purchasing and waste problems
minimal effect to immunoreaction	legal problems
Radiation counting well established	**Expensive production**
	Negative public attitude

Environmental reasons have become one of the most important driving forces toward non-radioisotopic techniques. A strong public attitude has grown against the use of radioisotopes even though the amounts used normally cause very minimal health hazards to the user. However, stricter safety regulations have been made concerning the purchase, use, storage, and disposal of radioactive material, and even stricter legal restrictions can be expected in future.

The expanding use of immunoassays, not only in specialized laboratories but also at doctors' offices, at the bedside, in patients' homes, in less developed countries, in agricultural field conditions, etc., requires simpler techniques made possible only with non-radioactive labels. Economic reasons are related to the shelf life of reagents, problems with the storage and delivery of kits, and the limited batch sizes in production.

One very important reason to develop non-isotopic techniques is the increasing demand for simpler assays and automated assays, assays that can be mechanized and which require less frequent standardization. On the other hand, the development of simple homogeneous assays was long considered impossible with radioisotopes. Recently, however, homogeneous radioimmunoassays have also been developed, assays which are based on β-emitting isotopes detected by the use of scintillation particles (either polymeric or inorganic crystals). The short distance penetration of β particles in aqueous solution is used in those "proximity" assays where the proximity phenomenon diminishes the need for physical separation (139). The use of short lifetime radioactive isotopes renders their use difficult in automated systems, however, and the homogeneous RIA hardly can find such extensive applications as, for instance, the fluorescence polarization based assay has achieved in the field of therapeutic drug monitoring.

Another approach toward automation has been the development of remote immunosensors, where, for example, fluorescent probes and evanescent wave excitation have found applications (Chapter 8.5) and where enzymes or enzyme-labeled reagents are used.

Improving the assay performance and especially increasing the sensitivity are very important reasons for developing labels with higher specific activity than radioactive isotopes have. The specific activity of a labeled antibody is the major factor limiting the sensitivity of noncompetitive assays. The detection limit of ^{125}I and ^{125}I-labeled antibodies is around 5 to 10 amols. Increasing the labeling level beyond one atom of ^{125}I per IgG may not offer any advantage due to the radiolytic damage caused by iodine. Radiolytic damage can significantly reduce the immunoreactivity of labeled antibodies, which is manifested as a rise in nonspecific binding and a reduction in specific binding (236, 237). It is only through the use of non-isotopic labels that it has been possible to demonstrate the importance of the high specific activity of labeled antibodies in determining immunometric assay sensitivity. It is now clear that whatever arguments have been used in the past in favor of non-isotopic techniques, in the future they will be the automatic choice on the basis of assay performance (238).

4.2. ALTERNATIVE LABELS

A great number of substances and detection techniques have been applied in immunoassays. Almost any compound which can be detected with high sensitivity and which can be firmly attached to the ligand without grossly altering its binding properties has been tested as an alternative to radioisotopes. The field of immunoassays is huge, both in respect to variations in compounds to be measured and in respect to concentration ranges, which may vary from millimolar to subpicomolar. The very optimal label should cover most of the applications and the wide concentration range of analytes present in biological samples. It sets a very high demand for the desired system, and covering the whole field of immunoassays may be a quite unrealistic demand for a single technique. Some general requirements could, however, be listed:

Sensitivity. In order to exceed the sensitivity of radioisotopic tracers, the alternative label should enable the labeled reagent to be detected at concentrations down to 10^{-15}–10^{-18} mols. The detection system should be relatively simple, rapid, and inexpensive. It is worth remembering however that the sensitivity of assays is not solely determined by the detection sensitivity of the label, but rather the properties of the immunoreagents—for example, the retained affinity and low nonspecific binding of the labeled antibodies.

Coupling Properties. In order to be used for assays of many different compounds, the label used needs to be coupled to immunological reagents. The coupling should not alter the immunological properties of labeled antigens, affect the affinity or specifity of labeled antibodies, or decrease the signal produced.

Homogeneity. For simple homogeneous assays, the extent of immunoreaction has to be monitored without physical separation of the reaction components. The label used needs to enable the monitoring either via a change in signal level upon immunobinding, via susceptibility to signal modulation, or via physical or optical properties, like fluorescence polarization.

Stability. The short shelf life of radioisotopes (^{125}I) is one of the most serious limitations of those labels. The alternative label should enable storage of labeled reagent for extended periods of time. Stable signal levels from assay to assay and from day to day are required for automated or mechanized immunoassay systems to decrease the need for frequent standardization. The optimal label should be inert against effectors derived from samples, like coloric compounds or quenching agents, endogenous enzymes or enzyme inhibitors, etc.

Unsusceptibility to Environmental Factors. One very strong benefit of radioisotopic labels is their robust detection, which is not affected by any compounds present in samples or assay buffers, nor physical conditions like temperature or pH. Alternative labels introduced are often quite sensitive to those factors, which must be taken into consideration in choosing the label and detection system.

Clinical Applicability. To be useful in routine clinical use—or preferable even at doctors' offices or at patients' homes—the label introduced should provide robust practical detection and be susceptible for automation.

Safety. The biological hazard caused by radioisotopes has caused the strong public—and also legal—opposition to the use of radioisotopic techniques. The alternative label should be nontoxic and safe and should not involve dangerous reagents nor cause waste problems.

Availability. To be widely accepted both in research and in clinical routine, the labeling reagents should be generally available, the labeling reaction should be mild and easily optimized for each particular immunoreagent, and the labeling should be highly reproducible.

4.2.1. Enzymes as Labels

Enzymes are biological proteins which catalyze specific reactions. The high detection sensitivity of enzymes is based on the high turnover number of the enzyme-catalyzed reaction, which produces a very efficient amplification effect; on average one enzyme molecule is able to produce up to 1,000 molecules of colored, fluorescent, or luminogenic product per second.

Enzymes were coupled to antigens and antibodies in 1966 by Avrameas and Uriel (239). The first enzyme immunoassays were reported in 1971 (180, 220, 221, 240, 241). These were primarily solid-phase assays for large antigens. However, the entry of enzyme immunoassays—and non-isotopic assays in general—into the clinical laboratory began in 1974 with Syva's (Syva Co., Palo Alto, CA) first EMIT assays, which were homogeneous "enzyme-monitored immunoassays" (242). Since then separation-based (heterogeneous) EIAs have rapidly gained wide application, first in the field of microbiology and virology, but later also in routine clinical assays for large antigens.

The determination of the amount of enzyme-labeled reagent which was bound during immunoreaction has traditionally been made by the use of substrates producing colored products upon enzymatic reaction. This detection principle has the advantage that results also can be determined visually in semiquantitative assays, even though photometric detection with automated instruments is more often used. Since photometric determination does not offer the highest possible detection sensitivity, a general tendency prevails toward fluorometric or luminometric detection principles (see Chapters 7.6 and 9), and even radioactively labeled substrates have been adopted in highly sensitive EIA (243). Regardless of the detection system applied, these assays can be characterized as enzyme immunoassays, even though discrepancy prevails within the terminology. Sometimes methods are described according to the detection system rather than the actual label.

The choice of an enzyme to be used as a label for immunoassays follows the same rules as the choice of labels in general: high sensitivity, stability during storage, insensitivity against interfering compounds present in samples, biocompatibility, easy coupling, and availability. Alkaline phosphatase (ALP), β-D-galactosidase (βDG) and horseradish peroxidase (HRP) have been the enzymes in a great majority of EIA applications so far. Several types of substrates and detection systems have been developed for their use. Table 4.2 summarizes some examples of sensitive detection systems for those enzymes. In some cases the ultimate sensitivity of a single enzyme molecule detection has been reached, but in general the detection sensitivities are around amol levels, and the detection of enzyme "molecules" is often more sensitive than the detection of radioisotopes (e.g., the ^{125}I detection limit is around 2–10 amols). Also, in some reported EIAs the actual assay sensitivity has exceeded those of RIA or IRMA. It is, however, worth emphasizing that the actual assay sensitivity reached is much more dependent on an appropriate separation system and the application of high affinity and low nonspecific-binding labeled antibodies than the detection limit of a single label molecule.

Enzymes have the general advantage of a high amplification of the signal, which results in high sensitivity for the label detection. A wide range of substrates has been developed for enzymes which facilitate their detection with different systems—or even manually. On the other hand, the signal obtained is very much dependent on incubation time, temperature, and other physical and chemical conditions in substrate incubation. Enzymes can also be sensitive to interfering substances in samples, such as endogenic enzymes or inhibitors. Enzymes are proteins with a relatively large molecular weight, up

Table 4.2. Sensitivity Limits for Some Enzymes Used in EIAs

Enzyme	Substrate	Detection System	Detection Limit/Incub. Time	Reference
Alkaline phosphatase	4-Nitrophenylphosphate	Photometric	10,000 amols	244
	4-Nitrophenylphosphate	Photometric	50 amols	245
	4-Methylumbelliferyl-phosphate (4-MUP)	Fluorometric	0.5 amols	245
	4-MUP	Fluorometric	1 amols/100 min	246
	^{3}H-AMP	Scintillator	0.01 amols/90 min	243
Peroxidase (horseradish)	o-Phenylenediamine	Photometric	25 amols/100 min	247
	4-Hydroxyphenylacetic acid	Fluorometric	2 amols/100 min	248
	3-(4-Hydroxyphenyl)-propionic acid	Fluorometric	0.03 amols/100 min	247
	Luciferin	Luminometric	0.125 amols	249
β-D-Galactosidase	2-Nitrophenyl-β-D-galactoside	Photometric	100 amols/100 min	246
	4-Methylumbelliferyl-β-D-galactoside	Fluorometric	0.003 amols/100 min	247
	6-Hydroxyfluoran-β-D-galactoside	Fluorometric	1 molecule	250
	2-Nitrophenyl-β-D-galactoside	Bioluminescent	0.002 amols/100 min	251

to 500,000 with βDG, which can cause steric repulsions. Their coupling to immunoreagents involves generally more complicated chemistry than the coupling of simple small molecules.

4.2.2. Luminescent Compounds

In a narrow sense, luminescence immunoassays could be characterized as assays based on the use of luminescent or luminogenic compounds as labels. The term is frequently applied also to immunoassays which are based on other types of labels, such as enzymes, substrates, cofactors, etc., where the detection is performed with a luminometer.

The term *luminescence* refers to all kinds of light emission from a compound in an electronically excited state except incandescence. In terms of immunoassays, the photoluminescent methods (e.g., those based on fluorescence, phosphorescence, or delayed fluorescence) are not commonly termed luminoimmunoassays, which accordingly cover only assays based on chemiluminescence (and bioluminescence as one type of chemiluminescence). Generally luminescence reactions are oxidative reactions involving a variety of organic molecules, the best known example of which is luminol.

Since the first specific binding assay of biotin, based on isoluminol-labeled biotin and chemiluminescence detection, described by Schroeder et al. in 1976 (252), the use of different types of luminescence immunoassays has rapidly expanded to various fields of immunoassays. In addition to—and in combination with enzyme immunoassays based on fluorescence or luminescence detection—these methods can be described as photon emission methods. Photon emission methods possess the potential to replace radioisotopic methods with techniques of superior sensitivity (253).

Luminoimmunoassay techniques can be divided into three main categories: a) assays based on immunoreagents labeled directly with luminogenic substances such as luminol- or acridinium ester-derivatives (238, 254, 255); b) bioluminescence assays, which are based on labeling with bioluminescent enzymes, their substrates, or cofactors or by using coupled enzymatic reactions (256, 257); and c) chemiluminescent enzyme immunoassays which are based on chemiluminogenic enzyme substrates for measurement of, for example, peroxidases used as labels (258, 259).

Recently the development of new luminogenic labels and luminogenic enzyme substrates such as derivatives of dioxetanes (260) and so-called enhanced luminescence detection of peroxidase (261) have created highly sensitive immunoassays. The field of luminoimmunoassays is extensively reviewed (254, 255, 257, 259, 262–265). Luminescence and fluorescence are related phenomena, and the respective applications have common points also. For example, fluorescent compounds are sometimes applied as energy donors, mediators, or enhancers in luminescence reactions.

4.2.3. Fluorescent Labels

Fluorescence immunoassays (FIAs) are based on fluorescent tracers, immunoreagents labeled with fluorescent probes, or fluorogenic compounds. Despite the fact that fluorescent probes were actually the first sensitive reporter groups used to monitor immunoreaction (5, 6), fluorometric techniques were not applied in real quantitative immunoassays until 20 years later—actually not until the advent of radioisotopic techniques.

The development of fluorescence immunoassays has followed three main lines: a) the development of quantitative alternatives from the early established immunofluorescence (IF) tests; b) the exploitation of the sensitivity of fluorochromes to changes in their microenvironment to develop homogeneous assays; and finally c) the search for sensitive alternatives to radioisotopic immunoassays.

Since the introduction of β-anthracene labeled antibodies in determining of pneumococcus bacteria in 1941 by Coons et al. (5), IF staining techniques have found wide application as the histological technique for the localization of antigenic determinants in tissue sections, in identifying viruses and bacteria, in research of cell surface receptors, etc. Fluorescein was first introduced in 1942 (6), and the application of isothiocyanate coupling for fluorescein conjugation led to FITC (266), the probe which since 1958 has been the most widely applied fluorescent probe both in IF and in FIAs. The first rhodamine derivative, tetramethylrhodamine, was introduced in 1958, also for labeling antibodies for IF stainings (267). Since then an extensive search for new fluorochromes has created a great number of fluorescent probes applicable to different fields of research (see Chapter 7).

The question of standardization and quantification in IF was raised in the early '50s (268, 269). Goldman (270) used a photomicrographic camera in his semiquantitative IF of amebae in 1960. The next step to quantitative analysis was the development of microfluorometers, fluorometers which are based on fluorescence microscopes but rely on quantitative detection of the emitted light (188). Microfluorometers are composed of microscopic optics (e.g., inverted fluorescence microscopy), epi-illuminators, and aperture defined μ-volume determination of single cells or beads (271).

Standardization of substrates—solid matrixes for antigen immobilizations—was another objective in the development toward more quantitative IF. Microscopic cellulose beads, such as cyanogen bromide activated Sepharose (186) or agarose (188), were used as "defined-antigenic-substrate-spheres" (DASS) for microfluorometers. Another approach was the adoption of paper discs impregnated with antigen and fixed with ethanol. They were used as solid-phase and measured directly with a fluorometer (183) (soluble-antigen-fluorescent-antibody SAFA) test. The technique has been applied in the serodiagnosis of microbial infections, such as tuberculosis (184), trypanosomiasis (272), schistosomiasis (273), etc. Activated paper disc was also used in the first sandwich immunofluorometric assay (IFMA) of IgG by Aalberse in 1973 (185). In this assay the bound fluorescein labeled antibody was extracted from the solid-phase with NaOH solution before its quantitations with a fluorometer.

Development in IF technology led also to quantitative IFMA assays, which still are frequently applied in serodiagnosis (see, e.g., FIAX assays, Chapter 8.2.6), but also, on the other hand, to automated flow-cytometric analyzing systems, commonly applied for cell identifications, cell surface receptor analysis, determination of malignant cells, etc. (274).

The first competitive, separation-based fluoroimmunoassays (Sep-FIA) were developed in early '60s (275, 276), almost simultaneously with the introduction of homogeneous nonseparation FIA based on fluorescence polarization measurement (277). The Sep-FIA developed by Tengerdy (275, 276) were based on precipitation of FITC-labeled antigen or antibody in immunoreaction, whereupon either the free fraction or resuspended pellet was measured with a fluorometer. The same type of precipitation assay has been applied analogously to the Farr-assay with the use of FITC-labeled antigen (278).

The use of fluorescence anisotropy technique as a measure of Brownian rotational motion to follow immunological binding of fluorescein-labeled small molecular haptenic antigens to their antibodies was developed by Dandliker and his coworkers in the early '60s. The first applications were for the demonstration of penicillin allergy by measuring anti-penicillin antibodies with a fluorescein-labeled penicilloyl derivative (277, 279). The technique was also applied for measurement of anti-ovalbumin (280) and anti-conalbumin (281) antibodies. It was not until 1973, however, that the feasibility of fluorescence polarization measurement as the end point detection for competitive immunoassays was actually demonstrated by Dandliker et al. (282) for assays of hCG and penicillin, and by Spencer et al. (283) in assays of antitrypsin and insulin.

The fluorescence polarization technique fell into disfavor, however, primarily because of the lack of suitable instrumentation. Later on, after the development of automated systems for polarization assays by Abbott, it became one of the most widely applied FIA techniques in clinical routine, especially in the field of therapeutic drug monitoring (Chapter 8.3.1).

During the 1970s and 1980s, several homogeneous assay principles that relied on fluorescently labeled antigens were introduced, and some of them, such as assays based on fluorescence quenching or enhancement (Chapter 8.3.3) and fluorescence excitation energy transfer (Chapter 8.3.4) have also entered into the clinical kit market as commercial products.

The early fluoroimmunoassays and immunofluorometric techniques, which used conventional organic fluorochromes, could not offer a sensitive alternative to radioisotopic techniques, mainly because the sensitivity of fluorescence detection is limited by high background interference. It was not until the introduction of fluorescence enzyme immunoassays (ELFIA) and time-resolved fluoroimmunoassays that fluorometric techniques were able to compete with radioisotopic methods in terms of sensitivity and fluorometric techniques were able to offer a real alternative to RIAs and IRMAs.

4.2.4. Miscellaneous Labels

In addition to the labels described above, a great number of alternative labeling reagents have been proposed and tested for immunoassays. Some of them have not found any further applications, some of them have been applied in specified fields or types of assays, and some of them might have potential future prospects.

Erythrocytes and their agglutination in blood group typing were discovered in 1901 by Landsteiner, and agglutination is used as a type of immunoassay with visual detection. Hemagglutination and hemagglutination inhibition were introduced as a homogeneous immunoassay for antibodies and antigens by Stavitsky and Arquilla from 1953 to 1956 (122–124).

For labeling—or sensitization—erythrocytes are often stabilized with different cross-linking reagents like formaldehyde, glutardialdehyde, or sulfosalicylic acid. For conjugation, either direct absorption, tanned cell technique (284) or various covalent couplings, including diazo coupling (285), difluorodinitrobenzene (286), diisothiocyanates (287) or carbodiimides (288) are used.

Hemagglutination and hemagglutination inhibition assays are frequently used as simple tests for gravity by measuring hCG concentrations in urine at a sensitivity level of 1000 IU/L (289). It is a very simple assay system, but accuracy and precision suffer from the biological variations in the quality of erythrocytes.

Bacteriophages are used as labels in assays named *viroimmunoassay,* first described by Mäkelä in 1966 (290). He measured antibodies against a haptenic molecule by coupling the hapten with a bacteriophage. The detection is based on the plaque formation capability of phages on bacterial growth, inhibited by the reversible binding of anti-hapten antibodies to labeled hapten. Even though the assay is rather cumbersome and laborious, it has found some applications in assays of rabbit IgG, insulin, lysozymes, prostaglandin, and estradiol (291–295).

Particles are used as labels in various types of latex agglutination tests where the agglutination is quantitated either visually or by turbidimetry or colorimetry. Singer and Plotz in 1958 were the first to use suspension of small particles coated with IgG in their assay of rheumatoid factor (296). In latex agglutination tests, plastic beads of 0.1–0.8 μm diameter are applied, and agglutination can be followed by Mie-scattering determined with near infrared turbidimetry (297). Latex agglutination assays are primarily applied in serology—for anti-nuclear antibodies (298), for instance. In a "Visible Immunodiagnostic Assay" (VIA of Covalent Technology Co.), latex-labeled antibodies are bound to Stiq-samplers, and resultant Mie-scattering of immunocomplexes is determined by color change.

Another procedure for the quantitation of agglutinations was developed by Cambiaso et al. in 1977 (299). This variation is based on particle counting after agglutination and is named particle-counting-immunoassay (PACIA). A direct assay is suitable for large antigens, and an indirect inhibition type of assay is applied for haptens using polyhaptenic conjugates as cross-linking bridges between antibody-coated beads. The assay is applied, for example, for AFP (300), IgE (301), and digoxin (302). The technology has been automated and marketed as the IMPACT system (Acade SA, Brussels, Belgium), and the assay achieves sensitivities down to 10^{-15} mols (303).

The sol particle immunoassay (SPIA) is based on small colloidal metal particles (diameter less than 50 nm). The method was developed by Leuvering et al. (304), who used both silver and gold particles for simultaneous detection of human placental lactogen and human chorionic gonadotropin. A manual test based on unit-dose packages containing colloidal gold labeled antibodies was introduced for C-reactive protein (CRP) (Nycomed As, Oslo, Norway). The detection is based on the purple color formed within complex formation. SPIA differs from latex agglutination assays principally in that the colloidal metal particles are smaller and the detection can be performed by absorbance or atomic absorption spectroscopy. Colloidal gold particles are routinely used also in microscopic techniques (305), and particle-labeled immunoreagents are available from various sources. In combination with fluorescent probes these have also been applied in multiparameter analysis in flow cytometry (306).

Free radicals are used as labels in spin immunoassays. Leute et al. introduced a spin immunoassay technology for morphine determination in 1972 (307). Spin immunoassays are homogeneous immunoassays based on a change in the electron spin resonance spectrum of spin labeled antigen upon binding to its antibody. Free radicals used as labels include derivatives of nitroxides, such as N-oxides of piperidinium, pyrrolidinyl, or oxazolidinyl derivatives. It is applied mainly for therapeutic drugs under the name FRAT® (free radical assay technique) (308, 309).

Metals are used in immunoassays with a variety of different detection systems, including fluorescence or phosphorescence (Chapter 8.4), chemiluminescence, radioisotopic counting (e.g., ^{57}Co), differential pulse polarography, potentiometry, or atomic absorption spectroscopy. Cais et al. (310) introduced the name *metalloimmunoassay* to immunoassays relying on metallic labels, metallohaptens. They used iron- and manganese-labeled steroids determined by atomic absorption spectroscopy. Mariet and Brossier (143) synthesized Mn-labeled drug for immunoassay based on a separation with extraction and atomic absorption for detection. Fourier transform infrared spectroscopy has been applied with manganese-labeled hapten, nortriptyline, in a system named *infrared immunoassay,* where the detection is based on IR absorption at 2030 cm^{-1} (311). Lavastre et al. (312) synthesized cymantrenic acid (Mn)- and benchrotrenoic acid (Cr)-labeled drugs for MIA. Metallohaptens are measured also with electrochemical detection—for example, morphine labeled with ferrocene (313), lead (314), cobalt (315), or nickel (316).

CHAPTER

5

PHOTOLUMINESCENCE SPECTROSCOPY

Luminescence is one of the oldest analytical techniques, having first been described by Monardes in 1565. Sir David Brewster noticed the red emission from chlorophyll in 1833, and Sir G. Stokes described the mechanism of the absorption and emission process in 1852. He also introduced the term *fluorescence* in 1853, after the mineral fluorspar (calcium fluoride), which exhibits a blue-white fluorescence when exposed with ultraviolet radiation.

Luminescence phenomena is divided into several categories according to the energy source used for excitation of the luminescent molecule. If the exciting energy is from radiative particles emitted by radioactive isotopes, it is called radioluminescence. If the energy is derived from electric current (as, for example, in gas discharge lamps) it is called electroluminescence. If the energy is from a chemical reaction it is termed chemiluminescence, or bioluminescence in cases when the chemical reaction is catalyzed by an enzyme. When the excitation energy is provided by photons, it can be generally termed photoluminescence, which consists of fluorescence, phosphorescence, and delayed fluorescence.

Fluorescence is defined often according to the duration of emission—that is, the lifetime of the excited state—in order to distinguish it from phosphorescence. Because fluorescence decay time can sometimes be quite long, the distinction according to the electronically excited states involved in the process, and the preservation of electron spin, provides a more objective definition. Fluorescence emission involves energy dissipation between singlet levels, while phosphorescence emission involves triplet-singlet transition.

Fluorescence was introduced as the measured signal for immunoassays because of its inherent specificity; the signal measured is defined both by excitation and by emission wavelengths and can be even further specified by fluorescence lifetime (time-resolved techniques). The higher sensitivity obtainable in fluorometric determinations, as compared to photometric techniques, derives from the fact that fluorescence is measured against a zero background, and accordingly the emission can be integrated with a sensitivity of single photons. Normally fluorescence detection of a fluorescent compound reaches sensitivities in the range of 10^{-9}–10^{-14} mol/L. In practical routine work, fluorometric techniques are prone to interfering factors, which actually set the limits to the sensitivities obtainable.

Fluorescence and fluorometry are extensively used techniques in various fields of biomedical research. The principle of fluorescence and phosphorescence and their applications have also been reviewed in numerous textbooks and review articles (317–323).

5.1. EXCITED STATES

When a photoluminescent molecule absorbs light, its electrons will be raised from the lowest energy level to some of the excited levels. The dissipation of absorbed energy back to ground state may occur via nonradiative processes to produce heat, or the molecule might transfer the energy to another molecule. The molecule can also dissipate the absorbed energy in the form of an emitted photon. According to the route via which the emission occurs, the luminescence is named fluorescence, phosphorescence, or delayed fluorescence. The excited states are generally presented as energy level diagrams, originally described by Jablonsky (324) and schematically presented in the following pargraphs for different types of luminescent compounds.

5.1.1. Fluorescence

At the ground state of an unsaturated organic compound, the orbital at the lowest energy is occupied by two π-electrons with antiparallel spins, whereafter the ground state is called the ground state singlet. The ground state as well as the excited states are split in various vibrational sublevels, and further on to rotational levels (Fig. 5.1), which makes both absorbance and emission spectra in solution nonstructural. The fine structure of the levels can be determined only from samples in solid states, in crystals or frozen.

When a molecule absorbs light, one of its electrons from the highest occupied orbital is promoted to an unoccupied orbital. When the electron spin is preserved, the electron reaches some of the higher excited singlet states. The energy differences between the ground state singlet (S_0) and excited singlets (S_1, S_2) give rise to absorption spectra.

The absorbed energy is dissipated rapidly by vibrational relaxation (VR) to the lowest level of the singlet and by internal conversion (IC) to the lowest excited singlet. The eventual fluorescence occurs from the lowest vibrational sublevel of the S_1 level, and the electron may return to any of the vibrational levels of ground state (Fig. 5.1), giving rise to a typical transition distribution and fluorescence emission spectrum. Because the emission always takes place from the lowest excited level, the shape of the emission spectrum is independent of the excitation wavelength. If the vibrational levels are similarly

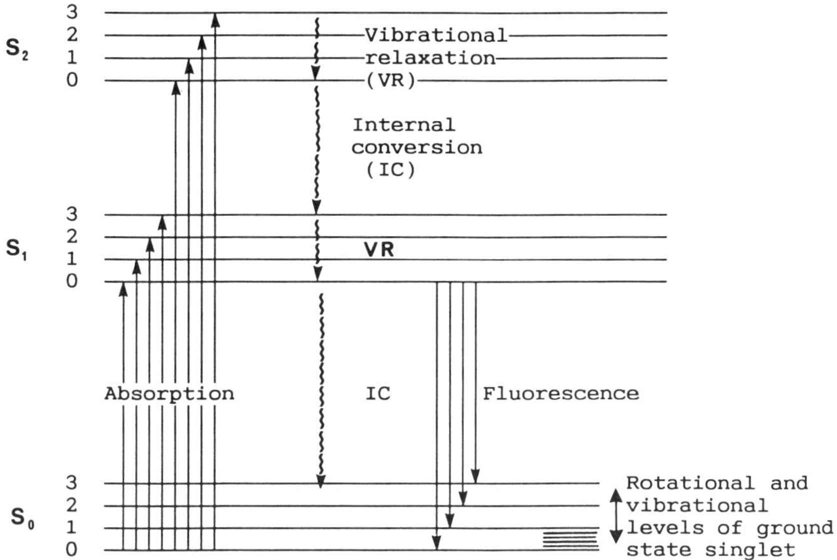

Fig. 5.1. Energy flow diagram for a fluorescent compound.

spaced in the ground state singlet and in the first excited singlet, the emission spectrum will partly be a mirror image of the absorption spectra, with 0-0 transition as the plane of symmetry.

5.1.2. Phosphorescence

Phosphorescence is characterized by emission from an excited level with reversed spin, called the triplet state. The triplet state was first identified as related to phosphorescence in 1944 by Lewis and Kasha (325). The conversion of an excited singlet with preserved spin to a triplet state with a change in spin angular momentum violates the classical law of conservation of angular momentum (it is "spin forbidden"). This transition is called singlet-triplet intersystem crossing (ISC) (Fig. 5.2), and it is generally very unlike transition. But because the transition to ground state is also "spin forbidden," the molecule will remain in the lowest triplet level a much longer time, hence producing a long decay time for phosphorescence. But phosphorescence also is a very unlikely process, especially in solutions at room temperature, due to the many competing processes; it may acquire thermal energy to go back to the S_1 state (delayed fluorescence), it may undergo intersystem crossing to isoelectric vibrational excited ground states, it can transfer its energy

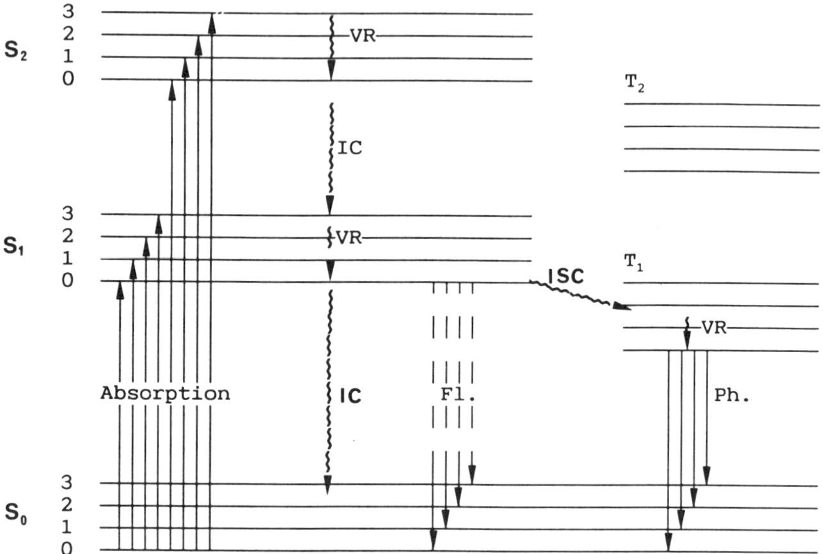

Fig. 5.2. Energy flow diagram for a phosphorescent compound. VR: vibrational relaxation; IC: internal conversion; ISC: intersystem crossing; Ph: phosphorescence emission.

to another molecule (e.g., dissolved oxygen), etc. Even though the triplet state is extremely sensitive to various energy transfer reactions and is easily quenched, relatively strongly phosphorescent compounds exist, and phosphorescence technique has been used in analytical chemistry and even in immunoassays (Chapter 8.4.4).

5.1.3. Delayed Fluorescence

Figure 5.3 outlines a postulated model for energy flow in the case of delayed fluorescence. After excitation, the excited singlet level is unloaded by singlet-triplet internal crossing, which efficiently diminishes prompt fluorescence. The molecule at the excited triplet state can further be activated to give an excited singlet by two mechanisms. The final product is fluorescence emission with a lifetime typical for phosphorescence.

Within the E-type (or eosin-type) of delayed fluorescence, the activation is derived from thermal energy. It is most often studied with eosin (326) but found also with proflavine, acridine orange, and anthracene (327).

In the P-type of delayed fluorescence, the activation energy comes from another molecule at the excited triplet state. It is called P-type because it is found with pyrenes (328). This T-T annihilation takes place when two excited

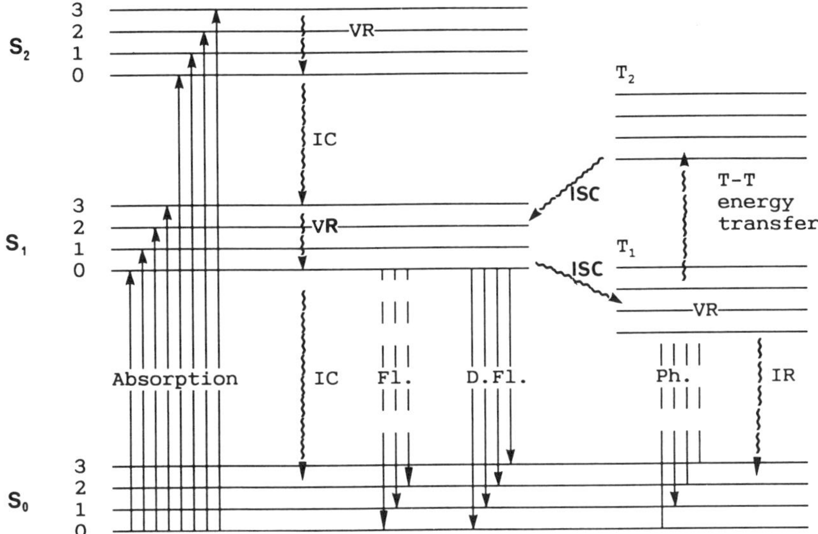

Fig. 5.3. Energy flow diagram for delayed fluorescence (D. Fl.).

molecules collide, form an excited dimer (excimer), and finally produce one de-excited molecule and one molecule at the excited singlet level. The donor and acceptor molecules can be the same or different. The mechanism resembles very much sensitized phosphorescence, first discovered by Terenin and Ermolaev in 1952 (329).

5.1.4. Photoluminescence of Chelates

Organometallic compounds and chelates produce their typical photoluminescence, sometimes with new interesting and useful properties. The luminescence produced depends on several factors, such as the paramagnetic properties of the metallic ion, the heavy metal effect, structural rigidity, and the optical properties of the ion and the ligand. The metal ion can quench the ligand, it can change the ligand structure, it can stabilize certain conformations, it can take part in electron transfer, it can accept energy from ligands or stabilize ligand triplet states, etc.

Depending on the relative position of the lowest excited singlet states, triplet states, and excited electronic levels of metals, four different types of chelates can be categorized (330).

Figure 5.4 shows a schematic energy flow with a chelate, where the excited metal level (M_1) is above both T_1 and S_1 levels of ligand. In these cases metal

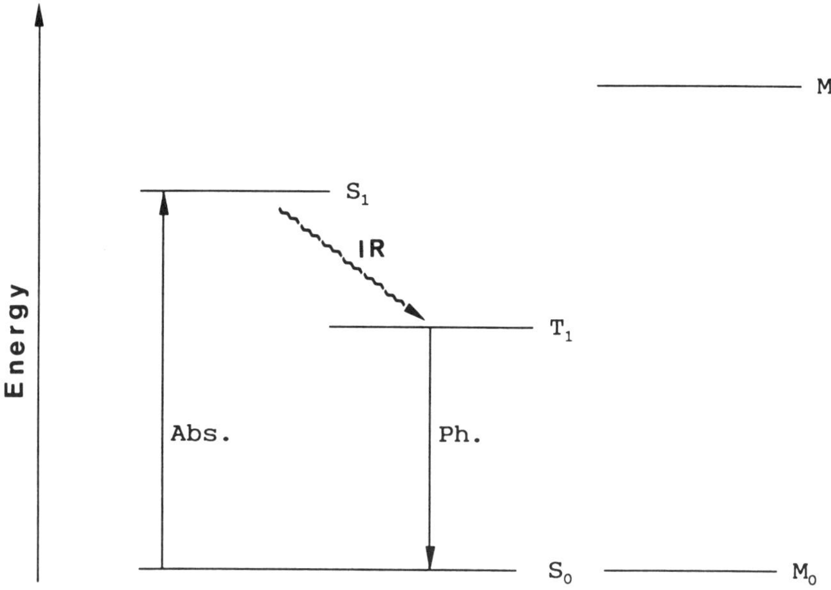

Fig. 5.4. Energy flow diagram for a phosphorescent chelate.

acts as an inert atom and may only affect the luminescence by stabilizing certain conformations of the ligand. These types of chelates can produce either fluorescence or phosphorescence and are formed generally with nontransition metals. Gd^{3+} has been applied as such a metal in the study of triplet levels of chelating ligands because it forms phosphorescent chelates; its own excited energy level is at so high a level that it cannot accept energy from organic ligands.

Figure 5.5 presents a typical energy flow for sensitized luminescence, where the chelated metal ion receives excitation energy from the ligand through the ligand triplet state. The chelated metal (typically tervalent lanthanide ions Tb, Sm, Dy, and Eu and also some chelates of Cr and Pt) efficiently quenches the ligand fluorescence and produces its typical ion luminescence characterized by d-d* of f-f* transitions. These types of chelates have a typical line type, long decay-time emissions which are also extensively applied in immunoassays (Chapter 7.4 and 8.4).

Figure 5.6 outlines energy levels for a typical transition metal chelate. The excited ion level located between the S_1 and T_1 levels of ligand efficiently quenches fluorescence and promotes intersystem crossing to triplet level. Such chelates (e.g., Pd and Pt-porphyrins) show high phosphorescence intensity in appropriate conditions and also have found application in phos-

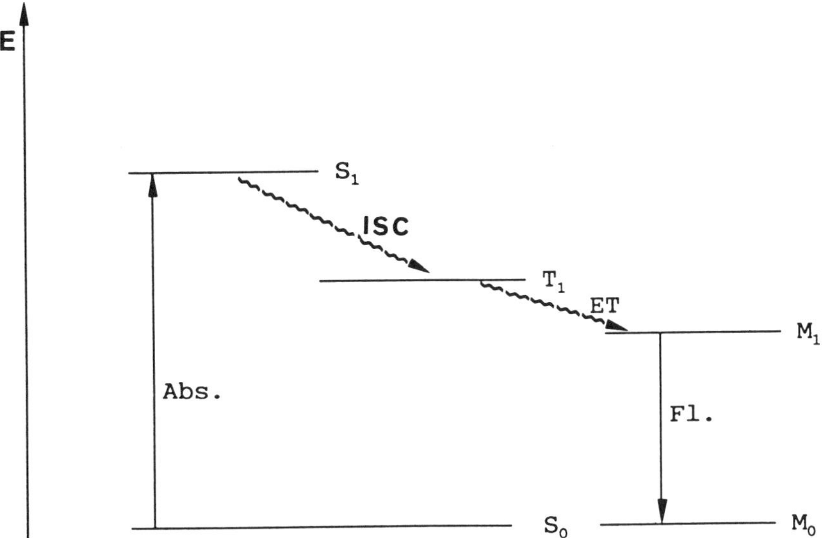

Fig. 5.5. Energy flow diagram for an energy-transfer type of chelate fluorescence.

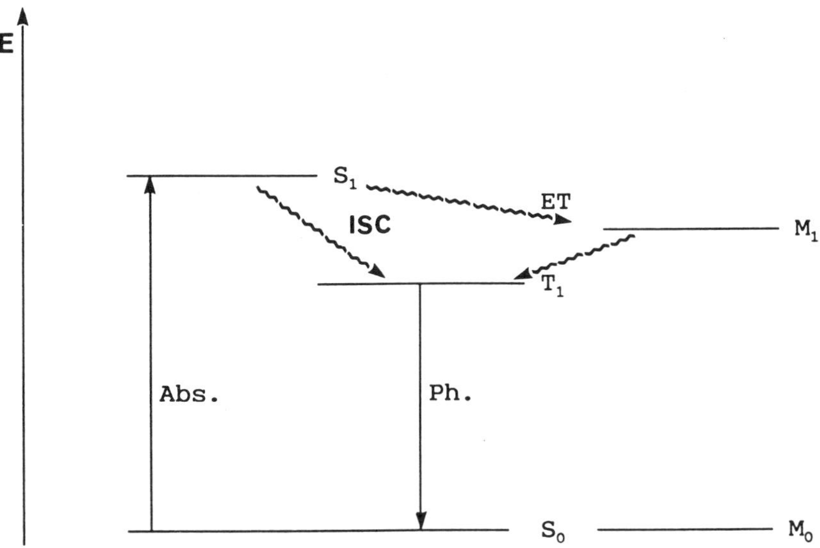

Fig. 5.6. Energy flow diagram for metal-sensitized chelate phosphorescence.

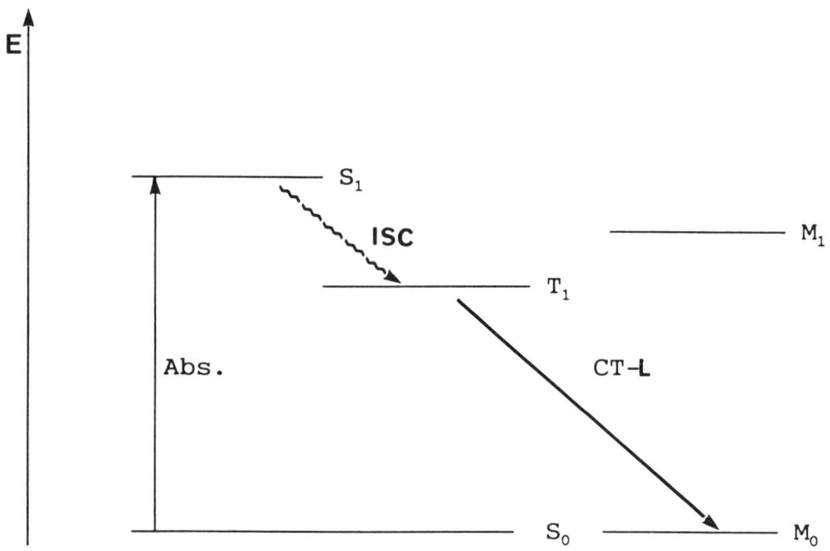

Fig. 5.7. Energy flow diagram for charge-transfer chelate fluorescence (CT-L).

phorescence immunoassays (Chapter 7.3.7 and 8.4.4). Metalloporphyrins also show a rarely existing fluorescence from the S_2 level. The S_2-S_0 fluorescence—which is called Soret fluorescence and excited by the "Soret" band (S_0-S_2), with absorption around 400 nm—has been found first with Zn and Gd tetrabenzoporphyrins (331) and can be seen also with Y, Lu, and Th porphyrins (332).

Figure 5.7 schematically depicts energy flow in chelates with metal-ligand charge transfer. Chelates of Ru, Os, or Ir with N-heterocyclic ligands show efficient charge-transfer luminescence with long decay times and Stokes' shifts. These chelates have been used as collectors for solar energy and recently also in immunological techniques (Chapter 7.4.6).

5.2. QUANTITATIVE FLUOROMETRIC DETERMINATIONS

Fluorometry is a very versatile technique, which allows not only qualitative or quantitative determinations of a fluorescent compound, but also the measurement of, for example, rotational movements, viscosity, polarity, or pH in the microenvironment of the probe, or distances between two groups.

There are several variables that can be measured from a single sample, such as molar absorptivity (ε), absorption and excitation maxima and spectra, emission maxima and emission spectra, quantum yield (Φ), decay time (τ), polarization level (p), or energy transfer between two fluors or a fluor and a quencher.

Absorption of light obeys a well-known Lambert-Beer Law (Eq. 5.1), where the light absorbed (I_A) is a function of initial light intensity (I_0), optical length (l), and molar absorptivity of the substance (ε);

$$I_A = I_0 - I_t = I_0 \times (1 - 10^{-\varepsilon lc}) \quad (5.1)$$

The intensity of fluorescence can be presented as a function of the total amount of light absorbed by the solution and the quantum yield,

$$I_F = \Phi_F \times I_A = \Phi_F \times I_0 \times (1 - 10^{-\varepsilon cl}) \quad (5.2)$$

where Φ_F is the quantum yield of emission. The fluorescence intensity is directly proportional to the concentration of the fluorescent compound, provided that the total absorptivity is small enough. Generally it is stated that the upper limit of linearity is at an absorption level of 0.05 or 0.02. Accordingly, the highest concentration of fluorescent compound to be measured (C_{max}) is

$$C_{max} = 0.05 \times (\varepsilon \times 1)^{-1} \quad (5.3)$$

When the concentration of the compound is low and absorbance is below 0.02, the fluorescence intensity can be presented by a simplified equation (5.4):

$$I_F = I_0 \times 2.303 \times \varepsilon \times c \times 1 \times \Phi_F \quad (5.4)$$

The quantum yield (Φ_F) is the proportion of emitted light as photons compared to absorbed light as photons and is presented either as a decimal (1.0 maximum) or a percentage (100% maximum).

$$\Phi_F = \text{Emitted quanta/Absorbed quanta} \quad (5.5)$$

Quantum efficiency also can be calculated from respective rate constants:

$$\Phi_F = k_f \times (k_f + k_d)^{-1} \quad (5.6)$$

where k_f is the rate constant for fluorescence and k_d the respective rate constant for deactivation processes.

The observed lifetime of the excited state, or the decay time of emission (τ_f), is a function of natural lifetime (τ_n) and quantum yield.

$$\tau_F = \Phi_F \times \tau_n \tag{5.7}$$

The decay time can also be determined as an inverse of rate constant ($1/k_f$). The fluorescence intensity at the time t can be calculated from an equation:

$$I_{Ft} = I_{Fo} \times e^{-t/\tau} \tag{5.8}$$

Equation 5.9 can be derived from Equation 5.8. It shows that the logarithmic intensity of fluorescence is a function of time with a slope of $1/\tau$.

$$\ln I_{Ft} = \mathrm{Ln}\, I_{Fo} - t/\tau \tag{5.9}$$

The polarization of fluorescence is generally presented in the Perrin equation:

$$1/P - 1/3 = (1/P_0 - 1/3) \times (1 + 3 \times \tau/\rho) \tag{5.10}$$

Rotational relaxation time (ρ) is around 1 ns for small molecules and about 100 ns for proteins. It is a function of viscosity (η), the volume of the molecule, the temperature, and the gas constant (R). Polarization is generally presented from horizontal and vertical measurements according to the equation

$$P_{meas.} = (I_V - I_H)/(I_V + I_H) \tag{5.11}$$

5.3. ENERGY TRANSFER

There are different forms of intermolecular energy transfer processes taking place between fluorescent molecules or a fluorescent molecule and a quencher. Some of the reactions, like T-T annihilation in delayed fluorescence, are described above. In a trivial mechanism, radiative energy transfer, the acceptor molecule simply absorbs the energy emitted by the donor, provided that the absorption of the acceptor overlaps with the emission spectra of donor.

There are various mechanisms for radiationless energy transfer between two molecules. In the resonance energy transfer or dipole mechanisms, first described by Förster in 1948 (333), there is no contact between the molecules, and energy transfer takes place at distances up to 100 nm. The rate of energy transfer is inversely related to the sixth power of the distance:

$$K_{et} = 1/\tau \, (R_0/R)^6 \tag{5.12}$$

Energy transfer requires overlapping spectra of the donor and acceptor and proper orientation of the oscillations of the molecules. It is dependent on the decay constant of the donor, and sometimes it is also "spin restricted" (some compounds are "T-acceptors" and some prefer S-level energy). Radiationless energy transfer is a common feature in nature—in photosynthetic pigments, for instance. It is also exploited in "tandem" conjugates to produce a larger Stokes' shift by coupling two fluors of overlapping excitation-emission spectra together. Dipole-dipole energy transfer has been applied as a "spectroscopic ruler" to study distances between two groups within a macromolecule (334). It is also applied in homogeneous "excitation transfer" fluoroimmunoassays (FETIA) (see Chapter 8.3.4).

In collisional energy transfer, the electronic clouds of acceptor and donor need to be in direct contact with each other. This type of energy transfer is diffusion controlled. An exciton migration happens only in solid crystals, where the energy is rapidly delocalized through the crystalline matrix.

5.4. SENSITIVITY OF FLUOROMETRIC DETERMINATION

Fluorometry is applied as a detection system primarily because of its inherent sensitivity. Theoretically, a fluorescent probe with high quantum yield and decay time of 5 ns could be excited up to 200×10^6 times per second and could produce about the same number of emitted photons. Even though this has not actually been achieved with any fluorescent probe, the utmost sensitivities of a single molecule detection have been demonstrated.

A detection of a single molecule in solution has been regarded as a formidable challenge, mainly because of the problems related to the numerous background sources present. Careful discrimination of the background derived from samples, solutes, cuvettes, and the instrument is required in order to obtain the highest possible sensitivity. Laser beams have played an important role in the search for ultimate sensitivity, partly because of the intensive excitation they provide and partly because of the high spatial resolution which enables miniaturization of the probed volumes. The emphasis in the development of single molecule detection is toward detection of a small number of molecules, not toward ultimate sensitivity in terms of concentration, which is often contradictory in the case of immunoassays.

Ishibashi et al. (335) were able to detect 20 pg/L amounts of fluorescein and riboflavin with nitrogen laser pumped dye laser excitation. According to them, higher sensitivities would require careful avoidance of all solvent derived backgrounds, including scatterings. Dovichi et al. (336) used flowing-droplet samples excited by an argon-ion laser to avoid background derived from windows of the cuvettes. They obtained a sensitivity of 8.9×10^{-14} M, which meant an average probability of less than one rhodamine in the probed volume of 11 pL. However, before they could attain an acceptable signal-noise ratio, an integration time of 1 second was needed, during which time 22,000 molecules of rhodamine 6G went through the focused volume.

Hirschfeld was able to visualize a single antibody molecule tagged with 80–100 fluoresceins (conjugated via a polyethyleneimine polymer) bound to a microscopic quartz slide in 1976 (337). He used an argon-ion laser with evanescent wave "darkfield" excitation at an energy level sufficient to bleach both the bound fluoresceins and the background and integrated the fluorescence from a surface area of 15×30 μm. Mathies and Stryer (338) have reviewed the item of single molecule detection and calculated the requirements for rate constants and quantum yields of absorption, emission, and photodestruction for a maximum theoretical sensitivity. They calculated that the maximum number of photons obtainable from one molecule of fluorescein is 3.7×10^4; for phycoerythrin, the number is 8.9×10^4. According to the calculations, single molecule detection would require a count rate of at least 10^5 photons per molecule, a decay time less than 1 μs, and Φ_D (quantum yield of photodestruction) less than 10^{-4}.

Phycoerythrin has been the fluorescent probe attaining the ultimate sensitivity of single molecule detection. Nguyen et al. (339) used argon-ion laser excitation in a flow cytometer using an excitation volume of 1.1 pL and were able to discriminate a fluorescence derived from 800 molecules of rhodamine 6G or a single molecule of B-phycoerythrin. Peck et al. (340) used autocorrelation to discriminate the fluorescence of a single phycoerythrin from a constant background. For the bulk solution they reached sensitivity of 1 fmol/L. Mathies and Peck (341) have presented a relatively simple general expression for optimized conditions for fluorescence detection taking into account molar absorptivity (ε), decay rate (τ), intersystem crossing rate (k_i), excited triplet state decay rate (k_t), and intrinsic photodestruction rate (τ_d).

The struggle for ultimate sensitivity is not very relevant for routine immunoassays, where detection is strongly blank-limited (342). In routine immunoassays, fluorometric detection is prone to various background sources, such as scatterings, endogenous fluorescences of sample constituents, reagents, cuvettes, and even instrument components. Fluorometric measurement also entails other problems, such as bleaching and quenching, which limit the development of more and more powerful excitations and labelings.

Increasing detection sensitivity has been the main goal in the development of more sensitive fluoroimmunoassays. The most used approach has been to apply various techniques to restrict background interference during the measurement. Another approach has been to increase the signal by choosing the proper environment or by applying a plurality of fluorescent probes tagged to one immunoreagent (polymeric labels; see Chapter 7.5).

5.4.1. Scattering

The scattering of excitation light from solvent, soluble molecules, proteins, aggregates, cuvettes, etc., is inevitably present in every fluorometric determination and can be the major background source with biological samples. Raleigh scattering derives from solvent molecules and Tyndall scattering from small particles. They have the same spectrum as excitation and do not have any lifetime. Scattering is especially problematic for fluorescent probes of short Stokes' shift and in assays where fluorescence is measured directly from a solid surface or from particle suspensions. High scattering also makes high demands on the filters used.

Some amount of incident excitation energy might be dissipated to vibrational and rotational movements of solvent molecules. The resulting scattering with apparent Stokes' shift is called Raman scattering. The energy loss in aqueous solution due to symmetric and asymmetric stretching is about 3380 cm^{-1} while that due to bending is about 1650 cm^{-1}. Scattering coming from cuvettes and solute molecules is present even in the purest solvent and may be the major background in "pure" conditions. Figure 5.8 shows scatterings measured from distilled water in a quart cuvette compared to the total emission obtained from 0.5 pM solution B-PE. The only way to obviate overlapping with Raman scattering is to choose a fluorescent probe with different (preferably longer) Stokes' shift.

5.4.2. Endogenous Fluors

Biological materials used as samples may contain a huge number of fluorescent components giving rise to high background fluorescence with a wide wavelength range (342). Serum or plasma, which are the most often used samples in clinical chemistry, contains proteins, hemin, NAD(P)H, bilirubin and albumin bound bilirubin, drugs, etc., causing a very high background level and even quenching or simple absorption of both excitation and emission of the probe used. Figure 5.9 shows the background fluorescence of

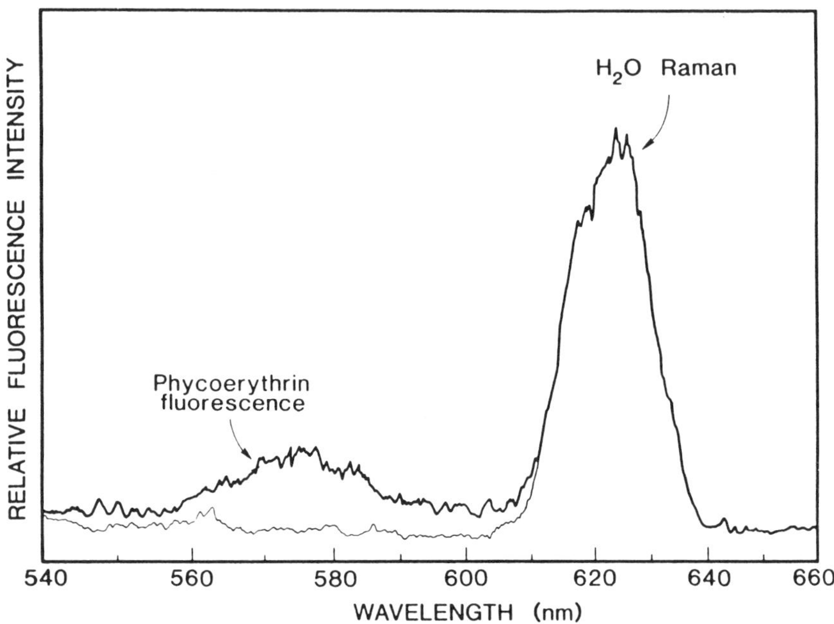

Fig. 5.8. Comparison of Raman scattering to the fluorescence intensity of 0.5 nM solution of B-phycoerythrin. (Reprinted from ref. 338 with permission.)

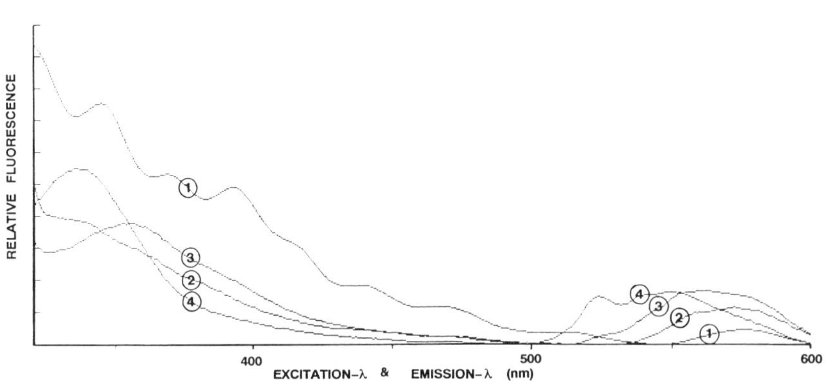

Fig. 5.9. Fluorescence background (synchronous excitation-emission spectra) 1/100 diluted human serum with Stokes' shift of 20 nm (1), 40 nm (2), 60 nm (3) and 120 nm (4).

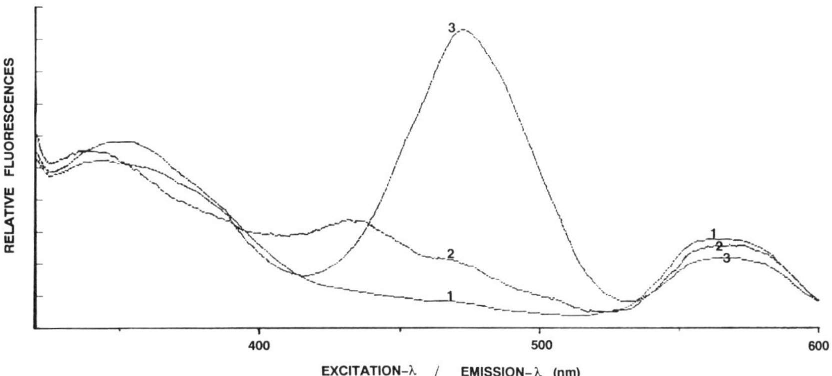

Fig. 5.10. Fluorescence background of normal (1), hemolytic (2), and icteric (3) serum samples.

diluted normal human serum for fluorescent probes with the Stokes' shift ranging from 20 to 120 nm. Normal serum contains various components with extended interference up to 600 nm.

Figure 5.10 depicts background fluorescences from serum samples with abnormally high concentrations of hemoglobin (hemolytic sample) or bilirubin (icteric sample). Protein bound bilirubin causes especially severe problems for the measurement of fluorescein because of their overlapping absorption and emission wavelengths. Increasing background levels have also been found from samples of uremic patients suffering from chronic renal failure (343), with excitation between 380 and 400 nm and emission between 440 and 460 nm. In addition to the absorption, quenching, and background fluorescence, serum components such as proteins cause a problem with some homogeneous assays (e.g., fluorescence polarization assays) by nonspecifically binding the fluorochrome-conjugated antigens (Chapter 8.3.1).

High background autofluorescence of cells in suspension or tissues, especially after fixation, has an intensity equal to the fluorescence of several thousand fluorescein molecules. Accordingly, background is a serious problem for IF staining techniques if high sensitivity is required.

Urine can also contain substantial amounts of interfering substances. Fluorescent compounds in urine (e.g., drugs) have been reported to cause false positive results in homogeneous FIAs if the cutoff value is stated from "normal" urine samples—for example, in screening illicit drugs (344, 345).

The endogenous fluorescence of the samples (serum, plasma, urine, etc.) and its background are a problem only for homogeneous FIAs, where the measurement of fluorescence takes place in the presence of all the sample constituents. Separation-based, heterogeneous assays do not have this problem, especially when solid-phase bound reagents are applied for an efficient separation. However, scattering from solid-phase materials—for example, from paper or microparticles—may cause as high or even higher background problems. On the other hand, many materials that are practically nonfluorescent in solution may show high fluorescence or even phosphorescence when bound to solid matrix. For example, most papers show extremely high fluorescence on UV excitation, and plastics as well as normal glass show luminescence with decay times from microseconds to milliseconds (346, 347). Thus, even in the heterogeneous assays, background luminescence characterized by materials used for solid phases or cuvettes remains. A careful choice of solid-phase material is needed for optimal detection sensitivity.

Equally careful choice of the materials used in lenses, mirrors, beam splitters, and filters is needed to restrict instrumental background. The photomultiplier tube is sometimes cooled to restrict the effect of photomultiplier dark current, especially in single photon counting.

5.4.3. Quenching

The quenching of emission can be a problem in certain fluorometric and especially in phosphorometric techniques. Quenching is directly related to various intra- and intermolecular energy transfer processes (see Chapter 5.3). Quenching can be categorized according to the energy transfer taking place. In trivial mechanisms, the quenching is related to absorption of the emission by the quenching compound. It requires that the absorption spectra of the donor molecule overlap with the emission spectra of the acceptor; relatively high spatial concentrations of these compounds also are needed. A short distance or exchange mechanism requires direct contact between the molecules, whereas in dipole-dipole energy transfer/quenching, the nonradiative energy transfer takes place through space (348).

Quenching can also be categorized according to the energetical status of the compound. In static quenching, the interaction between the fluorescent probe and quenching compound takes place when the fluorescent compound is at its ground state. In dynamic quenching, the respective interaction takes place during the time of the excited state.

Factors that increase intersystem crossing generally cause the quenching of fluorescence, and also total luminescence, as the triplet state is almost invariably unloaded by nonradiative transitions in solutions at room temperature (e.g., dissolved oxygen efficiently quenches RTP). Paramagnetic ions (e.g., Cr) and heavy atoms (e.g., iodine in erythrosin) increase intersystem crossing, resulting in decreased fluorescence and favored phosphorescence. Similarly, aggregation of fluorescent compounds, excimer formation, tends to favor phosphorescence. Excimer formation has been found at least partly responsible for the quenching taking place in carboxyfluorescein loaded liposomes (349).

Concentration quenching or inner filter effect has been noticed not only in liposomes, but also during the labeling of antibodies with more than one fluorescent probe of short Stokes' shift. It can be seen as a constant decrease in quantum yield with an increasing number of fluoresceins per IgG (Fig. 5.11), which actually results in the highest fluorescence being reached with a ratio of fluorescein:IgG of eight (350). On the contrary, inner filter quench-

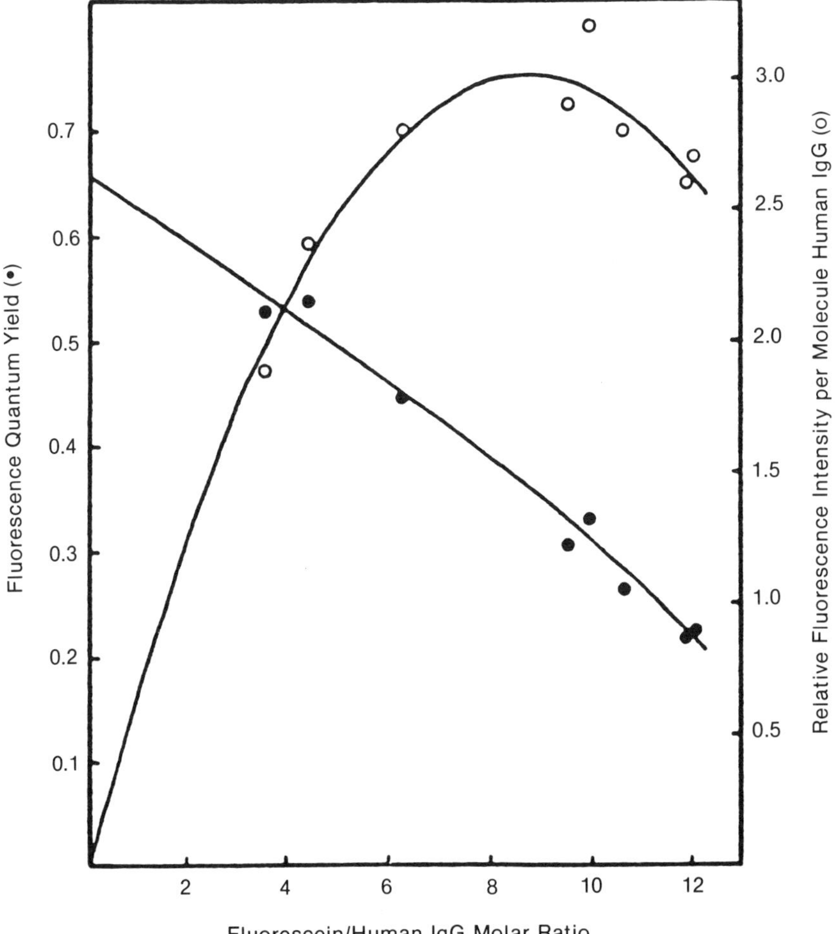

Fig. 5.11. The effect of labeling level to quantum yield (•) and the relative fluorescence (o) of fluorescein-labeled IgG. (Reprinted from ref. 350 with permission.)

ing is not a problem when the fluorescent probe has a long Stokes' shift, such as the chelates of europium. In such labeling the quantum yield was noticed to remain unchanged with labeling yields up to 28 chelates per IgG (Fig. 5.12) (351).

5.4.4. Bleaching

Bleaching, or fading, is the photochemical reaction causing fluorescence to decrease—fade—upon continuous excitation. Fading is recognized as a problem for all colored materials which lose their colors (e.g., in sunshine). The problem was described in 1794 and is primarily thought to involve oxidative reaction (352). The bleaching may be reversible, which means that during dark periods fluorescence may eventually be recovered, or it may be

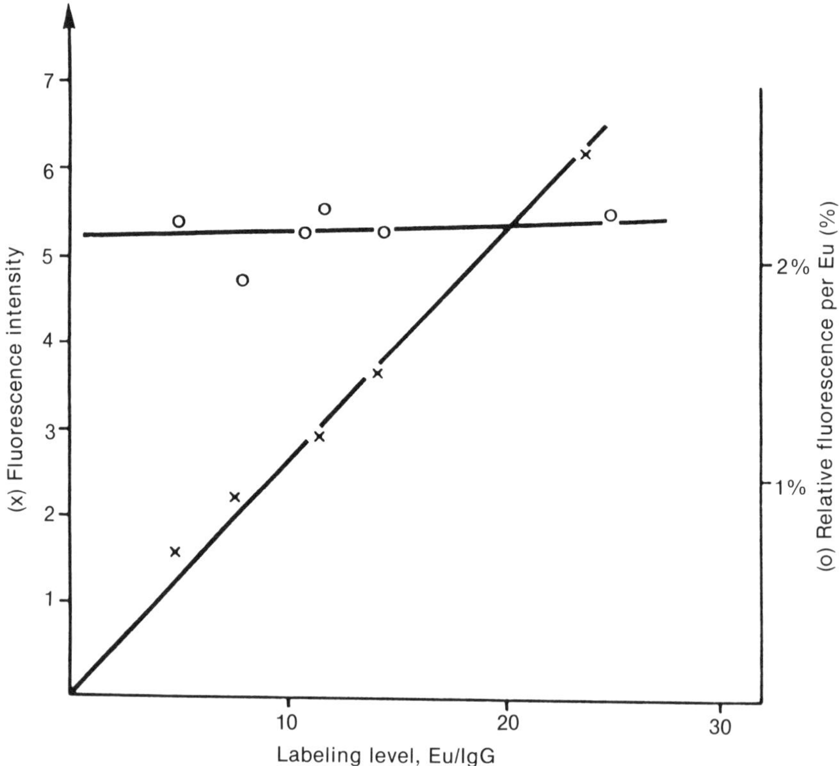

Fig. 5.12. The effect of labeling level to the relative fluorescence (O) and total fluorescence (x) of Eu-chelate-labeled IgG.

irreversible, a total photodestruction of the fluorescent entity. Bleaching is a major problem for microscopic immunofluorescence techniques (353); it prevents long manual observations, it may render photographic documentation difficult, and it can hamper comparisons and standardizations. Bleaching is generally not recognized as a problem in quantitative fluorescence immunoassays, however, mainly because of the apparently much less powerful and shorter excitations applied. It may become a problem when ultimate sensitivities are desired by using high intensity excitation (e.g., with lasers) and when several repeated measurements need to be applied and need to give constant readings.

Bleaching depends on the total amount or total intensity of excitation light used. Apparently it is also dependent on excitation wavelength and the environment of the probe. The rate of bleaching is related to the fraction of the total time that the molecule spends in an excited state. Accordingly, the efficiency of photodestruction, Φ_D, is directly proportional to decay time of the probe (338). The maximum number of photons that can be produced, n_F, can be presented as a function of the respective quantum yields (Eq. 5.13).

$$n_F = \Phi_F / \Phi_D \tag{5.13}$$

Fluorescein and fluorescein-labeled antibodies are about ten times more prone to bleaching than are rhodamine and rhodamine-labeled reagents (354). The bleaching, however, is not a simple reaction of the probe used, but it is strongly dependent on the excitation wavelength used and the environment of the probe. The bleaching of the fluorescent probe when it is bound to antibodies and used for staining a biological sample is strongly enhanced by the environment. In such systems, the dissolved oxygen and excitation light produced hydrogen peroxide are supposed to be involved in the bleaching by irreversible oxidation of the probe (354).

Because of the apparent damage bleaching causes, different ways have been introduced to overcome it. For example, prefocusing to the adjacent position of the sample, preferably with a longer excitation wavelength, can decrease the excitation time needed. Decreasing the excitation intensity with neutral filters (355) or by the use of pulsed excitation instead of continuous light (356) has been found useful in avoiding bleaching in some applications.

In microscopic IF techniques, various anti-fading agents are frequently applied, most often as a part of the mounting medium. Several compounds reportedly retard bleaching, even though published reports on the use of most of them contain contradictory results. Compounds used are mostly either reducing agents or radical scavengers, such as sodium azide, sodium iodide, polyvinylalcohol (PVA), polyvinylpyrrolidone (PVP) (353), sodium dithionite (357), N-propyl-gallate (358), dithiotreitol and dithioerythritol

(359), and 1,4-diazabicyclo [2,2,2] octane (DAPCO) (360). Böck et al. (353) tested several of the suggested agents and found positive effects only with sodium azide and sodium iodide. Krenick et al. (361) found phenylene diamine and N-propyl gallate efficient in protecting fluorescence from bleaching. Also, enzymes that can consume oxygen, like glutathione peroxidase with its substrate, glutathione, have been used as antifading agents (353).

Bleaching is not solely a negative phenomenon; it has found some useful applications too. Post- and preillumination has been used to bleach background in order to achieve better resolution in IF (362). Bleaching with an N_2-laser has been used to avoid serum (bilirubin) based background in fluorescence immunoassay (363). Hirschfeld used differences in the relative bleaching times to discriminate specific signal from background by "bleaching time-resolution" (364).

5.4.5. Background Elimination

Increasing sensitivity has been the goal in a great number of investigations done in the field of fluorescence immunoassays. Fluorescence detection is inherently very vulnerable to the background, which has been the major obstacle in developing sensitive fluorescence immunoassays. Background elimination is also needed to avoid matrix effects of samples and to make assays more robust by refraining the problems derived from samples of uncommon constitution. Of special concern are homogeneous assays of samples from severely ill patients which may contain abnormally high concentrations of intensively fluorescent substances. For example, serums of hepatic disorders may contain high concentrations of strongly colored and fluorescent compounds such as bilirubin (icteric samples) or hemoglobin (hemolytic samples). On the other hand, urine may contain colored and fluorescent substances related to drugs or renal dysfunction. In heterogeneous assays the background source can be different and accordingly other techniques have been created for its elimination. Basically, methods for background elimination can be divided into those derived directly from the assay's design, those applying chemical treatment, and those utilizing instrumental techniques.

In assay design, sample dilution is the most important factor, especially in homogeneous assays. The absorbing compounds in samples can cause attenuation of the excitation or emission signals by the inner filter effect. Generally, dilution of at least 1/100 has been used, but dilution down to 1/1600 or 1/2500 has been found appropriate in avoiding problems related to light absorption, background fluorescence, and nonspecific binding of the tracer to albumin (365).

Blank correction is an often applied technique in homogeneous FIAs.

The sample either can be divided into two aliquots or the blank value can be measured just prior to antiserum addition (366). Blank correction has also been made in separation FIA to eliminate effects caused by nonspecific binding of labeled reagents to albumin (367) or to the solid-phase used (368). The rate measurement of fluorescence intensity change in homogeneous assays (kinetic measurement) can also be used to avoid the effect of background level.

Various chemical methods have been applied in homogeneous assays to decrease background level. Extraction of the compound of interest from samples with an organic solvent has generally been applied in, for instance, steroid immunoassays mainly to avoid specificity and cross-reactivity problems. But the extraction can also be used to decrease the background derived from proteins and those substances that are insoluble to organic solvents. Solvents such as methanol and isopropanol have been used—for example, in fluorescence quenching immunoassay (369) and fluorescence polarization immunoassays (370)—to decrease background, to release the antigens from their binding proteins, and to avoid nonspecific binding of labeled antigens to albumin. TCA as a protein precipitating agent functions similarly (371). Other agents applied consist of proteolytic enzymes (pepsin) (367, 372), SDS (373), and various peracids (374) such as peracetic acid and persulfonic acid (375), which are applied in fluorescence polarization assays and also in fluorescence energy transfer assay (376). For urine samples, sodium iodide has proved effective (377). In commercial FPIA, TD_x of Abbott Laboratories, various methods are applied for avoiding sample interferences, such as dilution within assay, pretreatment with peracids, enzymatic treatments, or treatment with compounds under trade names such as Florisil® (378–380).

Physical methods also have been developed to eliminate background interferences. Windowless measurement of flowing samples by laser-beam excitation has been used in flow-through measurement to avoid scattering from cuvette materials (381). Various optical arrangements have been used for spatial filtering—for example, using refractive metal surfaces and measuring the resulting emission with a angle different from the excitation and its reflection (Fig. 5.13) (159).

As described above, specific bleaching of background also has been used to increase signal resolution. A "postirradiation" method has been used to bleach the background in pararosaniline-Feulgen DNA stained samples (382). Parola and Uzgiris (363) were able to decrease the background by 90% by the powerful pre-excitation of samples with a nitrogen laser, and Hirschfeld (364) used differences in bleaching times to discriminate rapidly bleaching components from slowly bleaching ones.

When the fluorescent probe has a narrow, line-type emission, as is typical with lanthanide chelates, it could in principle be distinguished from the more

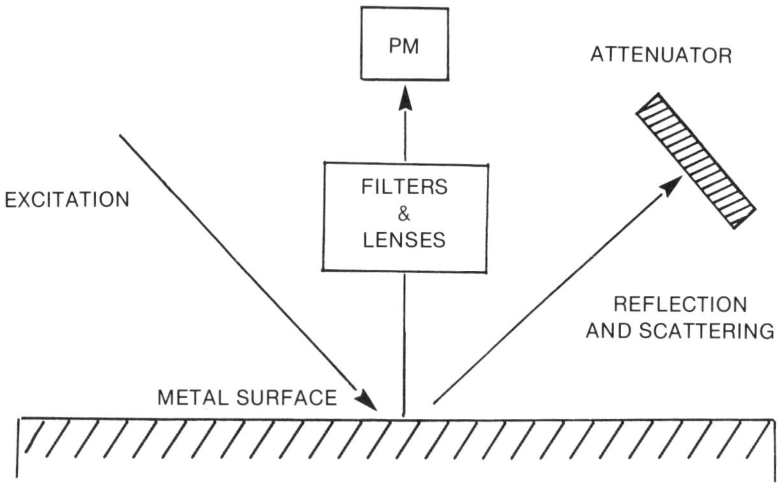

Fig. 5.13. Fluoroimmunoassay on reflective metal surface.

continuous background by measuring the emissions with three adjacent interference filters and subtracting the average background from the measured specific fluorescence (383). The principle has been tested by scanning the emission peak of a terbium chelate with a monochromator and calculating the peak area from its emission profile (384).

Time resolution with pulsed excitation and gated detection was introduced by Winefordner in the '60s (385, 386), and the principle is extensively applied in phosphorescence measurements. It also is perfectly suited for discriminating short-living fluorescence (background) from emissions of long duration. Mueller and Hirschfeld (387) used time resolution in 1977 to reduce background in fluorochrome staining. Time resolution was suggested as an efficient means to reject background in immunoassays by Wieder in 1978 (388) and Soini and Hemmilä in 1979 (342), provided that a fluorescent probe with a considerably long decay time could be developed. Since the development of labeling and detection systems for lanthanide chelates, time resolution has proved to be a very practical way to increase assay sensitivities by means of background elimination (Chapter 8.4). Frequency-domain fluorometry, or phase-resolved fluorometry, is another technique introduced to resolve specific fluorescence from background of different decay time. It can employ fluorescent probes with decay time differences even in nanosecond scales (389). That technique has found also some applications in the immunoassay field in techniques named phase-resolved fluoroimmunoassays (PR-FIA) (Chapter 8.4.4).

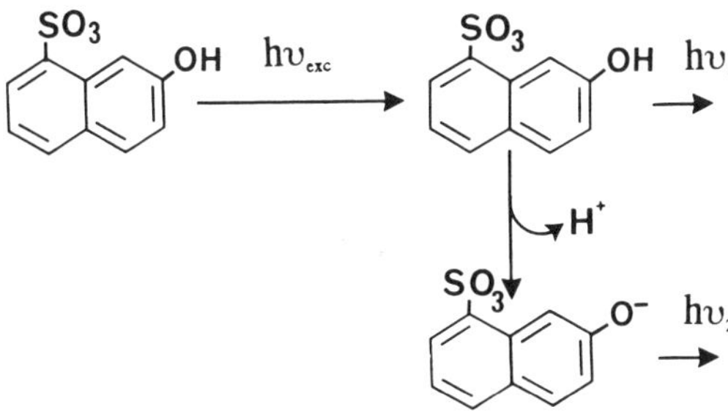

Fig. 5.14. Excited state proton transfer emission. (Redrawn according to ref. 390 by permission.)

5.4.6. Fluorescence Enhancement

Besides background reduction, optimization of the desired signal level can be used to achieve higher detection sensitivities. The most important factor, naturally, is the choice of the probe used, which should give the highest possible signal (high product; $\varepsilon \times \Phi_F$) in addition to good separation of the signal from disturbing backgrounds (spectral or/and temporal resolution). A generally applied approach is to optimize probe/analyte ratios or to use multiple labeling or polymeric labels (Chapter 7.5), provided that inner filter effects can be obviated (e.g., by using releasable probes). Because fluorescence is very sensitive to environmental factors, it is also possible to find optimal conditions for fluorescence measurement. Optimizing factors like pH, temperature, viscosity, effective ions, or detergents, drying, or the use of suitable solid carrier matrixes are common practice in phosphorescence measurement and also have found applications in some fluoroimmunoassays.

Increasing the Stokes' shift can also increase signal resolution. Increased Stokes' shifts have been found, for example, with fluorescent probes expressing excited state proton transfer. With those probes the excited compound is at another ionization level than the emitting compound (Fig. 5.14). For example, 2-naphthol-8-sulfonic acid, used in the fluorescence polarization immunoassay of phenytoin, has a Stokes' shift of 150 nm (390). Another approach is to exploit energy transfer by coupling two fluorescent compounds together with a chemical bond, whereby energy transfer efficiency is greatly enhanced. Such "tandem" conjugates were first described by Stryer (391). Coupling B-phycoerythrin and allophycocyanin together produces a "tandem" probe with high absorptivity at 545 nm ($\varepsilon = 2.5 \times 10^6$), 90% energy transfer, a Stokes' shift of over 100 nm, and emission at 660 nm (392).

In Sep-FIAs which resuspend the formed precipitate or release the labeled reagent from solid-phases into solution prior to measurement, the measurement diluent can be chosen both to give rapid suspension or release and also to give optimal fluorescence. Alkaline methanol solution is most often used in those assays with fluorescein or umbelliferones as labels.

Micelle forming detergents are used as one component in the enhancement of lanthanide ion dissociative fluorescence enhancement TR-FIAs (Chapter 7.4.3). Micelles have been used to enhance the fluorescence of organic fluorochromes (393, 394) and also have been applied in Sep-FIA with Lucifer Yellow as a label (395) and as signal modifier in homogeneous FIAs (396, 367). In addition to detergents, cyclodextrines have been tested as signal modifiers in homogeneous FIA of phenobarbital (398).

Removing water from solid surfaces prior to measurement is very often done in RTP, and it has also been done in some FIA applications to enhance fluorescence, especially with fluorescent lanthanide chelates.

5.5. ROOM TEMPERATURE PHOSPHORESCENCE

The widespread use of phosphorescence has been hampered by the inconvenient and time-consuming sample treatment required to avoid quenching. Traditionally, phosphorescence is measured from cryogenic glasses at low temperatures (at +77 °K) using suitable organic solvents. Phosphorescence in solutions at room temperature (RTP) is a rather rare phenomenon, because it is efficiently quenched in solution (e.g., by the dissolved oxygen). Various techniques are being developed to overcome the quenching problems, and accordingly phosphorescence is gaining more applications as a potentially sensitive qualitative, and also quantitative, analytical technique (399–401).

Certain structures in luminescent compounds favor phosphorescence—and often consequently quench fluorescence. For example, heterocyclic compounds show increased n-π transitions and can be phosphorescent. Some metals in chelates further increase the probability of n-π transition and enhance phosphorescence. Heavy atom substituents, such as iodines in erythrosin or bromines in eosin, increase the rate of internal conversion and molecular phosphorescence (internal heavy atom effect).

In techniques used for phosphorescence measurement, one of the most important methods is the increase of molecular rigidity, which can be achieved by, for instance, freezing or by immobilizing the compounds onto a solid matrix. Different solid matrixes, such as paper, silica, or alumina (TLC-plates), are applied (402). Drying the solid-phase and removing all moisture are generally required to obtain phosphorescence emission (403). The matrix holds the absorbed molecules rigid and restricts vibrational motions and nonradiative decay of the triplet state. Packing the compounds on the surface with added salts or sugars further inhibits molecular vibrations, and compounds are also protected from quenching by molecular oxygen (404). Avoiding the quenching caused by oxygen is especially important in applications of phosphorescence in immunoassays (PIA). In PIAs, deoxygenation has been achieved mainly by chemical treatment with sulfites (Chapter 8.4.4).

Solubilizing of the compounds with detergents, where the phosphorescent compounds are on the surface of detergent micelles, has recently been used for phosphorescence measurement of naphthalene, pyrene, and biphenyl (405). Similarly, cyclodextrines have been applied to increase RTP of hydrocarbons (406). Various heavy atoms, mainly metallic ions, have been used both with micellar systems and dried solid-phase systems to increase spin-orbit coupling of the excited state for increasing the rate constant of intersystem crossing (external heavy atom effect) (407, 408). Sodium iodide, 1,2-dibromoethane, silver, mercury, thallium, and lead have been used as such heavy atoms (406–409).

In immunoassays phosphorescence has evoked interest mainly because of its potential sensitivity and the possibility it offers to add temporal discrimination to spectral resolution in avoiding background interferences (similarly to time-resolved fluorometry and lanthanide chelates). This type of background rejection was suggested already in 1960s by Winefordner (385, 386) but was not widely applied in immunoassays until the 1980s with time-resolved fluoroimmunoassays.

CHAPTER

6

INSTRUMENTS IN FLUORESCENCE IMMUNOASSAYS

A fluorometric, phosphorometric, or luminometric detector is an indistinguishable part of the respective immunoassay method and it is actually becoming more and more integrated into the whole immunoassay system. Fluorometers or luminometers are also needed in enzyme immunoassays based on fluorometric or luminometric monitoring of the enzyme catalyzed reaction. The basic difference between luminometers and fluorometers (or phosphorometers) is the way excitation of the sample is performed, either by use of a chemical reaction or by means of light. Both the versatile systems used for excitation and the variability offered by photoluminescence emission determination make fluorometers more complex and dedicated instruments than luminometers. The range of fluorescence measuring devices used in immunological techniques range from fluorescence microscopes, flow cytometers, general filter- or spectrofluorometers, and plate readers or specialized FIA counters to totally integrated automated immunoassay systems.

The intention of the present chapter is by no means to try to cover all the instrumental aspects of fluorescence measurement, but rather to review some general trends of the technology and to discuss some items of special interest relating to, for example, excitation sources (lasers, fibers, evanescent waves) or special detection methods (polarization, photon counting, time resolution).

The early assays relied on the available research filter fluorometers or spectrofluorometers; subsequently, commercialized immunoassay systems employ special fluorometers designed for the required type of detection (e.g., plate fluorometers or polarization accessories). In the current immunoassay field, a very strong tendency prevails toward totally automated integrated systems, where the instrument does not only measure fluorescence but also performs sample treatment, dispensings, incubations, washings, and calculations of results. Another trend has started from manual microscopic immunofluorescence staining techniques (IF), and has struggled toward standardization, quantitation, and automation of IF. Within that field development has proceeded via quantitative microfluorometers to automated image analysis and pattern recognitions on one side, and automated flow-cytometric systems on the other side.

6.1. EXCITATION

The extent to which molecules are excited determines the amount of emission obtained, unless excitation energies exceed the saturation level. Bleaching the probes used with powerful excitation on one hand and the background interference it creates on the other hand set practical limits to the level of excitation, as do the economics of high-priced powerful lasers.

In the majority of FIA systems, final assay sensitivity is much more dependent on immunological factors, such as cross-reactivities of antibodies, replacement or nonspecific properties of labeled immunoreagents, and the background fluorescence level in the fluorometric detection, than on the power of the instrument. Therefore, conventional lamps are often perfectly satisfactory for FIA systems and are also used in FIA instruments.

A mercury gas discharge lamp has traditionally been used in fluorometers and fluorescence microscopes. It produces high output at 366, 415, and 435 nm, and wavelength range can be further extended by integral coating of the lamp with suitable phosphors (410). A low pressure mercury lamp is used, for example, in the IM_x automated immunoassay system of Abbott and in the MicroFLUOR™ Reader of Dynatech (Dynatech Laboratories Ltd., Billingshurst, UK). Short arc lamps (e.g., xenon) are most often used in spectrofluorometers because of their continuous spectral output (characteristic of high pressure xenon). Xenon flash tubes have been used as pulsed excitation sources in several commercial spectrofluorometers, phosphorescence detectors (pulse width of 1–10 μs), and time-resolved FIA fluorometers (e.g., ARCUS® and DELFIA® Fluorometers of Wallac Oy, Turku, Finland). Halogen lamps produce less efficient excitation, especially at UV, than do mercury or xenon lamps but have nevertheless been used in a number of fluorometers designed for FIA. In the automated system developed for Ames TD_A (SL-FIA of drugs), Optimate™ (Ames Division, Miles Laboratories Inc., Elkhart, IN, USA) a quartz-halogen lamp is used. Various types of halogen lamps are used in, for example, the Track XI® Fluorometer (Microbiological Associates Ltd, Billingshurst, UK), FIAX™ Fluorometer (International Diagnostic Technology, Santa Clara, CA, USA), Syva Advance (Syva Co., Palo Alto, CA), and Pandex Screen Machine™ (Pandex Laboratories Inc, Mundelein, IL, USA).

6.1.1. Lasers

Laser light is a result of a stimulated emission of the lacing material inside a cavity between two mirrors. The primary excitation, pumping, depends on the type of laser. Ion lasers are pumped with electric current, dye lasers with flash lamps, and diode lasers with electric current. Today lasers have evoked enormous interest as powerful light sources in chemical and clinical analysis also (411–415).

The use of lasers as excitation sources in fluorescence analysis has led to significant improvements in detection limits of many compounds. Sensitivities down to 1 pg/ml of fluoranthene (416) and 0.02 pg/ml (5×10^{-15} M) (335) or 1 pmol/L (417) of fluorescein have been achieved by excitation with nitrogen laser pumped dye lasers and 0.5 pg/ml of rhodamine B with argon-ion lasers (418). The ultra-high sensitivities of single-molecule detections are all achieved with use of powerful lasers as excitation sources (336, 337, 339, 340).

There are three salient features that distinguish lasers from conventional light sources: their spatial coherence, high degree of monochromaticity, and narrow temporal pulse width, if pulsed. When combined with extremely sharp focus, the high output can result in very high excitation intensities per probed volume or surface. The disadvantages of current lasers are often their high price, large size, and often quite limited wavelength selection (except with tunable lasers).

Of the various types of lasers, gas lasers have most frequently been used in immunological systems. An argon-ion laser, with its main output at 488 nm (other possible emissions are 514, 457, 465, 472, or 351 and 363 nm with specific mirrors), is well suited for the excitation of fluorescein and phycoerythrin and is routinely used in flow cytometers. A mixed gas laser, the He-Ne-laser, is small, cheap, and stable and emits light at 633 nm. It is primarily used for scattering analysis but also to excite, for example, allophycocyanin. He-Cd metal vapor lasers produce a moderate output at UV- and blue wavelength ranges (325 and 441.6 nm). Nitrogen lasers (337 nm) are very often used for excitation at UV and also for pumping dye lasers. As a pulsed excitation source, it is used in phosphorometers and time-resolved fluorometers and is perfectly suited for Eu-chelate excitation (Chapter 7.4). Yamada et al. (419, 420) achieved a detection sensitivity of 0.002 pM (2×10^{-15} mol/L) for a fluorescent Eu-β-diketonate chelate after excitation with a nitrogen laser. A nitrogen laser is commercially used in, for instance, a TR-FIA fluorometer, the CyberFluor 615™ Immunoanalyzer (CyberFluor Inc., Toronto, Canada).

Dye lasers contain solutions of fluorescent compounds in organic solvent, excited with flash lamps or lasers. Using mixtures of dyes and suitable filter selection, dye lasers can be tuned from near UV to near IR wavelengths. Because of the tuning possibility, dye lasers can excite organic fluorochromes of widely different excitation maxima. For example, a nitrogen pumped esculin laser has been used for the excitation of fluorescein with an obtained sensitivity of 2 ppt (421). Dye lasers are used in combination with argon-ion lasers for multiparametric analysis in flow cytometers.

Near IR emitting semiconductor lasers, laser diodes, have recently been developed mainly for telecommunication and data handling. These lasers are small, compact, reliable, and relatively inexpensive. The wavelength selection of the current laser diodes is mainly restricted to red and IR radiation (414, 415, 422). Intense research is going on to develope laser diodes for visible and UV excitation; such compact lasers might well replace lamps and other lasers in the near future. IR-emitting laser diodes, such as GaAlAs (800 nm), as well as some solid state lasers, such as Nd:YAG (1064 nm) also have evoked interest as excitation sources in FIA because of the low background caused by near IR excitation (423). Their use is hampered by the scarce existence of fluors which can be excited at such a long wavelength. Imasaka et al. used visible light excitation produced by a semiconductor laser in a fluorometric detection of compounds absorbing at near IR and obtained detection limits of 4×10^{-12} M for rhodamine-800 (excited at 670 nm) and 1.3×10^{-13} for oxazine (424). The same authors have used a 20 mW laser diode (780 nm) for an ELFIA of insulin by using an IR emitting fluorogenic substrate system composed of the quenching of indocyanine green fluorescence by peroxide produced by the enzyme (425). Chelates of Nd and Yb have reportedly been used as IR excited fluorophores in an FIA (426), however, without further scientific applications.

The high spatial resolution of lasers, their easily attainable perfect focusing, is a feature applied in flow cytometers, both to analyze scattering and to excitate various fluorochromes attached to cell surfaces (427). Spatial resolution is also used in various scanning devices and confocal microscopes. Kaufman et al. (428) used argon-ion and He-Cd lasers for excitation in their "flying spot" scanning fluorescence microscope. Small volume excitation with an argon-ion laser is also used in a nonseparation FIA based on fluctuation analysis of the microbead bound fluorescence and the freely diffusing fluorescence of unbound fluors in a system introduced by Nicoli et al. in 1980 (429). An inexpensive He-Ne laser (543.5 nm, 0.75 mW) has also been utilized to construct a simple fluorometer, which excites samples through the bottom of reaction cuvettes (430).

The third salient feature of lasers—pulsed lasers—is their narrow temporal pulse width. Pulsed lasers are extensively used in time-resolved fluorometric techniques in time scales from picoseconds to milliseconds. Those short pulses are generated by four main techniques (431, 432). In pulsed excitation the pulsing source can be an electric field (N_2-laser), flash lamp, or pulsed nitrogen laser (dye lasers). In Q-switching, either rotating mirrors, electro-optical shutters, or absorbing compounds are used. Mode locking produces very short pulses, and cavity dumping is achieved by using, for example, semireflective mirrors. An early example of the use of a pulsed laser for highly sensitive detection was the work of Lytle and Kelsey (431), who used a cavity-dumped argon-ion laser for time-resolved fluorometry to obviate scattering related background.

6.1.2. Fibers

Highly light transmitting optical fibers were developed mainly for telecommunication purposes, but they also provide a convenient means to conduct light in fluorometers (432). By using fibers for excitation and transmitting emission, even a normal spectrofluorometer, such as a Perkin Elmer spectrometer, can be converted into a microplate reader.

Vo-Dinh et al. (433) used bifurcated fiberoptics to construct a portable sensitive plate fluorometer used for ELFIA. Remote immunosensors are generally also made of fibers, which are either coated by their distal end using an evanescent wave (wave guide) for excitation, or coupled to cuvettes made from semipermeable dialysis membrane (Chapter 8.5). Also a fluorescence lifetime instrument with multi-frequency phase-modulated technique has been constructed with fibers (434).

6.1.3. Evanescent Wave Excitation

Attenuated total reflection (ATR) or *total internal reflection fluorescence* (TIRF) are terms describing the applications of an evanescent wave. They are well suited to the study of molecular interactions on a liquid-solid interface, such as the immunological binding of labeled antigens or antibodies on coated surfaces (435).

When excitation light propagates in a transparent matrix of high refractive index, n_1 (e.g., glass or quartz), and encounters the interface with aqueous solution (with lower refractive index, n_2), it undergoes total internal reflection for incidence angles greater than the critical angle (Fig. 6.1). The critical angle, Θ, depends on the ratio of the refractive indexes according to the equation

$$\Theta = \sin^{-1}(n_2/n_1) \tag{6.1}$$

Regardless of the 'total' reflection at the surface, an electromagnetic field called an evanescent wave penetrates a small distance into the liquid medium (Fig. 6.1). This evanescent wave can be used to excite molecules that are near the surface. The evanescent wave intensity I_z decays exponentially with distance z from the surface:

$$I_z = I_O e^{z/d} \tag{6.2}$$

In Equation 6.2, d is the factor which is dependent on excitation λ, the refractive indexes, and the critical angle. The rapid decay of an evanescent wave results in only a very small volume near the surface being excited. That phenomenon has been exploited by various technologies in immunoassays.

Hirschfeld (337) applied laser excitation with an evanescent wave in a

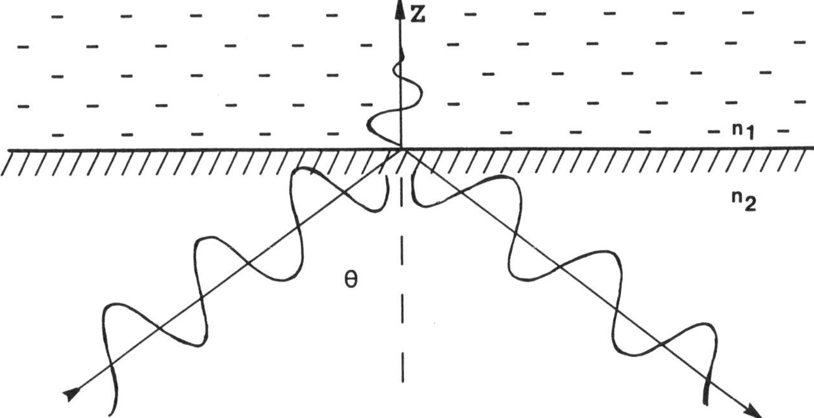

Fig. 6.1. Evanescent wave (Z) excitation of samples in solution (optical density n_1) with waveguide (optical density n_2).

quartz slide to detect a single fluorescently labeled antibody bound to the probed surface. He has also exploited the small volume excitation in a "virometer" (436, 437), where DNA-stained virions were excited by "darkfield" excitation and determined by fluctuation analysis, by separating the fluctuation caused by rapidly moving free fluorochromes from slowly diffusing labeled virions. The same TIRF principle was used to determine the fibrocytes in microscopes in 1961 by Ambrose (438).

Small volume excitation has also been used in the homogeneous "space-resolved" fluoroimmunoassay of morphine by Kronick and Little in 1975 (439, 440). They used a He-Cd laser (442 nm), a quartz plate coated with morphine derivative, FITC-labeled antibodies, and TIR.

Thompson and Axelrod (441) applied TIR, fluorescence correlation spectroscopy, and aperture defined microvolume detection in the study of the binding and dissociation kinetics of rhodamine-labeled antibodies to insulin-coated surfaces. Hlady et al. (442) used the intrinsic fluorescence of the proteins in their study of protein binding to surfaces by applying TIRF.

The evanescent wave in fibers has been used in remote waveguide immunosensors, based on free distal end coated with antibodies (443) (Chapter 8.5).

6.2. DETECTION

The emission emanating from an excited sample is quantitated generally with photomultiplier tubes after selection of the desired wavelength. The signal is amplified, and the resulting signals are determined as electric current (analogy) or as pulses (photon counting). Wavelength selection is generally achieved by suitable filters; for the most part, monochromators are used only in spectrofluorometers. The proper selection of filters is important for resolving the desired signal from interfering scattering.

To some extent the instrumental noise level can also affect the obtained result in assays requiring high detection sensitivities. The dark current of a PM tube can be omitted by cooling it (generally performed in time correlated single photon counting). With pulsed excitation sources, instrumental background can be determined utilizing the dark period for its measurement (e.g., Ames Fluorostat fluorometer).

In FIA fluorometers the detection is developed to satisfy the demands set by the particular assay type. The detection may be steady state detection or kinetic detection; it can be polarization measurement in fluorescence polarization assays, phase resolved in frequency domain systems, time resolved in TR-FIA, etc. The fluorescence can be measured from cuvettes, disposable tubes, microtitration wells, flow cuvettes or flowing droplets, microparticles in suspension or on a filter membrane, membrane surfaces or dried plastic surfaces, etc.

In immunofluorescence the results are traditionally recorded visually or by photographic film. In quantitative IF and in image analyzing systems, the emission can be screened with a PM tube or with systems named silicon intensified target cameras (SIT), video-intensified fluorescence microscopy (VIFM) (444), video-enhanced light microscopy (445), or a cooled charge-coupled device (CCD) (446).

6.2.1. Standardization

Standardization of measurement has become a major problem in the quantitation of IF techniques, but instrumental standardization is also necessary for FIA fluorometers. Generally in FIA fluorometers, excitation source fluctuation is eliminated by feedback control, taking samples from excitation light with a reference detector. In spectrofluorometers the reference system may contain concentrated rhodamine for quantum corrected excitation.

Standard samples as beads, films, or solutions are routinely used in fluorescence microscopes and flow cytometers and also in fluorometers. Uranyl glass was the first and is the most frequently used inorganic fluorescent standard material (447, 448), but europium doped crystals (449, 450) or glass fibers (451) are also used in microfluorometers and in a FIA fluorometer (410). Dye impregnated particles are standard in PCFIA of Pandex Screen Machine and in flow cytometers (452) beads labeled with FITC and TMRITC are generally used.

6.2.2. Polarization

Fluorescence polarization was used in immunoassays in the early 1960s by Dandliker (277, 279, 280), but it did not achieve wide acceptance as clinical routine technology until almost 20 years later, mainly because of a lack of suitable instrumentation. Although polarization filters and accessories were available for most research fluorometers, these did not satisfy the demands of routine clinical instruments, where a large number of samples needs to be processed quickly and in a reproducible way. Also, data processing is needed for result validation.

In polarization measurement, the polarization level, p, is calculated from parallel and antiparallel components of emission (compared to excitation) according to the formula

$$p = (F_V - F_H)/(F_V + F_H) \qquad (6.3)$$

where F_V and F_H present the vertical and horizontal emission intensities. The value p can vary between 0 and 0.5, and in a good instrument it can be determined with a precision of 1 mp (milli-p), which gives a maximum theoretical dynamic range of 500 to the polarometer. Kelly et al. (453) described a digital, photon counting polarometer containing a rotating polaroid sheet (90 rpm). A similar instrument was developed by Japan Immunoresearch Co. (Takasaki, Japan) containing a spinning polarizator (1800 rpm) (454).

In 1981 Popelka et al. (455) and Jolley et al. (456) described an automated polarometer which uses disposable tubes as cuvettes and also performs single tube blank corrections. The instrument contains liquid crystal and a polarizer for adjusting polarization detection levels. This combination has the advantage that the polarization level can be rapidly changed by an electric field. The instrument has sensitivity of 0.1 nmol/L of fluorescein and measures polarization with an accuracy of 1 mp. Since the introduction of TD_X, AD_X, and later on an automated system, IM_X by Abbott, fluorescence polarization assays have become one of the most widely applied FIA techniques, used especially in therapeutic drug monitoring, screening for drug abuse, and also in assays of some haptenic hormones (Chapter 8.3.1).

Recently several other polarization assay systems have been introduced. Kobayashi (373) used an IBF 129 polarization fluorometer (Kowa Kizai Ltd., Japan) in his assay of cortisol. In addition to research fluorometers, Perkin Elmer has introduced the PFI-20 Drug Screening System, which contains an autosampler and flow cell for polarization measurement (457). As a homogeneous assay FPIA can also be easily adapted to existing clinical chemistry analyzers, such as the Roche-Diagnostics FPIA (Roche Diagnostic Systems, Nutley, NJ, USA) and the Cobas Bio or Cobas Fara autoanalyzers.

6.2.3. Time-Resolved Detection

Time resolution in emission detection adds another dimension to photoluminescence spectrospcopy: time. Originally it was used in phosphorometric instruments to determine faint phosphorescence from cryogenic samples even in the presence of prompt fluorescence. It is also used to determine the luminescent lifetimes for various compounds and recently has been used as a technique for "time-filtering" the desired fluorescence from a mixture of luminescences of varying decay times (background rejection; see Chapter 5.4.5). The instrumental designs used for time resolution vary from mechanical or electrical phosphorometers to time-correlated single-photon detectors to time-resolved integration detectors to phase-resolved instruments.

The early phosphorometers were constructed using continuous light sources and mechanical choppers, such as rotating cans, for producing the pulsed excitation and "gated" detection (458). These types of phosphorometric accessories were also used in commercial spectrofluorometers for the measurement of phosphorescence. Weissman in 1942 used a phosphorometer where a high pressure mercury arc lamp was pulsed with a rotating disc for the determination of long lifetime europium chelate fluorescence (459). Mechanical phosphorometers suffer from the disadvantage of limited speed and the inconvenience in changing delay and window times, which are determined by the chopper model and speed.

Later on pulsed excitations and electronically gated detections led to more versatile instruments applicable to a wider range of decay times (386). Flash tubes are the most frequently used excitation sources for pulsed excitation in phosphorometers, but lasers—because of their high peak intensity—have also been used, for example, for detecting some drugs by heavy atom enhanced phosphorescence analysis (460). In pulsed excitation instruments, time-resolved detection can be achieved either by phototube gating (a PM tube turned on after the decay of the excitation pulse) or electronic gating (i.e., integrating photons with a predetermined time window or following the emission with multichannel detector) (461, 462). Pulsed excitation and gated detection are also used in commercial research fluorometers (Perkin Elmer LS 5 and LS 50 fluorometers of Perkin Elmer Ltd, Beaconsfield, Bucks, UK; Fluorolog-2 Spectrofluorometer from Spex Industries Inc., Edison, NJ, USA; and PTI LS-100 Luminescence spectrofluorometer from Photon Technology International Inc., South Brunswick, NJ, USA), instruments designed for measuring both short and long decay time fluorescences and phosphorescences. The PTI instruments contain a xenon flash tube for decay times over 10 μs, and H_2, D_2 or N_2 gas filled gated metal lamps (1.5 ns pulses) for decay-time analysis down to 200 ps.

Time-resolved fluorometries with pulsed excitation and gated detection (e.g., with boxcar integrator) are also used to achieve higher sensitivities in fluorometric determinations (410, 463). Extensive reviews of the applications of time-resolved fluorometry were recently published by, for example, Soini and Lövgren (464) and Fernandez (465). Lytle and Kelsey (431) used a pulsed laser and gated detection to overcome problems related to scattering background in the fluorometric detection of fluorescein and riboflavin. Sensitivity improvements were 100- to 1000-fold when compared to conventional fluorometric detection. Yguerabide et al. (466) used nanosecond fluorometry in their study of antigen-antibody interaction with a dansyl derivative as the fluorescent probe. In 1974 Sacchi et al. (467) used nitrogen laser excitation in time-resolved fluorescence microscopic detection to detect pararosaniline sulfate stained DNA.

Schneckenburger and Unsöld (468–470) have studied the sensitivity improvements in fluorometric analysis employing nanosecond scale time resolution. They used a cavity-dumped and mode-locked argon-ion laser, at 364 nm, or a dye laser in a time-resolved microfluorometer for detecting methanobacteria and methyl-umbelliferone ($\tau = 3.0$ ns) at a concentration of 5×10^{-16} M. Figure 6.2 demonstrates the improvements in signal-noise ratio they obtained after eliminating the effect of scattering.

In order to exploit the maximal benefit from time-resolved detection, the specific fluorescence should clearly differ from disturbing background sources by its duration (τ). Haugen and Lytle (471) have studied the benefits of time resolution by excitating with mode-locked argon-laser fluorochromes of decay times varying from 0.7 ns to 700 ns (acridinium orange, rose bengal, rubrene, and Ru-tris-bipyridine). Pyrene derivatives, which have somewhat longer decay times (100 ns) (472) than the average background noise of biological materials, have been tested in a number of time-resolved systems. Knopp and Weber (473) utilized the long decay fluorescence of IgM-pyrene conjugates in 1969. They used a free running spark lamp, fast photomultiplier, and oscilloscope to detect the delayed emission. Lovejoy et al. (474) have studied rotational movements and segmental rotations of antibodies by measuring time-resolved anisotropies from mixtures of pyrene and antipyrene antibodies. Wieder suggested (388) the use of pyrene derivatives as labels for a time-resolved fluoroimmunoassay. Pyrene derivatives have not, however, gained wider applications in FIAs due to practical problems relating to insufficiently long τ.

The development of chelates expressing the energy-transfer type of long lifetime fluorescence, or even phosphorescence, and techniques for their use in immunoassays has created a demand for developing time-resolved fluorometers for routine immunoassays. In the TR-fluorometer developed by Wallac Oy (Turku, Finland), a xenon pulse lamp (1000 Hz) is used for excitation of a fluorescent Eu-chelate solution within microtitration strip wells, and emission is integrated by rectangular (1230 Arcus™) or through mea-

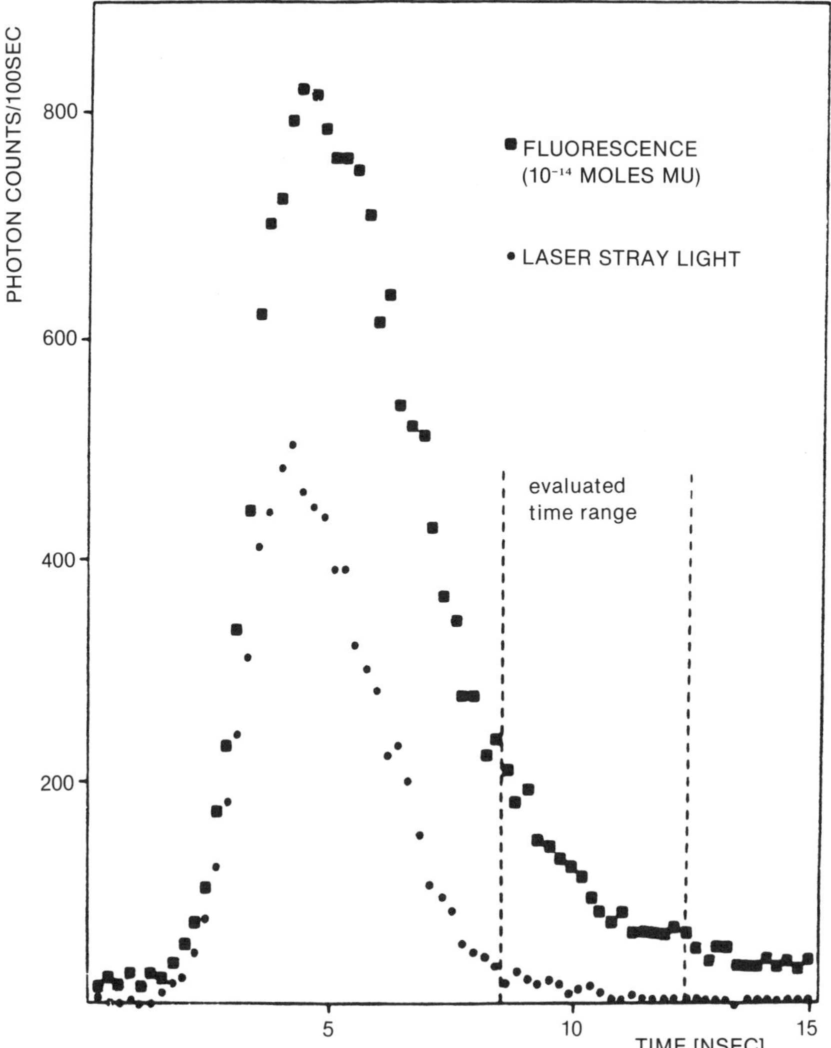

Fig. 6.2. Time-resolved fluorometric determination of 4-MU. (Reprinted from ref. 469 with permission.)

suring (1232 DELFIA Fluorometer and 1234 Research Fluorometer) optical arrangement with a predetermined time window (400–800 μs) (253, 475) (Fig. 6.3). In a system used by CyberFluor (Toronto, Canada) nitrogen laser epi-illumination (20 Hz) is used to excite the bottoms of white microtitration strips and emission is integrated from the dried surfaces by front-phase

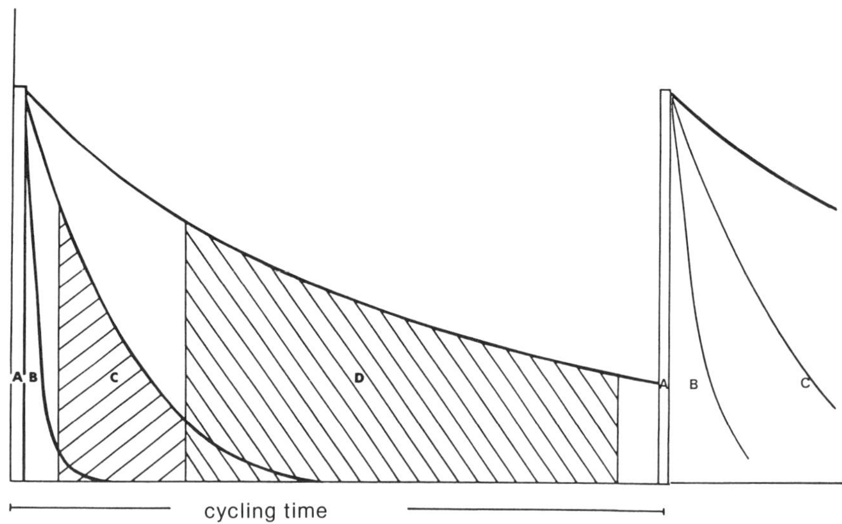

Fig. 6.3. Principle of time-resolved fluorometry for discrimination of scattering (A) and short decay-time background (B) from longer decay-time emissions (C and D).

optical arrangement. Since those instruments and related assay systems were introduced, TR fluorometers have rapidly achieved expanding applications as a highly sensitive detection system for immunoassays (Chapter 8.4).

The development of fluorescent probes on long decay times has also created a need to develop time-resolved fluorescence microscopes. Tanke et al. (476, 477) have used a modified Leitz Orthoplan epi-illuminating microscope attached to a xenon flash lamp and rotating disc to arrange suitable delay and recording time windows for time-resolved visualization of Eu-phosphor-particle stained samples.

Phase-resolved fluorometry, or frequency-domain fluorometry, is another basic technology applied to utilize decay-time differences in fluorometric determinations (478). Instead of pulsed excitation, in phase-resolved fluorometry the sample is excited with sinusoidally modulated light with modulation frequency ω and modulation depth m_{ex}.

$$E_t = A\, m_{ex} \sin\omega t \tag{6.4}$$

Depending on the decay time of the sample, the emission, F_t, is both demodulated and phase shifted by angle Φ (Fig. 6.4).

$$F_t = A\, m_{ex}\, m \sin(\omega t - \Phi) \tag{6.5}$$

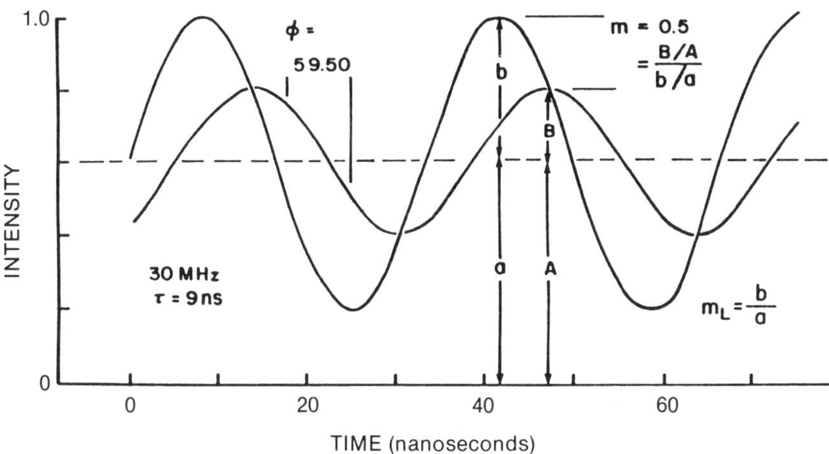

Fig. 6.4. Principle of phase-resolved fluorometry with modulated excitation (b) producing demodulated and phase-shifted emission (B). (Reprinted from ref. 478 with permission.)

This technique is especially suitable for determining decay times, even in time scales of nanoseconds and from samples of several components of differing decay times (479). Emission lifetime can be calculated independently both from m and Φ.

$$\tau_p = \tan\Phi/\omega \tag{6.6}$$

$$\tau_m = 1/\omega(1/m^2 - 1)^{1/2} \tag{6.7}$$

Phase-resolved fluorescence intensity, PRF, involves measurement of fluorescence at different phase angles, Φ_D. Unwanted background can be eliminated from PRF by selective nulling—adjusting the detector angle out of phase with interfering emission (e.g., scattering) or using a modulation frequency resulting selective demodulation of the undesired signal (480, 481). Phase-resolved technique is applied also in some research fluorometers—for example, in the SLM series of Aminco spectrofluorometers (Aminco, Urbana, IL)—for determining decay times ranging from 1 picosecond to 1.6 millisecond by applying modulation frequencies ranging from 10 kHz to 2 GHz.

PRF has been used to study anisotrophy and decay-time changes on the binding of toluidinenaphthalenesulfonic acid (TNS) to apomyoglobin (482). Bright and Litwiler (483) used single frequency phase-resolved fluorescence with bifurcated fiberoptics for quantitation of mixtures of fluorescers of varying τ. By using small probed volumes they also included fluctuation analysis to reject the rapidly fluctuating, unmodulated background.

Although present PRF has not been able to achieve very high sensitivities, it has been also applied to some FIAs (Chapter 8.4.4).

6.3. RESEARCH FLUOROMETERS

The early investigations of FIA relied on the use of existing research filter or spectrofluorometers. More or less all existing commercial research fluorometers were used during the technological development of FIAs, and quite a number of instruments have been constructed for polarization measurement. In the following discussion are some examples of the research instruments which have been used for FIAs.

The Turner filter fluorometer, Model 111 (J. K. Turner Ass., Palo Alto, CA) was used in the very early quantitative FIAs (184, 484). Aalberse used a Locarte fluorometer equipped with a flow cell in a SAFA test in 1973 (185). Aminco-Bowman fluorometers (American Instrument Co., Silver Spring, MD) were used in early SL-FIAs (485) and in fluorescence polarization immunoassay (FPIA) (19). SLM fluorometers, such as the Model 4000 polarization fluorometer (SLM Instruments, Urbana, IL), are used in several FPIA research applications (486, 487).

Perkin Elmer fluorometers LS 2B, 20, and the automated PFI-20 system which contains an auto sampler, polarizators, and flow cell cuvette (Perkin Elmer Ltd., Beaconsfield, UK) are used for numerous FPIA applications (344, 457, 488–490). The PE-1000 filter fluorometer was the detector in a number of separation FIAs (Sep-FIA) of drugs (371, 491), Perkin Elmer MPF-3L in an IFMA on microtitration plates (492) (where the bound fluorescein-labeled antibodies were eluted from surfaces and measured with a flow cell), and the MPF-2A in an assay of salivary albumin performed with microbeads as solid-phase by measuring the beads in suspension (493).

O'Donnell et al. (494) used a Varian model SF-330 spectrofluorometer (Varian Instrument Div., Palo Alto, CA) in their Sep-FIA after redissolving the antibody-precipitated fluorescent antigen prior to measurement. The Spectro Glo (Gilson Medical Electronics Inc., Middleton, WI) filter fluorometer has been employed in a number of IFMAs based on measuring microbeads in suspensions (192, 495, 496). Dual-beam differential fluorophotometers, the Shimadzu RF 510 and 520 (Shimadzu Seisakusho Ltd., Japan), are utilized in, for instance, fluorometric EIAs (209, 497) and in a Sep-FIA (498) using polystyrene balls as solid-phases. An MKI spectrofluorometer of Farrant Optical Co. (Valhalla, NY) was the detector instrument in IFMAs for serum antibodies published by Gillis et al. (499, 500), and the

IBF model 129 polarization fluorometer (Kowa Kizai Ltd., Japan) is used in a number of FPIAs (370, 373, 501, 502).

Further on research fluorometers such as the Spex Fluorolog (Metuchen, NJ) and Fluoripoint spectrofluorimeter (Baird-Atomic Ltd., Braintrac, Essex) have found some applications in FIAs. A Kontron spectrofluorometer SFM 25 with a 10 μl flow cell is used as the detector in substrate-labeled, homogeneous FIA (SL-FIA) (503) and a Schoeffel FS 970 filter fluorometer as the flow detector in continuous flow, "hit-and-run" FIA (504). Legros et al. (505) used a Jobin-Yvon Type 3D spectrofluorometer in their liposome-mediated complement lysis assay of serum antibodies, and Bacigalupo et al. (506) employed an FP 550 spectrofluorometer (Japan Spectroscopic Co., Tokyo) in a Sep-FIA of progesterone. An example of another principle of quantitation of immunoreaction is the detection of fluorescence signals in ELFIA by recording the emission with photographic film and quantitating with a densitometer (Bouzard CDM3 densitometer, Paris) (507).

6.4. MICROFLUOROMETERS

Recent development in immunofluorescence microscopy and microfluorometers takes IF nearer actual quantitative immunoassays, and the borderline between IF or QIF (quantitative IF) and IFMA has become vague. The development has led to assay designs very similar to IFMA techniques with "artificial" solid-phases, standardized procedures, and quantitative determinations of the produced emission. Quantitative measurement of the fluorescence of microtitration plates, beads, or cells is performed in QIF with microfluorometers developed specially during the 1970s by Prof. Ploem and his group (271, 508).

Much effort is expended in developing microscopes capable of measuring fluorescence intensity in terms of defined units (509–512). Standardized results also require standardization of staining techniques. Systems have been developed to standardize solid-phase antigen preparations by using soluble antigen preparations attached to "artificial" surfaces such as cellulose beads (defined antigen substrate spheres, or DASS) and cellulose discs (soluble antigen fluorescent antibody, or SAFA) (Chapter 8.2.2). The strong bleaching of fluorescence which is encountered in IF techniques also causes problems when standardized quantitative determination is desired.

The arrangement of sample excitation depends on the sample material used. Inverted microscopes with epi-illumination optics are often employed when using microtitration plates as solid-phases. The aperture-defined microvolume (ADM) method was developed for the automatic scanning of beads on microtitration plates (513). It has been applied also for automated measurement of enzyme activities using a microfluorometer (514). The CytoFluor 2300 system of Millipore Co. (Bedford, MA) is a scanning microplate fluorometer devised for quantitative measurement of cells (cell phenotyping, cytotoxicity assays or immunoassays). The cells on a membrane-bottom plate are measured through the bottom.

Fluorescence microscopes used in IF can be converted for QIF measurement by installing a photometer for emission quantitation. Laser scanning microscopes, low-magnification field microscopes, and a combination of scanning electron microscopes and TV-based image analysis systems have also been employed (508). Haaijman and Wijnants constructed a microfluorometer from a Leitz Orthoplan microscope by using pneumatic components to automate testing of a large number of QIF samples (515). A Leitz MPV-II fluorometer equipped with inverted optics for microplates is also used in a number of QIF assays (186, 188, 516). A Reichert microscope, with epi-illumination and a microphotometer equipped with a PM tube, is used in QIF by, for instance, van Dalen et al. in 1973 (188) and Knapp and Ploem in 1974 (517). Fiebach et al. used a Fluoval fluorescence microscope (VEB Zeiss, Jena, GDR) in a microfluorometric IFMA of bovine leukemia virus detection (518). Zeiss microscopes equipped with an epi-illuminator and a photometer are utilized also in several QIF experiments (449, 508, 510). Hart et al. (519) used laser-based computerized image cytometry, constructed from a Zeiss universal microscope, fiberoptic cable, argon-ion laser, and CCD camera, to detect HIV-infected cells after *in situ* hybridization. Ueki et al. (520) used an Olympus single beam microfluorometer to measure antinuclear antibodies bound to a human leukocyte nucleus by quantitating fluorescence from ten randomly chosen nucleoli by the use of a magnified image with a PM tube. Microfluorometers are also used as detecting instruments in a number of "normal" IFMA techniques (158, 516).

Besides the direction toward quantitative analysis of IF, another basic tendency is to develop automated image analysis and programs for pattern recognition for histological and pathological samples (521). In image processing the fluorescence patterns are divided into pixels, digitalized (Digital Image Fluorescence Microscopy) and processed with recognition programs (444, 522). In image processing, video cameras and CCD cameras can be used as primary detectors (523).

One of the future ideas introduced by Ekins et al. (524) is a technique he named "ambient analyte microspot multi-analyte immunoassay," which utilizes, in its preliminary format, a laser scanning confocal microscope

(Zeiss confocal microscope or Bio-Rad Lasersharp) to quantitate microspot bound fluorescences from a multiplicity of tiny coated spots.

6.5. FLOW CYTOMETERS

Flow cytometers can be considered the second generation of particle counters able to perform elaborate automated multiparametric analysis from a suspension of cells or particles and which are even able to sort cells according to predetermined properties. Flow cytometers have achieved extensive applications in different areas of clinical research, such as hematology, immunology, oncology, and microbiology (427, 525–528). In addition to "particle counting" (i.e., analysis of the size and shape of particles by the scattering they produce), flow cytometers apply numerous staining techniques including immunological staining with fluorescently labeled antibodies (as used in IF, QIF, and IFMA) to determine various parameters of cells.

In flow cytometers the analyzed cells or particles migrate through a thin capillary. Detection parameters such as scattering, absorption, and emissions are recorded with lasers. Analysis can utilize the number, size, volume, shape, or granularity of cells, their DNA or RNA content, the number of viable cells, receptors, or antigens on their surfaces, and so on. A flow cytometer is able to complete multiparameter analysis of 5,000–10,000 cells/second.

Flow cytometers contain generally one laser, but two lasers are also used, especially for multiparametric studies. A He-Ne laser (633 nm) is primarily used for analysis of scattering, but it works also for the excitation of long-λ excited probes (e.g., allophycocyanin, A-PC). An argon-ion laser (488 nm) is the most frequently employed laser and it is perfectly suited for the excitation of fluorescein and is also used for excitation of phycoerythrin. Multicomponent fluorescence analysis can be performed with a single laser, but more efficient resolution is obtained with dual-laser excitation, (e.g., by combining argon-ion with some dye laser) (529). Woronicz and Rice (530) used an argon-ion laser (488 nm) for FITC- and phycoerythrin-labeled antibodies, a rhodamine 6G dye laser for Texas red-labeled streptavidin and A-PC-labeled avidin, and an argon-ion laser, tuned to UV, for excitation of monochlorobimate (used to stain intracellular glutathione).

The flow cytometer market is covered by a few companies and instruments, such as the FACS 440 (Becton-Dickinson, Mountain View, CA), Epics (Coulter Epics Div., Hialeah, FL), or Spectrum™ (Ortho Diagnostic Systems Inc., Westwood, MA). Flow cytometers are extensively used in immunological investigations, in the study of the function of the immunosystem and its cellular populations, for studies of B- and T-cells, cell-surface antigens, or receptors, and so on. Analyzing those parameters on cells can require double label IF techniques with dual lasers (529).

The use of flow cytometers in quantitative analysis of noncellular immunoassays has only recently begun to be exploited. For example, the ability of flow cytometers to discriminate and selectively analyze particles of varying sizes offers potential for developing simultaneous multiparameter assays by using microbeads of different sizes (531, 532). This principle is applied in, for example, dual-label IFMA of serum antibodies against two viruses, which utilize latex particles of 5 and 7 μm sizes and phycoerythrin-labeled streptavidin as a detecting reagent for biotinylated anti-human IgG (65). The dual-emission detection facility provided by flow cytometers is also used for dual-label immunoassays by simultaneously using phycoerythrin- and fluorescein-labeled antibodies (533) or fluorescein- and rhodamine-labeled antibodies (534, 535).

Flow cytometers can also be used as automated detectors for microbead based IFMAs (97, 536) applied, for instance, for serodiagnosis of HIV infection (537). On the other hand, flow cytometers with powerful lasers and flowing droplet detection are used to achieve high sensitivities for the measurement of free soluble fluorochromes. Attogram amounts of rhodamine are detected with a "FACS" instrument (538). Lisi et al. (539) introduced a nonseparation IFMA based on the use of microbeads as solid-phase, which relied on the ability of flow cytometers to determine the particle associated fluorescence specifically, triggering the detection by analyzing the scattering caused by particles and hence obviating the need for physical separation.

In addition to flow cytometers, continuous-flow, flow-injection, and liquid-chromatographic instruments have sometimes been used in FIAs, either for the separation of bound fraction from free or as flow-through detectors for fluorescence measurements. Flow-injection analysis with immunoreaction cuvettes containing immobilized antibodies (or antigens) are used in, for example, a two-site immunoluminometric assay (ILMA) employing acridinium ester as the chemiluminescent label (540), and in Sep-FIA with carboxyfluorescein loaded liposomes as carriers of labels, lysed with detergent prior to fluorescence quantitation (172, 541). Lim et al. used stopped-flow injection analysis for a homogeneous fluorescence energy transfer assay (FETI) (542). Lidofsky et al. used HPLC, with a flowing-droplet detector and laser excitation (He-Cd at 325 nm) for highly sensitive detection of the condensation product of p-hydroxyphenylacetic acid, the fluorogenic substrate of HRP (543), and an argon-ion laser for detection of fluorescein used as a label in Sep-FIA (544). Allain et al. utilized HPLC and a fluorescence flow detector to automate SL-FIAs of theophylline and valproic acid (503) and Hosotsubo et al. used HPLC with a gel filtration column for separation in Sep-FIA of human IgG (545, 546).

6.6. FIA FLUOROMETERS

Besides the applications described above, where various research fluorometers have been applied for fluorescence measuring, the majority of FIA methods consist of complete systems containing both immunochemical procedure and the related instrument, optimized—and also restricted—to the kits produced by the same company. In the FIA field there exist considerably less open systems and general FIA fluorometers, as compared to, for instance, radioisotopic techniques, where instruments are primarily manufactured by companies which do not produce the respective assay kits. For EIA there also are numerous microtitration plate readers equipped with filters suitable for most of the frequently used enzymatic substrates. The number of enzymes and the available fluorogenic substrates used in ELFIAs are relatively limited, which makes it possible to have general plate fluorometers for those assays that employ microtitration plates as solid-phases.

6.6.1. Plate Fluorometers

Microtitration plates are gaining expanding use as solid-phase manifolds for EIA and FIA techniques performed in batches. The exception is the automated "random access" immunoassay systems where the tendency is toward unit-dose reagent cartridges. Analogously to EIA photometric readers, there also are generic fluorescence based microplate readers on the market for fluorescence based EIA, ELFIA.

Microplate fluorometers are based on either front-phase, through measuring, or right-angle optical arrangements (right angle only when wells are measured as single strips). Front-phase (epi-illumination) fluorometric design was used already in microfluorometers developed for microtitration plates (Chapter 6.4). They are generally based on semireflective, dichroic mirrors, which reflect excitation light but let through emission light. This optical system may also avoid the problems arising from inner-filter quenching in the case of a high concentration of fluorescent compounds (547). Epi-illumination is primarily used in present plate fluorometers, and the optical arrangement benefits the possibility of using black or white microtitration plates to restrict plastic background fluorescence (black plates) or to increase the efficiency of emission collection (white plates). Table 6.1 lists some examples of plate fluorometers used in immunoassays. The MicroFluor™ Reader (Dynatech Laboratories, Billingshurst, UK) and the Titertek Fluo-

Table 6.1. Plate Fluorometers Applied in Immunoassays

Instrument	Manufacturer
MicroFluor™ Reader	Dynatech Laboratories
Titertek Fluoroscan™	Flow Laboratories
FluoroFast™ Fluorometer	3M Diagnostic Systems
Auto FP-1 Fluorometer	Fuji Revio Co.
Microplate Fluorometer	Allergenetics
MTP-12F Fluorometer	Corona Electronics Co.
Microplate Fluorometer	Japan Spectroscopy Co.
CytoFluor 2300	Millipore Co.

roscan™ (Flow Laboratories, Irvine, UK) are used in numerous ELFIA applications and the FluoroFast™ fluorometer of 3M Diagnostic Systems (Mountain View, CA) in FAST™ allergy tests. The Screen Machine™ of Pandex Laboratories (Mundelein, IL) applies front-surface detection of microbeads captured on a surface of filters attached to bottoms of microtitration wells (548). The time-resolved fluorometer CyberFluor 615™ (CyberFluor) measures Eu-fluorescence by time resolution from the dried bottoms of white microtitration plates (74).

The through-measuring arrangement is applied in, for example, the DELFIA Fluorometer (Wallac Oy, Turku, Finland), designed for time-resolved measurement of fluorescent Eu-chelates in solution, while right-angle optics is used in the ARCUS Time-Resolved Fluorometer (Wallac Oy, Turku, Finland), which measures microtitration plates divided into single strips (475).

An increasing number of immunoassay methods are utilizing fluorescence as the detecting principle in the field of enzyme immunoassays, and it can be predicted that the number of plate fluorometers will likewise increase in the near future. Accordingly, the list of plate readers in Table 6.1. will certainly not be complete.

6.6.2. FIA Fluorometers

Most commercial FIAs have been developed in close collaboration with instrumental development, and the resulting methods form more or less complete systems. Accordingly, the instruments developed are adapted to the specific requirements of existing assay technique and may not be suitable for other techniques, and sometimes even research applications are excluded due to elaborate technologies difficult to handle for those who want to make in-house methods.

Table 6.2. Fluorometers Developed for Heterogeneous FIAs

Instrument	Type of assay	Manufacturer
Fluoromatic™	FIA	BioRad Laboratories
IDT FIAX® -100	FIA	International Diagnostic Technol
FIAX 400	FIA	Whittaker Bioproducts Inc.
Screen Machine™	FIA	Pandex Laboratories
AmeriFluor	FIA	American Diagnostics
Immpulse®	FIA	Sclavo Inc.
Track XI® System	FIA	Microbiological Associates Inc.
Immunostics™	FIA	Seward Laboratories
AutoFluor II System	FIA	California Immunodiagnostics
MicroFluor™ Reader	ELFIA	Dynatech Laboratories
Fluoroscan™	ELFIA	Flow Laboratories
FluoroFast™	ELFIA	3M Diagnostic Systems
CyberFluor 615™	TR-FIA	CyberFluor Inc.
1230-Arcus™	TR-FIA	Wallac Oy
1232-DELFIA®	TR-FIA	Wallac Oy

Table 6.2 lists some of the currently existing FIA fluorometers (heterogeneous) and Table 6.3 the respective fluorometers designed for homogeneous FIA applications.

A separation-based FIA system was developed in BioRad Laboratories (Richmond, CA) that utilized polyacrylamide beads as solid-phases (ImmunoBeads™), and a photon counting, microprocessor controlled fluorometer for automated fluorometric detection (Fluoromatic™) (549, 550). International Diagnostic Technology (Santa Clara, CA) has developed a dual-beam filter fluorometer, the IDT FIAX™ 100 Fluorometer, for measuring

Table 6.3. Instruments Designed for Homogeneous FIAs

Instrument	Type of assay	Manufacturer
Syva Advance™	FETI	Syva Co.
Fluorostat™	SL-FIA	Ames-Division of Miles
Optimate	SL-FIA	Ames-Gilford
Abbott TD_x	FPIA	Abbott Laboratories
Abbott TD_A	FPIA	Abbott Laboratories
Abbott IM_x	FPIA	Abbott Laboratories
IBF-129	FPIA	Kowa Kizai Ltd.
Perkin Elmer PFI-20	FPIA	Perkin Elmer Ltd.
Focus™	FPIA	Source Scientific Systems Ltd.

specially designed stick samplers (Stiq™) attached with coated cellulose acetate or nitrocellulose discs. It is primarily used for serological tests of circulating antibodies (Chapter 8.2.6). The Track XI® Fluorometer (Microbiological Associates Inc., Bethesda, MD) is a front-surface fluorometer optimized for measuring fluorescence from the company's spongelike Collimune® three-dimensional matrix attached to Track-manifold (551). The Immunostics™ Fluorimeter (Seward Laboratories, London, UK) is developed for Sep-FIAs utilizing magnetizable particles as solid-phases.

Syva (Palo Alto, CA) has marketed the Syva Advance™ filter fluorometer, an automated fluorometric system for fluorescence energy-transfer immunoassay, FETI (552). The instrument consists of sample and reagent compartments, a pipetting system, a flow cuvette, and a dual-beam fluorometer. The Fluorostat™ is a ratio-correcting filter fluorometer developed for Ames TD_A kits, which employ the homogeneous SL-FIA principle (553, 554). The instrument operates with a cycling halogen lamp and uses the dark period for correcting instrumental background sources, such as photomultiplier dark current and stray light. Fluorescence polarization detectors form the basis for the Abbott TD_X, TD_A, and partly also the IM_X systems (see Chapter 6.2.2.), which represent different levels of automation of FPIAs.

6.7. AUTOMATION

Today immunoassay automation is a major trend in instrumental and technological development. A rapidly growing number of totally or partially automated immunoassay systems have entered the market, and it can be anticipated that numerous new systems will appear during the 1990s.

The reasons for increasing automation arise from the advantages automated systems can provide, such as improved precision, savings in time and labor, savings in reagents and even in costs when only singlicates are needed without frequent standardization, and the better suitability, especially of "random-access" analyzers, to clinical routines. In addition front-end automation can avoid the danger encountered when handling infectious samples, and automated systems can increase the total through output of samples. Disadvantages of such automation relate to the high price of complicated instruments and reagents delivered as unit-dose packages. A totally automated instrument also forms a closed system, a "black box," not applicable for research and "home cookers."

The main objectives in the adaptation of assay techniques for automated systems include the search for more rapid assays (achieved with more rapid antibodies, shorter diffusion distances, higher temperatures, etc.), the increased stability of tracers, signals, and standard curves, ready-to-use reagents (unit-dose packages for random access analyzers), one-point calibration using complete standard curves from instrument memory, reduced sample volumes, front-end automation, centralized data handling capabilities, and universal bulk reagents such as buffers.

The main approaches toward automated immunoassays have been the development of a simple, manual test which does not require complicated assay steps nor instruments, the adaptation of existing homogeneous assay techniques to existing chemistry automates, the mechanization of heterogeneous batch-type immunoassays, and totally automated random-access immunoassays. The role of fluorescence can be seen in the number of fluorescence-based techniques used and in the tendency to involve fluorogenic substrates and fluorometric detection with automated EIAs. The future will show whether immunosensors are forming a new generation of automation suitable for on-line monitoring of immunologically analyzable compounds.

6.7.1. Why Has Success in Automation Been So Elusive?

The above question was raised by Rosemary Polsky-Cynkin in a recent article about automation (555), and it describes well the difficulties encountered in the 1970s and 1980s in the struggle toward automated immunoassays. Compared to routine clinical chemistry, the automation of immunoassays has not become the norm in the clinical laboratory to the same extent. The problems relate to the complexity of immunoassays, the inherent instability of standard curves (especially with radioisotopic labels), and costly instrumentation. Also, the technique routinely used at that time was competitive RIA, which is relatively robust and simple, and the availability of multiwell gamma counters made the evaluation of results automated and easy. However, the advent of noncompetitive assays, assays that require more assay steps from one aspect, and the general tendency toward non-isotopic assays from another aspect are changing the situation.

The early automated radioimmunoassay systems were unsuccessful, mainly because of the complexity of the techniques and the instability of reagents. One such automated continuous flow RIA system was introduced by Ismael et al. in 1975 (556). The described "Southmead System" was based on competitive-binding RIA on Sepharose beads as solid-phase and on-line filtering through membranes prior to counting. Numerous other automates have also been introduced, based on either continuous-flow or discrete systems, such as the Squibb-Gammaflo, Ventrex-Centria, Micromedics Systems-Concept 4, Becton Dickinson-Aria, and Vitek-KinetiCount.

The development of solid-phase separation systems for heterogeneous immunoassays was a premise for automation, because it relieved assays from centrifuges. The advent of immunometric assays, on the other hand, increased the complexity of assay technologies, involving more steps and critical washings, which increased the demand for automation. Finally non-radioisotopic assay techniques were able to provide stable labels, signal levels, and standard curves that can be stored for future use. Accordingly, current automates rely primarily on EIAs with photometric, fluorometric, or luminometric detection, and on FIAs.

6.7.2. Manual Tests

Diagnostic immunoassays which are simple to perform and do not require complicated instruments have become increasingly popular and in certain respects diminish the need for developing dedicated automates for those analytes. Simple manual tests are mainly used as "outside lab" or "near patient tests" in doctors' offices, at the bedside, in patients' homes, in the field, etc. Traditionally those assays utilize immunoassay technologies that produce visible responses, such as agglutination or colored reaction products. Analytes such as human choriogonadotropin (hCG) are frequently analyzed as a pregnancy test, lutropin (LH) for ovulation detection, urine proteins for kidney function, and various microbes (e.g., streptococcus) for infections.

The simple tests rely primarily on solid-phase chemistry and methods such as prosthetic group labeling, apoenzyme reactivation, enzyme channelling assays for homogeneous EIAs, multilayer film techniques, latex particle immunoassays, colloidal gold labels, liposome entrapped dyes, etc. The following chapter contains some examples of those simple test systems developed so far.

DOT-ELISA is a manual test system which uses minute amounts of antibodies or antigens as spots on a nitrocellulose filter. The response of the immunoassay is a precipitated colored enzyme substrate, detected by a naked eye (557). The Abbott Test Pack Plus system is based on a thin-layer membrane (nitrocellulose) containing colloidal selenium-labeled drugs, captured in the reaction zone by immobilized antibodies forming a color to the capture zone (558). The Directigen™ test system of Becton Dickinson Diagnostics (Instrument System, Towson, MD) is composed of ColorPak™ test packs containing reagents labeled with dye-entrapped liposomes. The Clearview chromatographic system (Unipath Ltd., Bedford, MA) is based on the agglutination of blue latex particles. The CARDS™ test pack from Pacific Biotech Inc. (San Diego, CA) is an EIA with monoclonal antibodies attached to a membrane. Other techniques introduced include Immunoconcentration™, ICON (Hybritech Inc.) (559), the Immunochromatographic Test (Syntex Medical Diagnostics, Palo Alto, CA) (560) and a microparticle capture test on a glass fiber (561) or Ektachem slides, techniques which are used, for example, in therapeutic drug monitoring (562). Because of the qualitative nature of the response and the somewhat limited sensitivity these systems achieve, their application will be limited to relatively few analytes.

6.7.3. Chemistry Automates

Homogeneous immunoassays, because of their simple technical performance, can be automated with a number of existing clinical chemistry analyzers, provided that they can be equipped with suitable detectors. For example, the homogeneous EIA of Syva Co., EMIT®, is automated with a number of analyzers, such as Cobas® Bio and Cobas® Fara (Hoffman-La Roche), Dacos (Coulter Electronics Inc.), Demand (Cooper Biomedical), EPOS (EM Diagnostic Systems Inc.), Hitachi analyzers (Boehringer Mannheim GmbH), Multistat® (Instrumentation Laboratories Inc.), RA-1000 (Technicon Instruments Co.), and Kone Program (Kone Oy) (563).

Roche Diagnostic Systems (Nutley, NJ) has developed its own FPIA kits to be measured with Cobas centrifugal analyzers—for example, FPIA of quinidine (564), procainamide, and NAPA (565), theophylline, tobramycin, phenytoin, phenobarbital, carbamazepine (566), and vancomycin (567). Cobas Bio and Fara centrifugal analyzers are also used for SL-FIAs (TD_A Ames) of drugs (568). The Perkin Elmer PFI-20 system has been specifically developed for the automation of existing FPIAs and is used, for example, in testing for methamphetamine using LIDIA based, single reagent FPIA (489).

Technicon Autoanalyzers are used for automated SL-FIA of theophylline (569) and the continuous-flow fluorescence quenching immunoassay (FQIA) of gentamicin (366). Spencer et al. (283) furnished a Technicon autoanalyzer with a flow-cell polarization detector for FPIA of insulin. SL-FIAs (TD_A) of the drugs theophylline and gentamicin are automated with a Multistat III centrifugal analyzer (Instrumental Laboratory, Lexington, MA) (570).

Even though homogeneous assays are easy to automate with existing instruments, the homogeneous principle restricts those applications mainly to small molecular weight analytes and invariably to analytes present at considerably high concentrations. To be generally applicable within the whole area of immunoassays, the automated system needs to process more complicated heterogeneous, separation-based assays, because heterogeneous assays are the only way to measure analytes requiring high sensitivities.

6.7.4. Mechanized Immunoassays

Heterogeneous immunoassays consist of several laborious steps, the performance of which may be critical to the results obtained (such as washings), and have therefore created the need for the mechanization of these steps. If the steps are further integrated within one instrument so that the procedure

Table 6.4. Mechanized Immunoassay Systems

Instrument	Assay system	Manufacturer
IM_x	TD_x / FPIA	Abbott
IM_x	MEIA/ ELFIA	Abbott
Stratus®	Radial partition ELFIA	American Dade Div.
Screen Machine™	Particle Concentration FIA	Pandex Laboratories
Amerlite™	Enhanced Luminescence EIA	Amersham Int.
Amerlite PC	Enhanced Luminescence EIA	Amersham Int.
Syva Advance™	Fluorescent EMIT, FETI	Syva Co.
Immpulse™	FIA	Sclavo Inc.
Optimate™	SL-FIA	Ames-Gilford
Photon Era™	EIA	Hybritech
ELISA Processor	EIA	Behring Diagnostics
Labotech®	EIA	Chemilia
CAP System	ELFIA	Pharmacia Diagnostic
FAST System	ELFIA	3M Diagnostics

does not require manual operations, the system may be classified as automated. However, that classification is rather arbitrary, and differentiation has mainly been made according to the order of analysis: batch-analyzing instruments and random-access analyzers.

Table 6.4 lists instruments and assay systems performing batch-type automated analysis, including both heterogeneous and homogeneous assay principles.

The Stratus system of American Dade (a division of Baxter Health Care, Miami, FL) is a totally automated batch-analyzing instrument using the ELFIA principle. The system employs normal competitive assays, sequential addition competitive assays, and noncompetitive two-site assays (571). The instrument contains dispensers for the automatic addition of samples and reagents. The standard curve is stable for two weeks, and sample processing time is about seven minutes. The ELFIA is performed on glass fiber solid-phase, the washing with the enzyme substrate solution (4-MUP) results in the elution of unbound reagent from the detection area ("radial partition"), and fluorescence is determined kinetically (5 measurements per second) with a front-surface fluorometer (dichroic mirror).

Abbott has launched a totally automated batch-analyzing system, IM_x, which employs two assay principles: microparticle capture ELFIA ("MEIA") for large antigens and for analytes requiring high sensitivity, and TD_x FPIA for haptenic antigens (410). MEIA is based on alkaline phosphatase (ALP)-labeled antibodies, microparticles as solid-phase attached to a glass fiber matrix, and 4-MUP as the fluorogenic substrate, measured kinetically with a front-surface fluorometer. The system has already been widely used and evaluated (Chapter 9.2.2).

The Syva Advance is an automated instrument dedicated for Syva's proprietary homogeneous FIAs, FETI and EMIT (EMIT by utilizing the fluorescence detection of the enzymatic substrate NAD(P)H). The instrument contains sample and reagent cuvettes, dispensers, and a flow-cell fluorometer for kinetic measurement.

The Optimate instrument has been developed in collaboration between Ames and Gilford and is aimed for Ames TD_A SL-FIA kits. The system consists of an aspirator, sample carousel, dispenser, reagent valve, diluter, and both a photometer and a fluorometer. The batch analyzer can be used for both SL-FIA and chemical analysis.

The Pandex Screen Machine and PC-FIA function with microbead solid-phases and immunoassays in microtitration wells equipped with filter bottoms. The instrument performs reagent additions, incubations, separations by filtration through, washings, and readings.

Automated Sep-FIAs also have been developed by using coated surfaces in the Immpulse™ system (572), where the instrument does the pipetting, washing, reading, and calculating. The Amerlite system employs EIA with luminometric detection of the peroxidase activity. The assay is also partially automated with an instrument containing an incubator and workstations for dispensings and washings.

One way to automate the existing batch-analyzing systems is to construct a robotic system to handle all assay steps. For example, DELFIA® analytes of TSH, T3, T3, PL, FSH, hCG, and cortisol are automated with a robotic system by Sasaki and Ogura (573).

6.7.5. Random-Access Automates

Random-access immunoassay systems are totally automated systems, in which individual samples and analytes can be loaded in the instrument in random order, and the instrument takes care of assay performances for each sample individually. The number of random-access automated systems is rapidly growing, and at present several new systems are introduced every year. The majority of the present systems rely on EIA, and an increasing number utilize fluorogenic substrates (primarily 4-MUP for ALP detection). These systems generally use bar-coded unit-dose reagent cartridges, but some of the systems work with bulk reagents.

Dry reagent technology is accordingly important for the technology, in order to produce very stable and reproducible reagent packages to ensure stable signal levels and stable standard curves (574). Dry reagent technology and ligand displacement principle (LIDIA) are developed for homogeneous

Table 6.5. Random-Access Automated Immunoassay Systems

Instrument	Technology	Solid-phase	Manufacturer
ES 600/300	EIA Photom.	Coated tube	Boehringer Mannheim
Affinity	EIA Photom.	Coated tube	Becton-Dickinson
PK 300	EIA Photom.	Beads	Olympus
Oasis	EIA Photom.		Sensor Diagnostics
SR1	EIA Photom.	Magnetic beads	Serono
Pulse FIA	EIA Photom.	Magnetic beads	Beckman Instruments
Biotrol 7000	EIA Photom.	Magnetic beads	Biotrol Diagnostics
Quartus	EIA Photom.	Magnetic beads	Mitsui Pharmaceut.
Immuno-1	EIA Photom.	Magnetic beads	Technicon/Triton
ACS:180	LIA	Magnetic beads	Ciba-Corning
ImmuLite	EIA Lumin.	Ps. ball	Cirrus Diagnostics
	EIA Fluorom.	Surface	Kallestad
Photon ELITE	EIA Fluorom.	Magnetic beads	Hybritech Inc.
AIA 600/1200	EIA Fluorom.	Magnetic beads	TOSOH Co.
OPUS	EIA Fluorom.	Filter	PB Diagnostic Sys.
OPUS	FIA	Film	PB Diagnostic Sys.
VISTA	EIA Fluorom.	Magnetic beads	DuPont/Hitachi

SL-FIAs of theophylline (575), for instance. If premature immunoreaction is to be avoided, the components need to be dried separately—for example, by using organic solvent (576). Unit-dose reagent cartridges—named, for instance, dry reagent delivery modules (577)—contain either dried reagents or ready-to-use solution. Most often the unit-dose cartridge contains separate compartments for the coated surface (cuvette or beads) and labeled reagents, and the instrument takes care of dilutions, dispensing, reagent reconstitution, and the other steps required to carry out the heterogeneous assay.

Table 6.5 lists some of the random-access automates for which information was available during 1989 and 1990. This table very likely will go out of date rapidly as new systems and instruments enter the market.

The automated systems introduced so far differ from each other in the systems applied (EIA or FIA), the way reagents are delivered (unit-dose or bulk), the solid-phase materials employed (surfaces, matrixes, or beads), the analyte assortment, and through output times. A strong tendency can be recognized to apply EIA and to use magnetic beads as solid-phase and a fluorogenic substrate, 4-MUP, for ALP monitoring.

The ES 600 and ES 300 systems from Boehringer Mannheim are fully mechanized multibatch analyzers which function with photometric EIA (578). The systems use the Enzymum Test® System with reagents labeled with HRP and ABTS as the chromogenic substrate. The reagents are delivered in bulk, and the instrument is able to process 100–200 samples per hour (579). Becton Dickinson's AFFINITY is a fully mechanized random-access instrument (EIA) using reagents in unit-dose cartridges (ImmUnit™). The instrument can measure both absorbance (with a photodiode) and fluorescence (with a PM tube). Flow through is 40 samples per hour, the stability of the standard curve is two weeks, and a single analyte takes 15–30 minutes. The SR1 system of Serono Diagnostics uses Serozyme™ EIA, which is performed with anti-fluorescein coated magnetic particles (universal solid-phase for all assays), with FITC-labeled primary antibodies delivered in bar-coded ready-to-use cartridges, with ALP-labeled antibodies and phenolphthalein monophosphate as the chromogenic substrate determined kinetically. Sample processing time is about 30 minutes and through output 56 samples per hour. The Immuno-1™ Immunoassay System was developed in collaboration between Technicon Instrument Co. and Triton Biosciences (Alameda, CA). This system is also based on universal magnetic particle separation, ALP as a label, and photometric determination of ALP activity.

Two automatic systems use luminometric detection. The ImmuLite system uses ALP as a label and a dioxetane-phosphate derivative as the luminogenic substrate. The ACS:180 system of Ciba-Corning is based on a direct LIA with dimethylacridine labels (580). In this system the assays are performed using bulk reagents and polypropylene tubes as reaction cuvettes (not assay specific). Incubation times required for various assays are all adjusted to 7.5 minutes by stipulating the amounts of solid-phase antibodies and labeled antibodies.

The Photon ELITE is a random-access analyzer from Hybritech Inc. It uses magnetic beads (coated ferrite particles) as solid-phases, ALP-labeled reagents in unit-dose reagent cups delivered in dry form (Tandem-M-Pak™), and 4-MUP as the fluorogenic substrate measured kinetically with a front-surface fluorometer. Practically the same instrument (and assay technology) was later introduced as the AIA 600 and AIA 1200 systems by TOSOH Co. (Tokyo, Japan). In this system the crossover problem between samples is avoided by using separate pipetting tips for each sample. Incubation times are adjusted to 40 minutes for all assays. Magnetic particles are kept in suspension during the incubation by virtue of a changing magnetic field, and washing is performed by filtration (581).

VISTA™ is a benchtop, random-access analyzer based on DuPont's proprietary MagniSep™ chromium dioxide particles (582). Bar-coded Flex cartridges contain reagents for 32 assays, which are based on ALP as a label and its detection with 4-MUP as the substrate. The instrument is a joint venture of DuPont and Hitachi Ltd.

PB Diagnostic System Inc. (Westwood, MA; a joint venture of Polaroid Co. and Behringwerke) has introduced an immunoassay system named

OPUS™, which, similar to IM_x, incorporates two separate assay principles, heterogeneous Sep-FIA on a thin film layer and ELFIA on a filter matrix. Both assay kits are delivered as unit-dose reagent cartridges (583). Competitive Sep-FIA takes place on three-layer polysaccharide films (agarose) coated on a plastic support. The first layer beneath the plastic spreading layer delivers buffer substances, required detergents, or blocking agents; the second layer is an optical barrier where the scattering iron oxide particles hide the top layer from excitation. Excitation penetrates to the reaction layer through a transparent polyester film. The reaction layer contains immobilized low-affinity antibodies preincubated with rhodamine-labeled haptens. After the immunoreaction, the released tracer migrates through the thin barrier to the upper layers and is shielded from the excitation (584, 585). Large molecular weight analytes and analytes requiring high sensitivity, such as digoxin (586) (performed with competitive ELFIA with back-titration), are analyzed with ELFIA. ELFIA is performed on a glass fiber filter, similar to the ELFIA of the Stratus system. The filter matrix contains immobilized antibodies. Additional reagent wells in the cartridge contain labeled antibodies (ALP) and fluorogenic substrate (4-MUP). The unbound labeled reagent is washed from the optical window area simultaneously with addition of the substrate solution (587). The products evaluated are described in Chapter 9.2.3.

The Kallestad Immunoassay Analyzer (Chaska, MN) is a random-access automated system which will be introduced during 1990–1991. Like most of the automates described above, this is also based on ALP as a label, dry reagent delivery modules, and 4-MUP as the fluorogenic substrate. The 4-MU fluorescence produced by ALP is measured with an epi-illuminating fluorometer which has detection limits down to 0.96 nM of 4-MU (588, 589).

At present intensive development is going on, especially in commercial companies, to develop more automated immunoassay systems, and new automated systems are introduced one after another. The tough competition in the field has resulted in a bustle in launching new systems, and in some cases delays in introducing the promised systems are encountered. The near future will show whether automated immunoassay analyzers will actually change the whole clinical laboratory routine in the future, the same way chemistry automates are currently changing the routines of chemical analysis in clinical laboratories.

CHAPTER

7

PHOTOLUMINESCENT PROBES

The performance of any photoluminescence analysis is greatly dependent on the probe used. For example, the sensitivity achieved in fluorometric analysis depends on both the intensity of the produced signal and on its discernment from the background noise. In addition, quite many of the fluorescence-based immunoassay techniques rely on some specific property of the fluorochrome applied, and the use of a specific assay technique may require development of a suitable fluorescent probe for the purpose. On the other hand, the discovery of fluorescent probes with interesting new properties can create totally new perspectives for technological development.

7.1. APPLICATIONS OF FLUOROCHROMES

Fluorescent compounds, and organic fluorochromes in particular, are applied in diverse fields of routine life and science (590). Examples of the routine use of fluorescent dyes are materials used for dyeing cloth or the various fluorochromes applied as dyes or optical brighteners for plastics. Inorganic phosphors are used in television screens and as coating materials in lamps, for example. Various fluorescent compounds also form the basis of some lasers.

In biomedical sciences, fluorescent compounds are used, for instance, as liquid or solid scintillators, as stains for microbes and cellular compartments, and as fluorescent indicators in pH measurement, complexometric analysis, redox titrations, etc. In the field of biochemistry, fluorescent compounds are also used as fluorogenic reagents for primary amines and proteins, in the study of enzymes and other proteins (591), for staining DNA and RNA (compounds such as ethidium bromide and propidium iodide, Hoechst dyes, acridine orange, etc.), and proteins, for detecting cations (Ca^{2+}), and in the study of lipids and membranes (592, 593).

In the immunological field, fluorescent compounds are applied for labeling viable cells to be used as targets in assays of cell-mediated immunology. In addition to the widespread use of covalently coupled fluorochromes as marker substances for antibodies or antigens in FIA, IFMA, IF, and flow cytometry, the strong immunogenicity of fluorescein is utilized in the production of anti-fluorescein antibodies, which are employed as a part of a universal catching system in IRMA (594) and ELFIA (595), and as an immunogenic signal amplifier in EIA (596). Fluorescent compounds, and especially the change in their fluorescence properties upon binding to antibodies, have been utilized in the study of antibody-antigen reaction since 1964 (280). For example, dansyl-group (5-dimethyl-aminonaphthalene-1-sulfonamido group) has been used as a polarity sensitive probe in a study of the structure of antigen-combining sites of antibodies (597).

Fluorescent compounds also function as energy mediators and enhancers in numerous chemiluminescence reactions. Fluorescein can enhance the luminescence quantum yield of a dioxetane reaction from 0.000013 to 0.00048 (598). Anilinonaphthalenesulfonic acid (ANS) is used as an energy acceptor for the chemiluminescence reaction between peroxide and peroxy-oxalate used in EIA with glucose oxidase as the label (599). Perylene has also been applied as an enhancing energy mediator for the same reaction (600). Patel and Campbell used fluorescein as an energy acceptor for isoluminol chemiluminescence in a homogeneous energy transfer immunoassay technique (601).

7.2. REQUIREMENTS SET FOR FLUORESCENT PROBES

The main requirement for a fluorescent probe is its detectability in required conditions—which is the prerequisite for any sensitive fluorometric analysis. Detection sensitivity depends on two factors: the relative fluorescence intensity of the probe (the product $\varepsilon \times Q$), and the contrast, that is, the discernment of the emission from background noise with respect to the wavelengths or the decay time (602). Other requirements are related to the behavior of the probe or the labeled reagent in immunological applications during storage, assay, or detection. Table 7.1 lists some of the general requirements set for fluorochromes to be used in immunoassays.

In addition to the general requirements mentioned above, many techniques impose their own specific demands. FPIA requires a fluorescent probe with τ longer than the Brownian motion of the free antigen but shorter than the rotational time of antibodies. TR-fluorometric applications, on the other hand, require probes with τ which is substantially longer than any background fluorescence. Fluorescence quenching and enhancing immunoassays utilize fluorochromes which are sensitive to changes in their microenvironment, such as changes in pH, viscosity, or polarity taking place upon immunoreaction. SL-FIAs and ELFIAs need fluorogenic enzyme substrates, which are derivatives of fluorescent compounds derivatized with suitable enzymatically cleavable bonds, which renders them practically nonfluorescent. FETI assays require two compounds having overlapping emission and

Table 7.1. Requirements for Fluorescent Probes to Be Used in Immunoassays

High relative fluorescence	$[\varepsilon \times Q] > 10{,}000$
Spectral or temporal resolution	long Stokes' shift and/or long τ
Hydrophilicity	good solubility of reagents, low affinity to serum proteins or solid-phase surfaces
Negative net charge	low nonspecific binding to coated surfaces
Photostability	long-term stability of reagents and avoiding of bleaching in IF
Easy coupling	retained immunoreactivity of labeled antibodies
Small size	no steric hindrance

absorption spectra to facilitate the energy transfer between them. Double-label assays, on the other hand, require probes with clearly differing emission lines to diminish mutual interference in their determinations, and polymeric labels function properly only with fluorescent probes with a long Stokes' shift in order to overcome inner-filter quenching.

7.3. ORGANIC FLUORESCENT PROBES

Organic fluorescent probes covalently coupled to antibodies have been used as markers in immunological research since 1941 (5, 6). Even today, most FIA technologies rely on organic fluorochromes, many of which have long been known, but new derivatives have recently been introduced.

The development of new fluorochromes with desired properties is hampered by the complexity of the fluorescence process. Currently available data are not yet sufficient to allow any definite generalizations in regard to the relationship between the molecular structure and fluorescence. Fluorescent organic compounds are generally highly conjugated, forming planar, rigid structures. The rigidity of the molecule decreases the probability of vibrational deactivation, hence increasing fluorescence quantum yields. Extensive π-conjugation and π-π^* transition favors fluorescence. The $n\pi^*$-type transition (heterocyclic compounds) is more prone to quenching due to intersystem crossing, and those compounds are generally less fluorescent but may exhibit phosphorescence in suitable conditions. Substitutions such as Br, I, NO_2, or CHO function as triplet sensitizers causing quenching of fluorescence, but on the other hand such compounds (e.g., erythrosin and eosin) can exhibit phosphorescence. Suitable substituents in aromatic structure can be used to make the parent compound less fluorescent (used as energy acceptors and quenchers in FETI) in order to produce bathochromic shift or to create phosphorescent compounds.

Numerous review articles describe the use of fluorescent compounds in biochemical and medical research. Chen and Scott (603) have written an extensive "atlas" of the fluorescent spectra of probes used in biochemistry. Kanaoka (591) reviewed the use of fluorescent probes in the study of enzymes, including the use of SH-reactive fluorochromes for modification of active sites of enzymes. Waggoner (592) reviewed the probes used in flow-cytometric and image-cytometric applications, including covalently coupled fluorochromes used with antibodies, in addition to noncovalent probes used for staining vital cells, membranes, and nucleotides, and for measuring enzymes (fluorogenic substrates). Detailed information about fluorescent probes can also be found in commercial catalogues, such as the catalogues of Molecular Probes Inc. (Eugene, OR) and Lambda Probes & Diagnostics (Graz, Austria).

Overviews of the use of fluorescent probes in FIAs are also included in several FIA reviews (342, 602, 604, 605). However, direct comparison of the properties of different fluorochromes is difficult if based solely on published data because of the high variations in the values presented. Often the fluorescence characteristics are strongly dependent on the conditions used and conjugation reaction applied. Small variations in the parent structure of the fluorochrome may have a decisive effect on the fluorescence achieved. A good example of the effects of substituents on the fluorescence of fluorescein derivatives can be found in, for instance, the articles describing the development of energy donor-acceptor pairs for Syva's fluorescence energy transfer immunoassays (350).

7.3.1. Fluorescein And Its Derivatives

Fluorescein, as an isocyanate activated intermediate, was the fluorescent probe used as early as 1942 by Coons et al. (6) in their microscopic IF test. Compared to their earlier IF experiments with β-anthracene, the green emission of fluorescein resulted in a better separation of the specific emission from the blue autofluorescence of cells. During the 1940s and 1950s, Coons et al. further optimized both the labeling procedures and immunological staining techniques for IF (606, 607). In 1958, Riggs et al. (266) introduced fluorescein isothiocyanate (FITC), which was prepared analogously to the respective isocyanate from aminofluorescein by using the less dangerous thiophosgene (liquid) instead of gaseous phosgene. Since then, FITC has been the reagent most commonly used in fluorescein labeling, but other derivatives, such as the dichlorotriazinyl derivative of aminofluorescein (DTAF) and the N-hydroxysuccinimide derivative of carboxyfluorescein (Fig. 7.1) also have been used for protein labeling. DTAF was originally

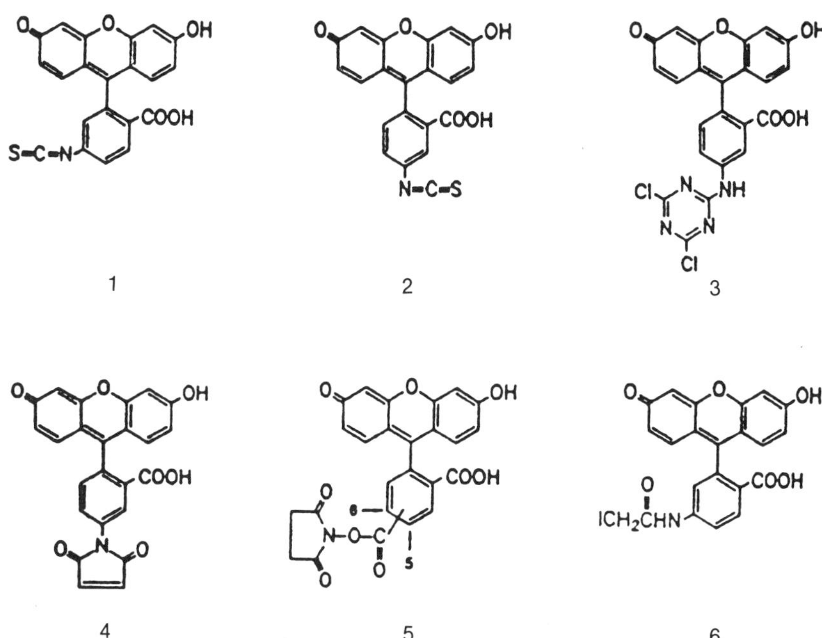

Fig. 7.1. Fluorescein derivatives used for protein labeling, 5′-FITC **(1)**, FITC **(2)**, DTAF **(3)**, N-maleimide derivative of aminofluorescein **(4)**, N-hydroxysuccinimide **(5)** and iodoacetamido **(6)** fluorescein.

introduced by Barskii et al. in 1968 (608) for labeling of antibodies. Blakeslee and Baines (609) have further developed the labeling procedures using DTAF. Its high reactivity also enables labeling sugars (e.g., dextranes) with fluorescein (610).

Fluorescein has retained its position as the most frequently used fluorescent probe in FIA and IFMA as well as in IF, QIF, and flow-cytometric applications. The reason for its superiority over most of the subsequently introduced probes relates to its high relative fluorescence intensity, high absorptivity, and quantum yield approaching unity in optimized conditions. As a well-known and thoroughly characterized fluorochrome, fluorescein has become the standard to which all new fluorochromes are compared. Some of the critical properties of fluorescein are tabulated in Table 7.2, and the fluorescence spectra obtained with FITC-labeled antibody are presented in Figure 7.2.

In spite of the high quantum yield of fluorescein as a free reagent in alkaline aqueous solution (0.85), its fluorescence level is considerably decreased (0.5–0.3) upon binding to proteins (611). The quenching of fluorescein

Table 7.2. Properties of Fluorescein

+	High relative fluorescence intensity, $\varepsilon \times Q \approx 61{,}000$
+	Excitation at 492 nm is well suited for many light sources
+	Green emission at 520 nm is at the efficient range of PM tubes
+	Reasonable water solubility
+	Negative net charge (dianionic form)
+	Small size
+	Highly immunogenic, easy production of anti-FITC antibodies
+	Low temperature coefficient, 0.0036/°C
+	No bleaching under normal fluorometric conditions
+	Suitable τ for FPIA
–	Polymorphic forms in some preparations
–	Short Stokes' shift, prone to interference by scattering
–	Inner-filter quenching limits practical labeling yield
–	Emission overlaps with that of albumin bound bilirubin
–	Affinity to serum proteins interferes with homogeneous assays
–	pH sensitivity
–	Quantum yield decreased upon conjugation
–	Bleaching problematic in IF

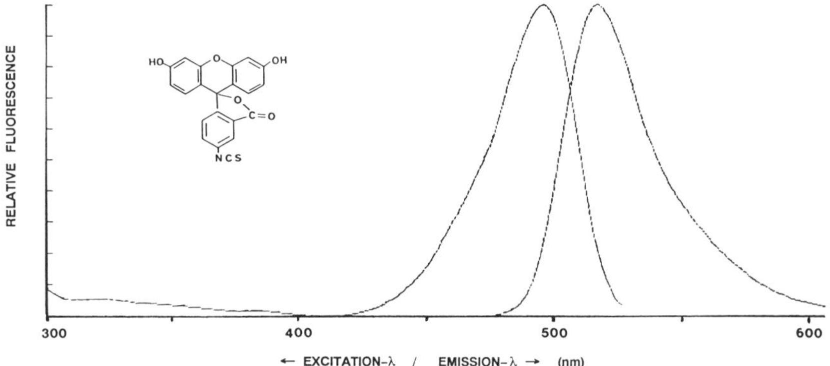

Fig. 7.2. Fluorescence spectra of FITC-labeled IgG.

upon binding to anti-fluorescein antibodies (612), which are easily produced because of the high immunogenicity of fluorescein (594–596), is exploited in various indirect quenching FIAs (Chapter 8.3.3). Its short Stokes' shift efficiently eliminates the attempts to increase signal levels by increasing the labeling yield beyond 5–6 FITC/IgG (613), which is the result of a strong inner-filter quenching (Fig. 5.11). With albumin, the labeling level of 5 FITC/protein produces the highest fluorescence intensity (196), and the optimum labeling yield for Fab ′ or IgG is around 2 or 4 FITC/antibody, respectively (496, 614). Thus, labeling with polyfluorescein can create real benefits only when special techniques are employed, such as excitation to total bleaching level used by Hirschfeld (337) or the use of releasable bonds and measuring the final fluorescence from free solution (615).

The overlapping fluorescence wavelengths of fluorescein and bilirubin (especially albumin bound bilirubin) lead to high background interference in homogeneous assays. In addition to the background interference, the affinity of fluorescein to serum proteins causes problems in homogeneous FIAs, and sample pretreatment is occasionally needed to avoid these problems.

A variety of derivatives of fluorescein have been synthesized, and also commercialized, for conjugating with antibodies or other compounds of interest. Isothiocyanate primarily reacts with aliphatic amines and can leave sulfhydryl groups unmodified (616). Iodoacetamidofluorescein can be utilized for labeling both SH-groups and NH_2-groups, and has been tested in, for example, FPIA of creatine kinase BB (617). DTAF is used in a number of FPIAs, and carboxyfluorescein as a N-hydroxysuccinimide ester in FETI, where fluorescein functions as an energy donor for tetramethylrhodamine-labeled antibodies (618, 619). 4 ′-(aminomethyl)-fluorescein was synthesized for coupling to haptenic antigens from the 4 ′-position of the ring, and is used in FPIA products of Abbott (620). The binding position at the phenolic ring produced chirality to the compound and hindered rotational freedom of the conjugate. Table 7.3 contains the fluorometric properties of the most frequently used fluorescein derivatives which have been applied in fluorescence immunoassays.

A large number of fluorescein derivatives have been synthesized and tested as energy acceptors for the basic fluorescein in fluorescence energy transfer assays (621, 622). Methoxy substituents at positions 2 ′ and 7 ′ produce a bathochromic shift of both excitation and emission λ, whereas methoxy substituents at positions 4 ′ and 5 ′ function as efficient quenching groups. Accordingly, 4 ′,5 ′-dimethoxycarboxyfluorescein is an optimal energy acceptor for fluorescein in FETI, because the energy absorbed is efficiently converted to heat and no secondary emission occurs.

Carboxyfluorescein (CF) is a noncovalent, hydrophilic fluorochrome used for labeling vital cells (e.g., cancer cells to be used as targets for cytotoxicity

Table 7.3. Fluorescein Derivatives

Fluorochrome	Exc. max (nm)	ε (L/M cm)	Em. max (nm)	Q	τ (ns)
Fluorescein (FITC, DTAF)	492	72,000 (66,000)	516–525	0.3–0.85	4.5
Carboxyfluorescein (CF)	492	73,000	514–518	0.87	
2′-Methoxy-CF	500		534	0.78	
4′,5′-Dimethoxy-CF	512	78,200		0.0004	
Tetraiodo-F (Erythrosin)	530	101,000	560_{Fl} 690_{Ph}	0.015 0.003	0.4 270,000
Tetrabromo-F (Eosin)	525	101,000	550_{Fl} 580_{Ph}	0.02 0.001	0.9
Calcein	490	83,000	520		

assays; see Chapter 10.2). The labeling of mammalian cells is performed with a nonpolar, nonfluorescent diacetyl ester of CF (CFDA), which readily penetrates cell membranes and becomes polar and fluorescent CF by the action of cell esterases. Polar dianionic CF cannot penetrate intact cell membranes, and leakage of CF takes place only when the membrane integrity is broken (623). Because CFDA is incorporated only to living cells, the staining technique can also be applied to counting viable cells (624). CF-labeled cells are also used for assays of cell-mediated and complement-mediated cytotoxicity (625, 626). These assays are based on either CF-release as a result of cytotoxic reaction, or the counting of the remaining fluorescent intact cells. Kolber et al. introduced another fluorescein derivative, acetoxymethyl ester of 2′,7′-bis (carboxyethyl)-5,6-carboxyfluorescein for use in cytotoxicity assays, a derivative which reportedly contributes to a simpler labeling procedure, more rapid release, and less spontaneous leakage (627).

CF is also the fluorochrome most commonly used in liposome-mediated immunoassays, used encapsulated into the liposomes. The CF concentrations used in liposomes are high enough (millimolar) to produce efficient self-quenching with subsequent fluorescence recovery upon liposome lysis. Thus, labeled liposomes can function both as signal amplifiers (Chapter 7.5.3) and as a label system employed in homogeneous assays (Chapter 8.3.5). Liposomes loaded with calcein, a derivative of fluorescein, are even more efficiently quenched due to excimer formation in the highly concentrated solution in liposomes (628).

The tetraiodo derivative of fluorescein, erythrosin, produces less intense fluorescence, due to the heavy atom quenching effect of the iodine substit-

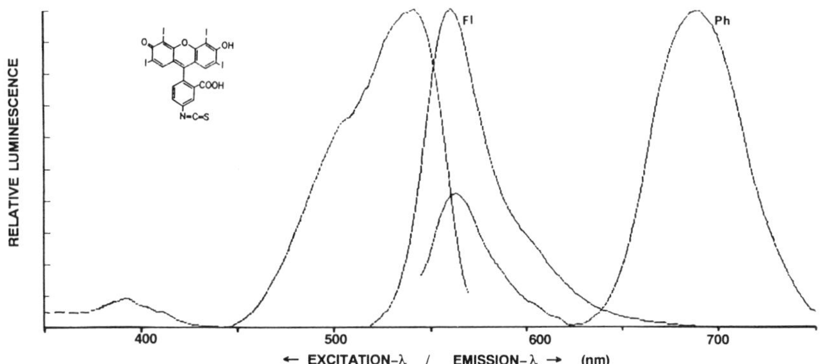

Fig. 7.3. Excitation, fluorescence emission (Fl), and phosphorescence emission (Ph) of erythrosin-labeled IgG.

uents. Under suitable conditions (on solid matrix or in de-aerated solution) erythrosin-labeled reagents may show reasonably strong RTP at 690 nm (Fig. 7.3). The phosphorescence of erythrosin-labeled haptenic antigens is used in phosphoroimmunoassays (PIA) (Chapter 8.4.4). The respective tetrabromo derivative, eosin, produces less strong phosphorescence, even though phosphorescence is recorded for both erythrosin- and eosin-labeled proteins (629). However, eosin is also used in a PIA and in an assay based on delayed fluorescence. Because of its low fluorescence, eosin is also applied as energy acceptor—and quencher—in FETI (Chapter 8.3.4). Figure 7.4 shows the fluorescence spectra of an eosin-labeled antibody.

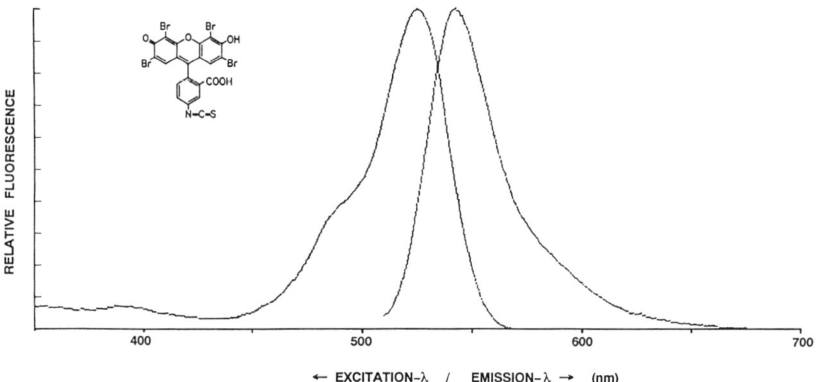

Fig. 7.4. Fluorescence spectra of eosin-labeled IgG.

7.3.2. Rhodamines

Rhodamines are derivatives of the same basic structure, xanthene, as fluorescein, but contain acylated amino groups in positions 3′ and 6′ instead of phenolic hydroxyls. Rhodamines have been developed in the course of an intense search for new alternatives to fluorescein, which would omit the drawbacks inherent with fluorescein. A major share of the research has been aimed at finding suitable counterparts for fluorescein for double-label staining techniques (i.e., probes that would have longer emission λ). A number of alternative structures have been found, many of which are commercialized and used in IF, flow cytometry, and also some FIAs.

Lissamine rhodamine sulfonylchloride (RB-200-SC) (Fig. 7.5), was originally introduced as an alternative fluorescent probe to fluorescein in 1958 by Chadwick et al. (630). In the same year Hiramoto et al. (267) introduced tetramethyl-rhodamine (TRITC) (Fig. 7.6). With the availability of these new fluorochromes, a number of tests were conducted to evaluate their usefulness as alternative, or complementary, probes for fluorescein in IF staining. For example, Brandtzaeg (631, 632) compared FITC with three different rhodamines, namely RB-200-SC, TRITC, and rhodamine-B isothiocyanate (RBITC) (Fig. 7.7), as labeling reagents for IgG and also studied their applicability in dual-label IFs.

A summary of the properties of rhodamines is presented in Table 7.4. The figures, which are based on various articles and catalogues again, show great variation, which might reflect the fact that those values have been measured under quite heterogeneous conditions. Primarily, rhodamines

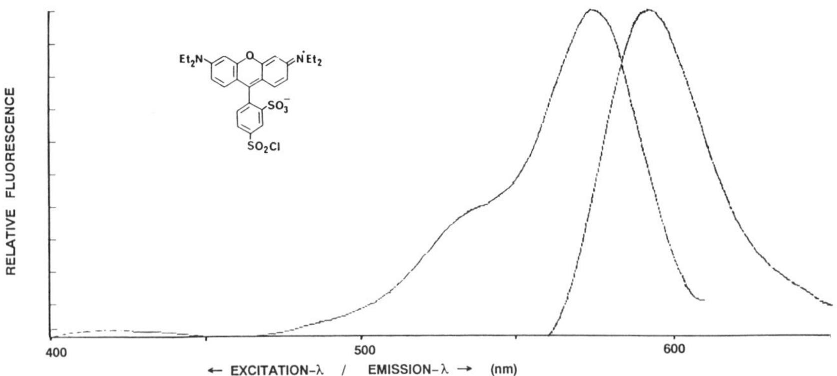

Fig. 7.5. Fluorescence spectra of lissamine rhodamine sulfonyl chloride-labeled IgG.

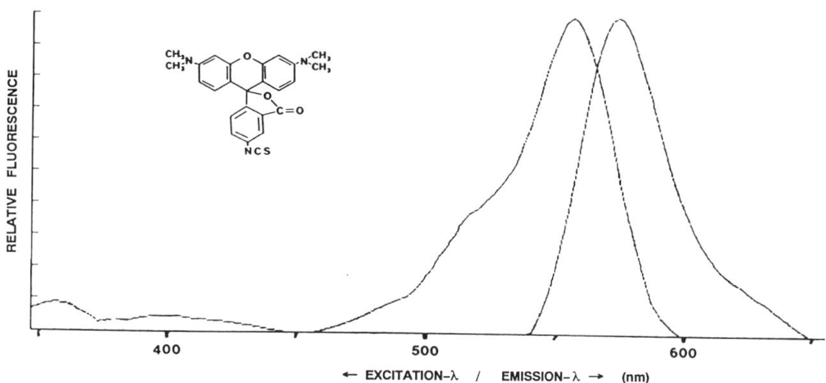

Fig. 7.6. Fluorescence spectra of TRITC-labeled IgG.

produce longer λ emissions than fluorescein but generally have lower quantum yields. Many of their applications are specifically based on the long λ emission.

TRITC is one of the most commonly used rhodamine derivatives, and has also found applications in numerous FIAs. Because of its absorption at the range where fluorescein emits, it can be used as energy acceptor for fluorescein in FETI assays (552, 621). Furthermore, it has been employed in *in situ* hybridization assays as a marker for the 3′-terminus of an RNA probe (634). The synthesis of TRITC tends to produce two isomers, a 5-substituted G

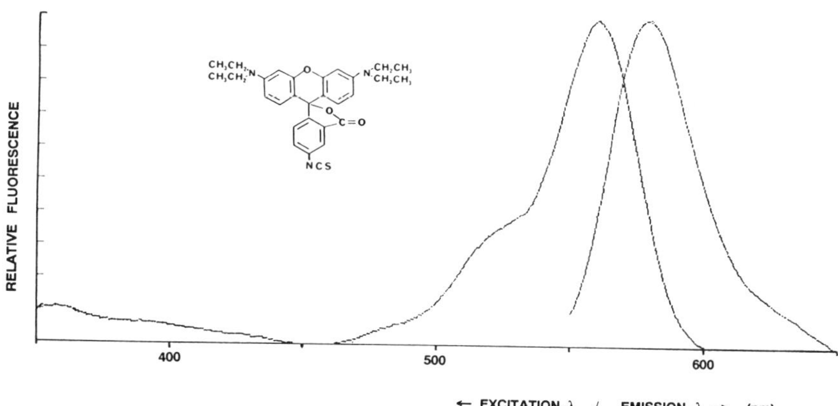

Fig. 7.7. Fluorescence spectra of RBITC-labeled IgG.

Table 7.4. Properties of Rhodamines

Fluorochrome	Exc. max (nm)	ε (L/M cm)	Em. max (nm)	Q	τ (ns)
RB-200-SC	550–560	80,000	575–585	0.04	1.0
RBITC	545–560	103,000	585		3.0
TRITC G	535–545	107,000	570–580		2.0
TRITC R	535–545	103,000	570–580		
XRITC	575	84,000	595–615		
Texas Red	595	85,000	615–620	0.3	
Rhodamine[a]	550		580	0.9	
Rhodamine-800	685	89,500	700	0.9	

[a]Rhodamine derivative patented by Arnost et al. (633).

form and a 6-substituted R form (635), also marketed as separate products by Molecular Probes Inc. Sulforhodamine and rhodamine-B have similar structures. They have been primarily used as antibody-labeling reagents in IF experiments. Sulforhodamine has also been applied as a marker loaded within liposomes in a Sep-FIA (636).

Texas Red™ (the trademark of Molecular Probes Inc.) is a sulfonyl chloride derivative of sulforhodamine 101, whose structure resembles that of the respective ITC derivative, XRITC. Texas Red was introduced by Titus et al. (637) as a more hydrophilic, activated derivative of sulforhodamine 101, as compared to XRITC, and it has since been used in flow cytometry for dual- and triple-label stainings, in many cases as a labeling reagent coupled to avidins. Moreover, Texas Red is used as an energy acceptor for suitable donor fluorochromes to form tandem probes with extended Stokes' shifts (e.g., DuoCHROME of Becton Dickinson formed by coupling B-phycoerythrin and Texas Red), and to form homogeneous assays with labeled antibodies or with DNA-probes (638). The long λ emission is also exploited to overcome problems related to the serum derived background (albumin bound bilirubin) in the phase-resolved FIA (PR-FIA) of human serum albumin (639). Figure 7.8 shows the structure of Texas Red and the fluorescence spectra of a Texas Red-labeled antibody.

Arnost et al. (633) have patented a new, hydrophilic rhodamine derivative which reportedly has a very high quantum yield (0.9). This rhodamine derivative has its excitation maximum at 550 nm and emission maximum at 580 nm. It is applied in an automated Sep-FIA system developed by PB Diagnostic System Inc. (584). Rhodamine-800 is an IR emitting fluorochrome which

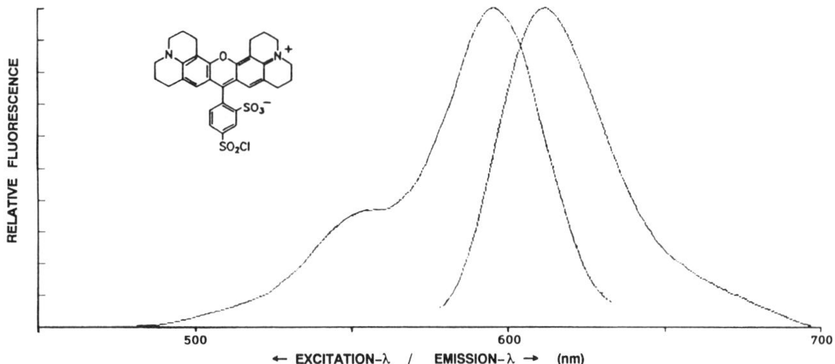

Fig. 7.8. Fluorescence spectra of Texas Red-labeled IgG.

might find applications in IR fluorometry. It has been measured fluorometrically with use of a semiconductor laser for excitation with a sensitivity down to 4 × 10^{-12} mol/L (424).

7.3.3. Polycyclic Aromatic Hydrocarbons

Unsaturated conjugated polycyclic hydrocarbons form the basic structure of most fluorochromes, many of which also contain heterocyclic parts in their structure. Some pure aromatic hydrocarbons have also been used as fluorochromes in FIAs after derivatization with groups making them more hydrophilic and enabling their coupling to immunoreagents. Derivatives of naphthalene, phenanthrene, anthracene, pyrene, and perylene have been used in special FIA techniques. A summary of the derivatives used is presented in Table 7.5.

Anilinonaphthalene sulfonic acids (ANS) and 5-dimethylaminonaphthalene-1-sulfonyl chloride (dansyl chloride) have widespread applications in basic biochemical research (590, 591, 603). As a polarity sensitive probe, ANS has been used in the study of membranes and protein surfaces. It is used, for instance, as a fluorogenic reagent in the measurement of serum albumin concentrations (640). The number of immunological applications of ANS is more limited, besides the use of ANS as a blocking agent in assays of thyroid and steroid hormones. In a homogeneous assay of anti-nuclear antibodies, ANS was used as a fluorescent label after coupling to nucleotides by carbodiimide reaction. In the assay its fluorescence is increased 12- to 35-fold in

Table 7.5. Properties of Aromatic Hydrocarbons Used in FIA

Fluorochrome	Exc. max (nm)	ε (L/M cm)	Em. max (nm)	Q	τ (ns)
ANS	370–380		470–480	< 0.8	16
2-Naphthol-8-sulfonamide	337	5,100	480	0.29	
Dansyl-chloride	340–350	4,300	510–560	0.03–0.3	14
Dansyl-protein	350–380		510–520	0.3	12
Dansylaziridine	340–355	4,500	495–525		
Anthracene-ITC	295, 357		460	0.6	29
Phenanthro-quinone	258, 312		390		
Pyrene-derivatives	340–345	40,000	375, 395	0.7	100
Perylene	450		545		

the course of anti-DNA antibody binding (641, 642). ANS has also been used as an energy acceptor in a chemiluminescence immunoassay based on peroxy-oxalate reaction (599).

Dansyl-chloride is a commonly used fluorochrome for amino-terminal amino acids in the study of the primary structure of proteins. An environmentally sensitive probe, dansyl-chloride, coupled to ε-amine of lysine, was used in the study of the antibody-antigen interaction as early as 1967 (597). In the interaction, antibody binding was manifested by the blue shift of dansyl emission and by the increase in its quantum yield from 0.027 to 0.9, with a concomitant energy transfer from protein absorption at 280 nm. The suitability of dansyl-chloride for labeling antibodies for IF tests has also been studied (611), but without further applications. Because of the relatively long decay times of dansyl derivatives, they could be suitable for polarization assays of relatively large antigens. The use of dansyl and dansylaziridine in FPIA of CK-BB failed (617) mainly because of the flexibility of the probe (sequential rotation decreasing polarization) and its sensitivity to serum background interference as a result of its relatively short emission wavelength. Bright et al. (643) constructed a regenerable fiberoptic immunosensor which was based on the fluorescence enhancement of immobilized dansyl-labeled Fab′-fragments upon binding of the respective antigen, albumin. Figure 7.9 shows the excitation and emission spectra of a dansyl-labeled antibody.

2-Naphthol-8-sulfonic acid as a sulfonamide derivative has evoked interest as a potential fluorescent probe for FIA because of its long Stokes' shift (140 nm), which is a result of excited-state proton transfer from the phenolic group after illumination. It has been tested in homogeneous FPIA (390) and in an indirect quenching FIA of phenytoin (644). 1-Amino-naphthalene-5-

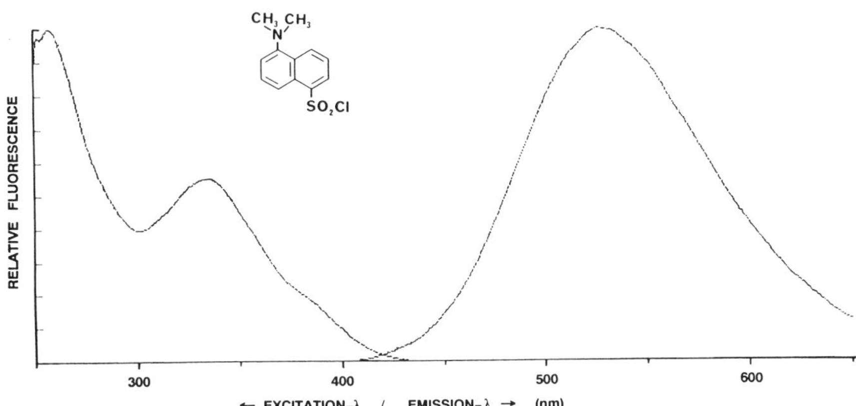

Fig. 7.9. Fluorescence spectra of dansyl-chloride-labeled IgG.

sulfonic acid is used for the fluorescent labeling of nucleotides via their triphosphates (645). Smolarsky et al. (646) utilized 1-aminonaphthalene-3,6,8-trisulfonic acid (exc., 337 nm; em., 480 nm; Q, 0.29) as a probe encapsulated in liposomes in the complement mediated homogeneous liposome immunoassay. In the liposomes the naphthyl derivative was efficiently quenched by the addition of a quencher, α,α'-bipyridine.

A phenanthrene derivative, phenanthrene-9,10-quinone, is used as a fluorogenic reagent for measuring arginine residues on proteins. Upon arginine binding it forms fluorescent (exc., 258 nm; em., 390 nm) phenanthroimidazole-2-amine derivatives (647). Bacigalupo et al. (506) utilized it for Sep-FIA of progesterone in an assay which, however, required quite complicated separation, redissolving, and extraction procedures to overcome protein-related interferences.

In the very first IF test, introduced by Coons et al. in 1941 (5), β-anthracene isocyanate was used as the fluorescent probe. Even though it was soon realized that the blue emission of anthracene (Fig. 7.10 and Table 7.5) produced poor resolution from the blue autofluorescence of tissues and cells (6), anthracene derivatives have nevertheless been tested in IF (611), and the reagent is commercially available for protein labeling. The 9,10-diphenyl derivative of anthracene is used as a fluorescent chemiluminescence amplifier in a thermochemiluminescence immunoassay based on luminescence of adamantylidene dioxetane (648).

Pyrene and its derivatives share the drawback of a relatively short emission wavelength, characteristic of most of the pure polycyclic hydrocarbons (Fig. 7.11), which efficiently diminishes their usability in FIAs. The feature which has raised considerable interest is the exceptionally long fluorescence

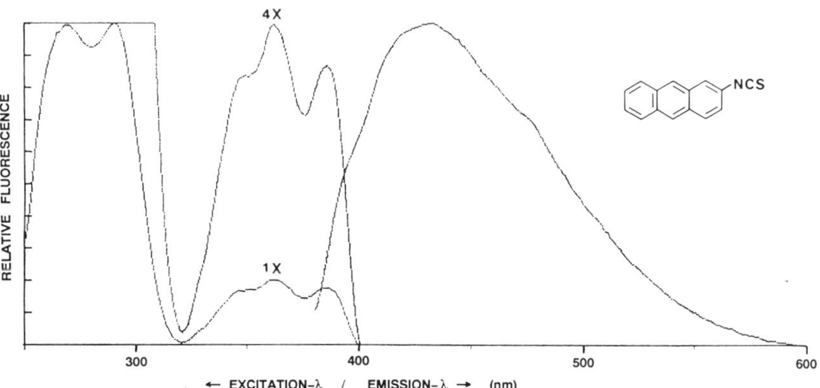

Fig. 7.10. Fluorescence spectra of anthracene (ITC)-labeled IgG. Excitation spectra are multiplied by factors 1 and 4.

decay time of the conjugates (Table 7.5), intended to be exploited in various types of time-resolved fluorometric assays. The conjugates most frequently used in immunoassays are formed with pyrene-butyrate or N-(1-pyrene) maleimide (472), but isothiocyanates also can be used for labeling of proteins (Fig. 7.11).

Lovejoy et al. (474) used pyrene as an antigen and a long lifetime fluorescent probe in the time-resolved anisotrophy study of the antigen-antibody binding reaction. Wieder suggested the use of a pyrene-butyrate derivative as a label for time-resolved fluoroimmunoassay in 1978 (388), and Morrison has

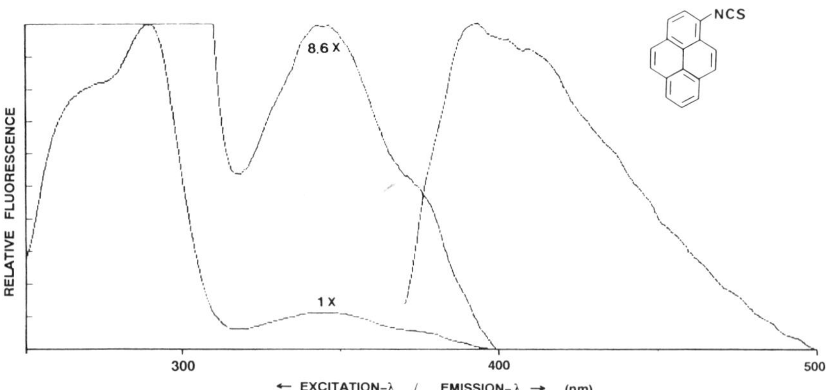

Fig. 7.11. Fluorescence spectra of pyrene-ITC-labeled IgG. Excitation spectra are multiplied by factors 1 and 8.6.

patented a time-resolved energy transfer proximity assay based on energy transfer from pyrene (excited with short laser pulses) to phycoerythrin and measured after a delay time in order to omit the background derived from the direct excitation of phycoerythrin (649). This time-resolved energy transfer assay with pyrene-butyrate conjugates as long decay-time energy donors has also been applied to an immunoassay of IgG (650) and homogeneous solution-hybridization assays utilizing a fluorescein-labeled DNA probe (651) or a Texas Red-labeled DNA probe as an energy acceptor (638).

Liburdy made use of the environmental sensitivity of a pyrene-maleimide labeled antigen (IgG) in the development of the fluorescence enhancement FIA (652, 653). Recently, pyrene derivatives have also found applications as labels in electroluminescence assays. Aizawa et al. (654, 655) developed a homogeneous electroluminescence immunoassay (EC-LIA) using pyrene-labeled human albumin in a fiber biosensor assay based on the antibody inhibition of ECL. Tromberg et al. (656) utilized a pyrene derivative, tetrahydroxy-tetrahydro-benzo[a]pyrene, as a tracer for benzopyrene FIA in an assay which was also performed on a fiberoptic immunosensor. Recently, sulfonyl derivatives of pyrenes have created interest as probes for micelles, as pH indicators, and as blue light emitting fluorescent probes for IF. Those derivatives reportedly show extremely high photostability (657).

The hydrophobicity of the larger aromatic hydrocarbons renders them impractical for tracers in immunoassays. Compounds such as perylene are highly fluorescent but scarcely soluble in aqueous solution. Molotkovsky and Bergelson (658) used 3-perynol-labeled lipids as fluorescent tracers for lipid interactions, the fluorescence of which was highly dependent on the polarity of their environment.

7.3.4. Coumarines

Derivatives of coumarines, such as 7-hydroxycoumarine, or umbelliferone, have been used in various types of immunoassays: as labels for antigens in homogeneous FIAs, as blue emitting fluorochromes in IF and flow cytometry, and as polymeric multi-coumarine labels for IFMA. Umbelliferone derivatives have found the widest applications as fluorogenic substrates for enzyme determinations (Chapter 7.6) used in ELFIAs (Chapter 9) and as fluorogenic substrates coupled to antigens in SL-FIA (Chapter 8.3.2).

The fluorescence intensity of coumarine derivatives is strongly dependent on pH. The effect of substituents on the fluorescence quantum yield and pH dependency has been studied for the development of probes for monitoring pH under physiological conditions (659). For example, the fluorescence of umbelliferone has been shown to be entirely dependent on the excitation of the phenolic form only (660). Goodwin and Kavanagh (661) found the highest fluorescence from the 3-acetic acid derivative of umbelliferone. The addition of electron accepting groups ($-CF_3$, $-CN$) to the position 4 of the coumarine structure resulted in a remarkable shift of emission to longer wavelengths (bathochromic shift) (605).

Table 7.6 shows the structures and fluorescent properties of some coumarine derivatives, and Figure 7.12 describes the fluorescence spectra of 4-methyl-umbelliferone (4-MU). Coumarine derivatives produce blue emission at 450–500 nm, which as such is less distinguishable from tissue autofluorescence than the emission of fluorescein or rhodamines. The blue emission,

Table 7.6. Fluorescent Properties of Some Coumarine Derivatives

Compound	Structure	Exc. max. (nm)	ε (L/M cm)	Em. max. (nm)
Coumarin (C)	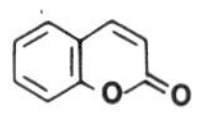	312		—
7-Hydroxycoumarin, Umbelliferone (U)	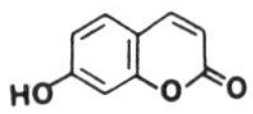 HO, O, O	325		465
4-Methyl-U (4-MU)	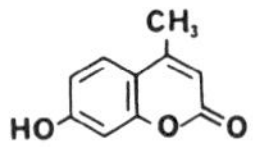 CH_3, HO, O, O	325	16,000	450
4-MU-3-acetate	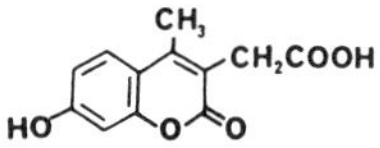 CH_3, CH_2COOH, HO, O, O	365		455
U-3-carboxylic acid	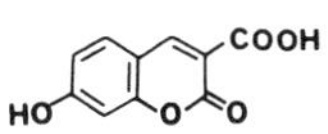 COOH, HO, O, O	400		455
7-Diethylamino-4-methyl-3-maleimidyl-coumarine (DACM)	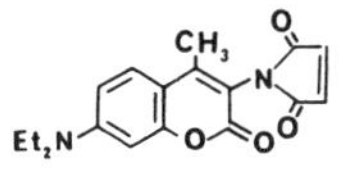 CH_3, O, N, O, Et_2N, O, O	390	24,000	480
7-Diethylamino-4-methyl-3-p(isothio-cyanatophenyl)-C	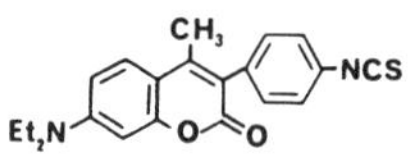 CH_3, NCS, Et_2N, O, O	383	29,000	416
7-Diethylamino-3-benzothiazole-sulfonylchloride-C	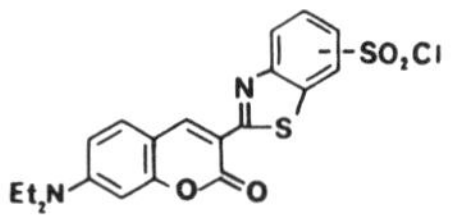 SO_2Cl, N, S, Et_2N, O, O	442		510
7-amino-4-methyl-3-acetic acid-C (AMCA)		355		450

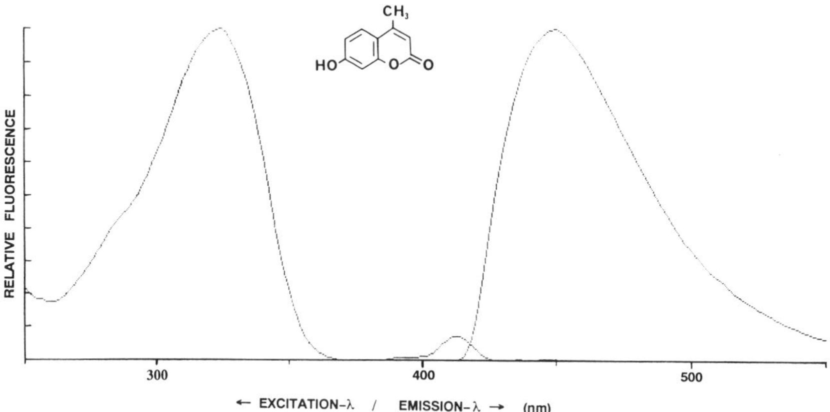

Fig. 7.12. Fluorescence spectra of 4-methyl-umbelliferone in buffer.

however, has been utilized as an additional signal in double/triple label IF and in respective cytometric applications. Especially amino, 7-diethyl- and dimethylamino derivatives (AMCA, DAMC) (Table 7.6) have been used as blue emitting staining reagents (662–664). For example, Staines at al. (665) used DAMC, coupled to avidin, as the third fluorochrome in a three-color IF with fluorescein and rhodamines as the longer λ emitters. Lambda Probes Inc. has developed a long λ emitting labeling reagent by replacing the coumarine structure with a benzothiazole group at position 3 (666).

The relatively large Stokes' shift of coumarine derivatives is exploited in Sep-FIAs and IFMAs when using polymeric labels coupled to antigens, or when using high labeling ratios in antibody labelings, thus avoiding the inner-filter problem encountered with, for example, fluorescein. Exley and Ekeke developed Sep-FIAs for steroids by using steroid tracers coupled to polylysine and labeled with up to 25 4-MU-3-acetic acid groups (667–669), or alternatively antibodies labeled by about 16 umbelliferone derivatives per IgG (667, 670). An umbelliferone-labeled polymer was used as a tracer in FIA by Chuang (671), but he dissociated the bound fluorochromes by periodate oxidation prior to the fluorometric determination.

Due to its properties as an environmentally sensitive probe, umbelliferone has gained wider application in homogeneous FIAs than in heterogeneous assays (except ELFIA). Li et al. (672) used the 3-carboxyamido derivative of umbelliferone by coupling it to theophylline, and they used the conjugate as a tracer for FPIA. Grossman tested 4-MU, among the other fluorochromes, in FPIA of CK-BB, but without success (617). Umbelliferones, and 3-substituted umbelliferones, form the basis of almost all published substrate-labeled FIAs (SL-FIA) (Chapter 8.3.2), in which either an ester bond, formed with a 7-hydroxy group, or the respective glycoside bond is utilized as the enzymatically releasable quenching linkage. Haptenic antigens are coupled to the fluorogenic substrate either via the same ester bond (673) or through 3-acetic acid (674).

7.3.5. Fluorogenic Amino Reagents

Fluorescamine, MDPF, and NBD-Cl (Fig. 7.13) are reagents which have been developed for the fluorogenic determination of primary amines, such as proteins, peptides, or amino acids, for example, after chromatographic fractionation. These have also been utilized in some fluorescence immunoassays. The fluorescent properties of the conjugates prepared with the reagents are presented in Table 7.7, and the fluorescence spectra of an NBD-Cl-labeled protein are shown in Figure 7.14.

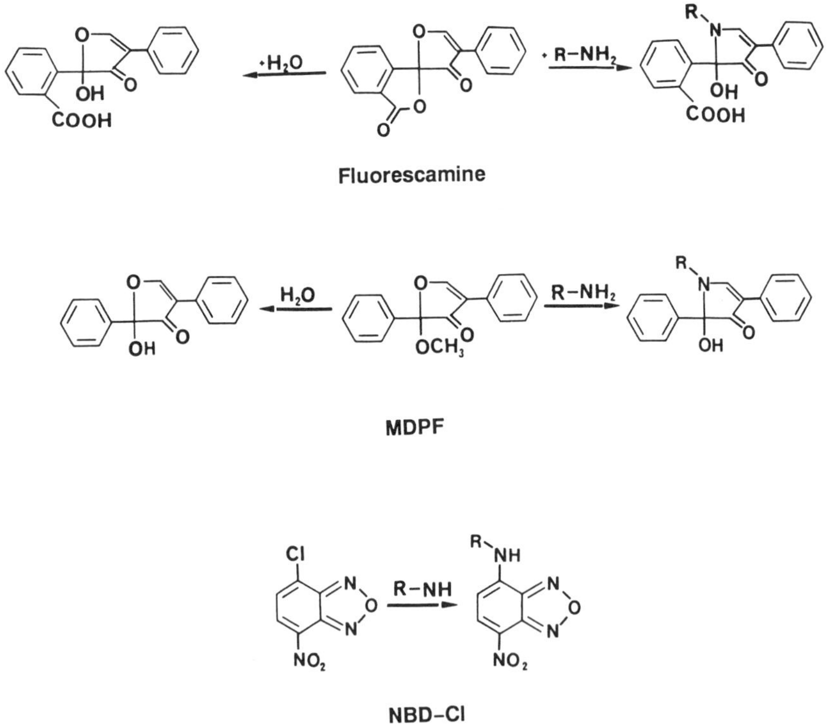

Fig. 7.13. Reactions of aminoreactive fluorogenic reagents fluorescamine, MDPF, and NBD-Cl.

Table 7.7. Fluorogenic Amino Reagents

Compound	Exc. max (nm)	ε (L/M cm)	Em. max (nm)	Q	τ (ns)
Fluorescamine	395	6,300	480	0.1	7
MDPF	290, 390	6,400	480	0.1	
NBD	470	12,900	550		

Fluorescamine and MDPF have also been studied in view of their possible applicability as labeling reagents for proteins and antibodies (675–677). Weigele et al. (675) supposed MDPF to be a superior labeling reagent for IgG for use in IF. Furthermore, Egwu and Kumar compared MDPF with FITC (678) and obtained a lower intensity, more rapid fading, and higher nonspecific binding with MDPF than with the respective fluorescein-labeled antibodies. Cukor et al. (679) tested MDPF as a label for antibodies in an allergic response test (specific IgE) and compared the results obtained with those of ^{125}I-labeled antibodies (RAST). However, tests with MDPF-labeled antibodies failed to give any acceptable results. Katsh et al. used fluorescamine as an amino reactive reagent in a chromatographic separation-based FIA applied for small amine-containing antigens (680).

Fluorescamine and MDPF have also been tested in various homogeneous assay principles. Miller et al. used a fluorescamine-labeled drug derivative as an energy donor for fluorescein-labeled antibodies in a FETI of nortriptyline (681). Fluorescamine and MDPF-labeled thyroxine have been tested in the fluorescence enhancement immunoassay of T_4 (682). Thakrar and

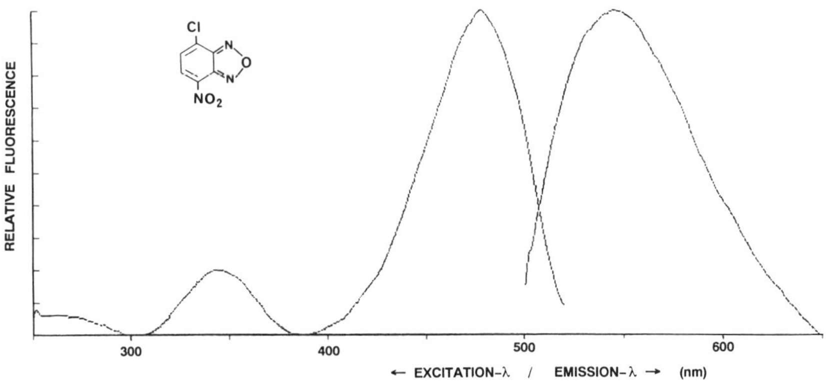

Fig. 7.14. Fluorescence spectra of NBD-Cl–labeled IgG.

Miller (683) compared fluorescein, fluorescamine, and quinacrine as energy donors (conjugated to albumin) for eosin-labeled anti-albumin antibodies. However, in their test fluorescamine gave the least sensitive assay.

NBD-chloride is primarily used for the detection of free amines (684), and seldomly in immunoassays. NBD-labeled estrogen and progesterone are tested as tracers for breast cancer in *in vitro* receptor assays (685).

These compounds share the benefits of many of the above described alternative labels in respect to the long Stokes' shift (nearly 100 nm) and thus avoid inner-filter quenching. The small size and relatively hydrophilic nature allow antibodies to be labeled with up to 20 fluors/IgG (677). The short emission near 500 nm, however, makes them more vulnerable to serum background interferences (682), which may have restricted their applicability in FIAs.

7.3.6. Miscellaneous Organic Simple Fluorochromes

In addition to the fluorochromes described above, numerous other simple organic fluorescent compounds have been tested and even used in immunological applications. For example, the following aromatic structures are extracted from the available literature describing the use of fluorescence in immunoassays—structures such as derivatives of aminonaphthalimine, stilbene, quinacrine, flavin, fluoranthyl, and squaric acid. Some examples of the derivatives used are shown in Figure 7.15, and their fluorescence properties are summarized in Table 7.8.

Lucifer Yellow, a derivative of disulfonaphthalimine, is available from many commercial sources as a free reagent, activated intermediate for protein labeling (e.g., as vinylsulfone, VS) and also as ready labeled proteins (antibodies, protein A, and avidins). The advantages of Lucifer Yellow over fluorescein relate to its longer Stokes' shift (Fig. 7.16), the hydrophilicity achieved with sulfonyl groups, and the stable fluorescence level unaffected by pH or coupling. Like most of the new fluorochromes, Lucifer Yellow found its very first immunological application as a fluorescent staining reagent in IF and flow cytometry; quantitative FIA applications are more limited so far. Bailey et al. (686) used Lucifer Yellow VS for labeling albumin for Sep-FIA. Kirk and Miller published the synthesis of Lucifer-Yellow-conjugated progesterone for use in FIA (687). Lucifer-Yellow-labeled testosterone and estriol have also been tested in the FPIA of those steroids (688), and labeled albumin has been tested as an energy donor for rhodamine-B-labeled anti-albumin antibody in the FETI assay of human albumin (689). The relatively long Stokes' shift of Lucifer Yellow can alleviate the problems caused by the direct excitation of the energy accepting fluorochrome in FETI assays.

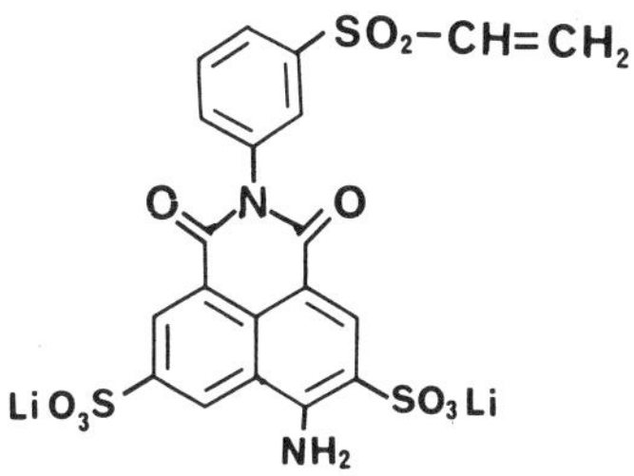

Lucifer Yellow VS

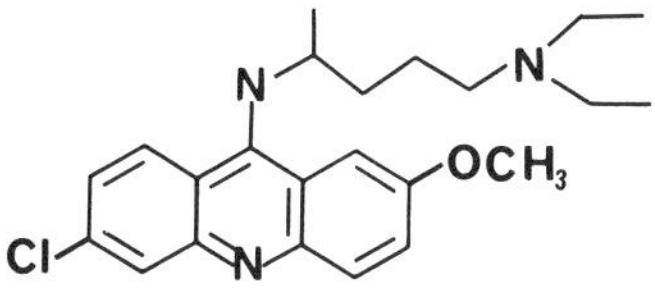

Quinacridine

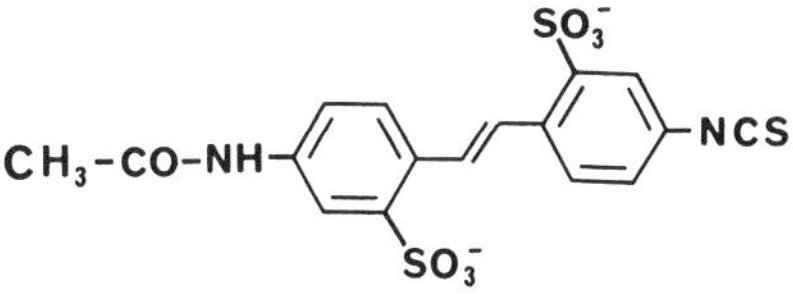

SITC

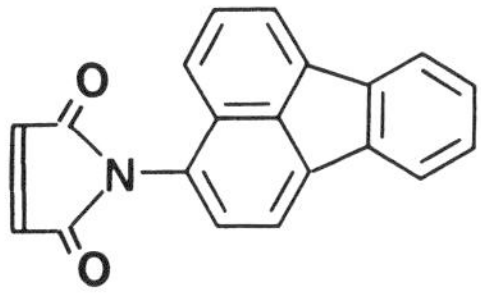

Fluoranthylmaleimide

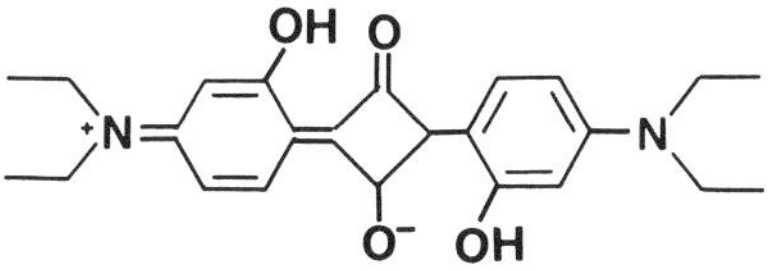

Squaric acid deriv.

Fig. 7.15. Structures of miscellaneous fluorescent probes.

4-Acetamido-4′-isothiocyanatostilbene-2,2′-disulfonic acid (SITS) (Fig. 7.15) is a fluorescent compound commonly used as an anion transport inhibitor. It has also been tested as a fluorescent marker for antibodies (611, 690). However, due to its blue emission at 430 nm, SITC was judged inferior when compared to fluorescein. On the other hand, the blue emission of SITS (as also some of the other above described fluorochromes) has found applications in two- and three-color stainings (691).

Fluoranthenyl maleimide (FAM) is an SH-reacting probe primarily utilized in the study of enzymes (591). As a medium-long lifetime fluorochrome it could find some use in FPIAs of large antigens. Parini et al. (692) synthesized some new fluorescent derivatives of progesterone, including the conjugate with FAM, and the authors pointed out their usefulness as tracers for FIAs.

Table 7.8. Miscellaneous Fluorescent Compounds

Compound	Exc. max (nm)	ε (L/M cm)	Em. max (nm)	Q	τ (ns)
Lucifer Yellow	430	13,000	540	0.2	3.3
SITS	320–350	40,000	430		1.3
Fluoranthenyl maleimide (FAM)	365	3,000	465	0.6	29
Quinacrine	420	9,000	490–505	0.1–0.4	4–13
Flavin	445		525		
Squaric acid[a]	636	366,000	653	1.0	
Indocyanine green	780	180,000	820		
Indocarbocyanine	555	130,000	568	0.03	
Indodicarbocyanine	548	215,000	670	0.06–0.13	
Indotricarbocyanine	750	200,000	780		

[a]Squaric acid derivative of reference 696, Figure 7.15.

Acridinium derivatives have provoked intensive research as luminogenic labels for chemiluminescence immunoassays because of their sensitive detection made possible by lower background than the respective luminol detection. LIA principles based on acridinium esters are commercialized and widely used, but acridinium derivatives have also been used as fluorogenic labels. Chen studied an acridinium derivative as a fluorogenic reagent for proteins (693), and Shibnev et al. as a reagent for peptides (694). Furthermore, it has been tested in the search for alternative fluorescent probes for antibodies (611). Thakrar and Miller (683) tested quinacrine mustard as an

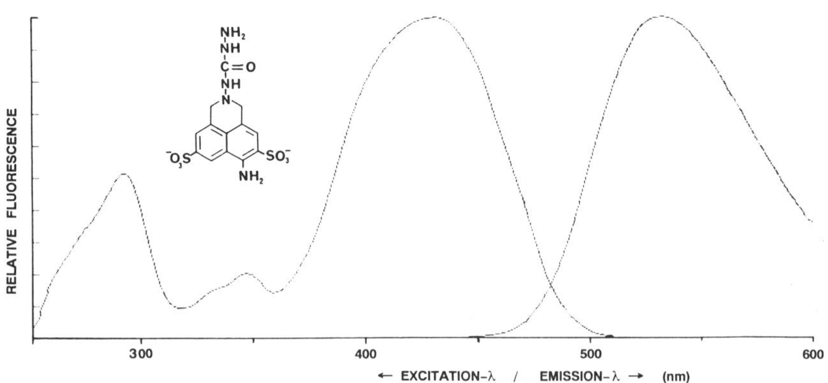

Fig. 7.16. Fluorescence spectra of Lucifer Yellow.

energy donor for eosin-labeled antibodies in the FETI of albumin. In the tested system, quinacrine gave results equal to those obtained with fluorescein.

From the natural coenzymes, NAD(P)H has been utilized both as a colorimetric and fluorometric substrate for detecting enzyme catalyzed reactions. It is also used as a fluorogenic substrate in ELFIAs. FMN-AMP coupled to theophylline is used in SL-FIA based on the use of nucleotide pyrophosphatase as a releasing enzyme (695). The distance between FMN and AMP in the substrate is small enough to produce an efficient quenching of FMN fluorescence.

Squaric acids and their derivatives form a scarcely studied group of fluorescent compounds which might have potential for probes in FIAs. Some of the derivatives synthesized by the Syva Co. (696) reportedly exhibit exceptionally high relative fluorescence intensities at long emission λ, a quantum yield approaching unity, and a high molar absorptivity (product $\varepsilon \times Q$ about 300,000), but a very short Stokes' shift (Table 7.8). Aniline squarate is tested in assays of digoxin, employing the FETI principle with antibodies labeled with a quencher, gallocyanine, and the Sep-FIA principle based on magnetic particles, in which the particle bound fraction of labeled digoxin is measured after detergent dissociation (696). The excitation of the tracers was performed with a He-Ne laser (633 nm).

Fluorophores producing long λ (or even at IR range) emission have attained interest for two reasons: the availability of inexpensive, reliable, and compact diode lasers well suited for their excitation and their fluorometric detection would be free of background problems. Rhodamine 800, thionine (em. 623 nm), methylene blue (em. 683 nm), nile blue (em. 672 nm), oxazine (em. 691 nm) (424), and indocyanine green (em. 820 nm) (422) are fluorescent probes available as such but not as activated reagents for conjugating with proteins. Different indocyanine dyes have also been coupled to antibodies and tested in IF and flow cytometry (697). Sauda et al. (698) used indocyanine green as a fluorescent probe for albumin determination in a system where albumin enhanced its fluorescence by binding it and hence avoiding the dimerization of the probe. The same group also developed an ELFIA employing the sensitivity of indocyanine green fluorescence to the quenching of H_2O_2. It remains to be seen whether these new structures will lead to the development of further applications in the field of quantitative immunoassays.

7.3.7. Porphyrins

Porphyrins are substituted tetrapyrrole structures in which pyrroles are coupled together with methylene bridges, forming cyclic conjugated structures with chelating inner cavities. They are found in a number of biological and synthetic pigments, such as hemin and hemin proteins (hemoglobin, myoglobin, cytochrome), chlorophylls, etc. The structure is very similar to that of open chain tetrapyrrole-bilins—which forms the light harvesting structures of phycobiliproteins—also utilized as fluorescent probes for immunoassays (Chapter 7.3.8).

Porphyrins exhibit strong fluorescence, optimally detectable in dilute hydrochloric acid (699). This fluorescence is very sensitive to impurities, and transition metal ions, for instance, can change it if chelated with the porphyrin. The photoluminescence properties of metallo-porphyrins greatly depend on the chelated ion, which may quench the fluorescence, enhance it, or create phosphorescent complexes. Generally, closed shell metal ions stabilize fluorescence and transition metal complexes stabilize triplet levels. For example, the ions Zn^{2+}, Cu^{2+}, Pd^{2+}, and Pt can produce phosphorescent metallo-porphyrins detectable at low temperatures, but Pd and Pt can exhibit phosphorescence even at room temperature in suitable solvents or even in an aqueous micellar solution (700, 701).

The salient feature of porphyrins is their typical strong absorption and excitation at relatively low λ, around 400 nm. This absorption, which derives from the electronic transition directly to a higher excited singlet level, generally called Soret band absorption, predominates with most porphyrins having a molar absorptivity around 100,000–300,000 (701) (Table 7.9). The strong absorption at the Soret band gives rise to a long Stokes' shift, the feature which makes porphyrins interesting alternatives for FIA.

Another feature, which has elicited interest, is the phosphorescence of metallo-porphyrins. Figure 7.17 shows the phosphorescence spectra of Pt and Pd coproporphyrines, recorded from a chemically deoxygenated micellar solution. They can even produce "Soret-phosphorescence" (i.e., emission emanating directly from a higher excited level) even though at a lower quantum yield than the respective emission from the lowest excited triplet level (332). The extreme sensitivity of phosphorescence to dissolved oxygen in aqueous solutions is used in the measurement of O_2 levels from biological systems with the use of Pd-coproporphyrin as a label (702). The relatively large size of the aromatic structure of the porphyrins renders them scarcely soluble and hydrophobic. The addition of negatively charged sulfonyl or carboxyl groups makes porphyrin structures more hydrophilic (703, 704), a feature which is of considerable significance for immunoassays.

The potential of porphyrins, with their high absorptivity, long Stokes' shift, and long λ emission, has been widely recognized and has resulted in a number of patents. Bio-Diagnostic Inc. has (705) patented a general procedure of using porphyrins as labels, including chlorophylls and porphins, and Hoffman La Roche (703) has patented the use of tetrakis-(4-carboxyphenyl)-porphin as a label for IFMA, exemplified by an assay of CEA. In addition, Savitsky et al. (706) have patented the procedure of using porphyrin-

Table 7.9. Luminescent Properties of Some Porphyrins

Porphyrin	Exc. max. (nm)	ε (L/M cm)	Em. max. (nm)	Q	τ (ns)
Coproporphyrin I	396	120,000	620	0.05–0.1	1.7
Coproporphyrin III	402		623	0.05	6
Pd-Coproporphyrin III	396	200,000	668_{Ph}	0.17	1,000,000
Hematoporphyrin IX	402		619	0.1	0.2
Protoporphyrin IX	410		633	0.07	1
Zn-Protoporphyrin IX	420		589		
Etioporphyrin I	400		625	0.09	
Pd-Etioporphyrin I	390		668_{Ph}		2,000,000
Pt-Etioporphyrin I	390		641_{Ph}		
Tetrakis-(4-carboxy-phenyl)-porphin	415		670		
Zn-Tetrakis-(4-carboxy-phenyl)-porphin	427	161,500	625 $792,804_{Ph}$	0.35 0.01	6 >5,000,000
Chlorophyll a	430		665		2–6
Chlorophyll b	453		650		

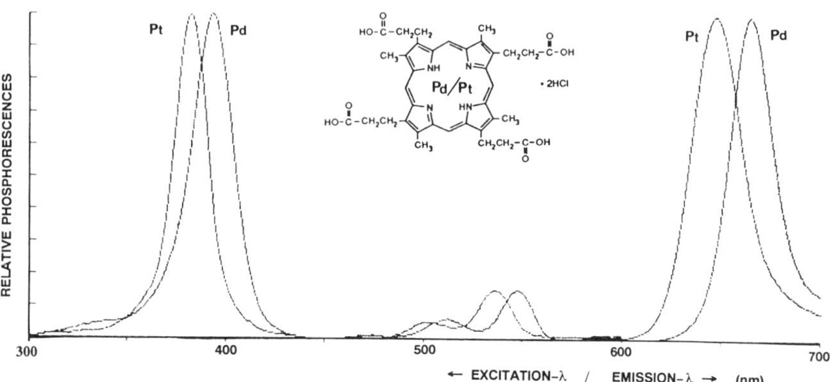

Fig. 7.17. Phosphorescence spectra of palladium and platinum coproporphyrins.

labeled immunoreagents on solid-phase FIAs by redissolving the tracer after the immunoreactions have taken place with the use of a detergent, a principle which in fact has been applied by the same authors with small modifications to phosphoroimmunoassay (see below). The high absorptivity and long Stokes' shift of, for instance, aluminum phthalocyanines are also recognized in the development of fluorochromes for flow cytometry (707, 708). Porphyrin derivatives have also been patented for use in chemiluminescent assays by the Fisher Scientific Co. (709), including the use of hemoglobin, cytochrome, catalase, myoglobin, or metallo-porphyrins. Becton Dickinson Inc. has patented the use of peridinin, a chlorophyll protein purified from dinoflagellates, as a fluorescent label for FIAs (710).

In spite of the numerous patents mentioned above, the number of actual applications of porphyrins in FIAs is so far limited. Hendrix has reviewed the properties of porphyrins which could have properties suitable for FIA (711), including coproporphyrin-III, hematoporphyrin-IX, protoporphyrin-IX, uroporphyrin-I, chlorophyll a, and chlorophyll b. Papkovsky et al. have tested the conditions for labeling monoclonal antibodies with coproporphyrin-I and also optimized the conditions for its fluorometric determination (712). Coproporphyrin-I–labeled RIgG was used as a tracer in Sep-FIA (713), and coproporphyrin-labeled antibodies in an assay of influenza-A virus antigen (714). Coproporphyrin-III–labeled anti-thyroxine was used as a tracer for the Sep-FIA of T_4 (715) and labeled digoxin in the Sep-FIA of digoxin (716).

Recently, the RTP obtained from metallo-porphyrins was utilized in a phosphoroimmunoassay (PIA) of anti-insulin antibodies (717). Pt-coproporphyrin, used as a phosphorescent label, produces strong phosphorescence in optimized conditions, having the product $\varepsilon \times Q$ of 34,000—considerably higher than obtained with, for example, erythrosin (≈80), the probe used in the majority of PIAs. The metallo-porphyrin-labeled antibodies were determined after dissociation of the label from solid-phases with a detergent and deoxygenation with the addition of sodium bisulfite.

An interesting *in vivo* application area of porphyrin-labeled antibodies is their usage as photoimmunotoxins in tumor therapy. Antibody conjugated porphyrin can function as a targeted *in vivo* cytotoxic reagent, which upon near IR irradiation (650 or 850 nm) produces singlet oxygen, which selectively destroys tumor cells (718, 719).

7.3.8. Phycobiliproteins

Phycobiliproteins are light harvesting proteins in the photosynthetic system of many species of algae (720, 721). They have an oligomeric protein structure formed from $\alpha\beta$-subunits, containing multiple bilin prosthetic groups (open chain tetrapyrrole structure). The bilins are well isolated from the external environment by virtue of the surrounding polypeptides. In the native environment phycobiliproteins are present in aggregates, called phycobilisomes, that lie near the chlorophyll centers and efficiently transfer the energy they absorb to photosynthesis. As large proteins which contain up to 30 bilin groups per protein, phycobiliproteins could be regarded as natural polymeric labels, but without the self-quenching problem encountered with artificially made polyfluorochrome clusters. The potential of the unique fluorescence of phycobiliproteins in immunology was realized in 1983 by Oi et al. (722), and since then those proteins have been utilized especially in flow-cytometric and IF applications, and an increasing number of quantitative FIA applications have also emerged (723, 724). Patents have been issued on the use of phycobiliproteins in immunoassays (391, 725).

The three main classes of phycobiliproteins—phycoerythrin (PE), phycocyanin (PC), and allophycocyanin (A-PC)—differ from each other primarily with respect to protein structure and pigment content (Table 7.10). The proteins are relatively stable and highly soluble. The bilin groups create high absorptivity, up to 2.4×10^6 with PE. Still, the phycobiliproteins can have a fluorescence quantum yield as high as 0.98 (722, 726). Accordingly, the relative fluorescence, the product $\varepsilon \times Q$ (up to 2,300,000) is higher than with any single fluorochrome and is even high compared to polymeric labels. The fluorescence of one B-phycoerythrin (B-PE) equals the fluorescence of about 30 fluoresceins or 100 rhodamines. Because of the high fluorescence efficiency of phycobiliproteins, the majority of the attempts to achieve single molecule detection have been made with B-PE (338, 339).

Table 7.10. Properties of Phycobiliproteins

Protein[a]	Molecular weight	Exc. max (nm)	ε (L/M cm)	Em. max (nm)	Q	τ (ns)
B-PE[a]	240,000	545	2,410,000	575	0.59–0.98	3
R-PE	240,000	565	1,960,000	578	0.82	
C-PC	72,000	620	580,000	650	0.51	2
	226,000		1,690,000			
A-PC	104,000	650	700,000	634	0.7	3
R-PC	103,000	618	760,000	634	0.7	2
B-PE/A-PC		545	2,410,000	660		

[a]Abbreviations used: B-PE = B-phycoerythrin; R-PE = R-phycoerythrin; C-PC = C-phycocyanin; A-PC = allophycocyanin; R-PC = R-phycocyanin; and B-PE/A-PC = tandem conjugate of B-PE and A-PC.

All phycobiliproteins emit at long λ, between 560 and 670 nm, but have short Stokes' shifts (Figs. 7.18, 7.19, and 7.20). Conjugates emitting with longer Stokes' shifts are produced by coupling two phycobiliproteins, B-PE and A-PC, together to form a tandem probe. In the tandem conjugate, B-PE absorbs the excitation efficiently at 545 nm and transfers the excited energy with 90% efficiency to A-PC, which emits at 660 nm (727). A respective tandem probe has been constructed also from B-PE and Texas Red and is marketed as DuoCHROME-labeled reagents by Becton Dickinson.

Because the emitting bilins are well protected inside the protein structure, the fluorescence is insensitive to changes in pH and collisional deactivations. Also, the photostability of B-PE is reportedly better than that of fluorescein (338, 728).

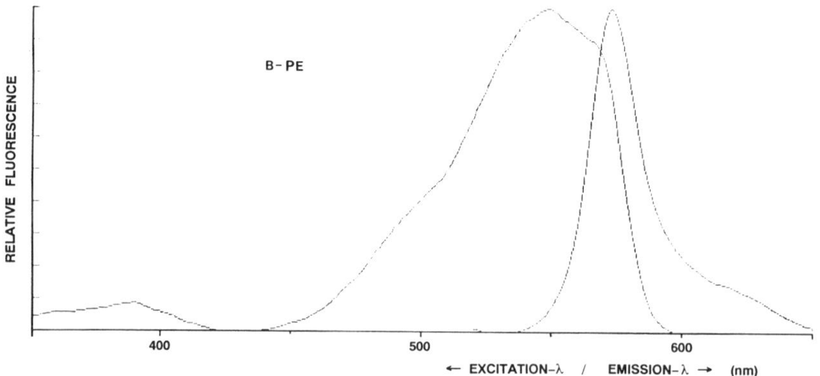

Fig. 7.18. Fluorescence spectra of B-phycoerythrin.

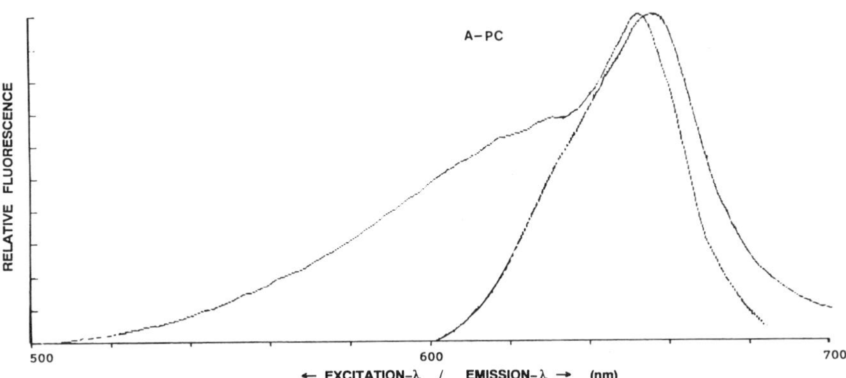

Fig. 7.19. Fluorescence spectra of allophycocyanin.

The drawbacks encountered with phycobiliproteins relate to their biological nature as proteins. Their coupling to immunoreagents, performed generally with heterobifunctional cross-linking reagents (723), is more laborious than with simple fluorochromes and involves elaborate purification and fractionation steps. Recently, however, already activated, SH-reactive derivatives of phycobiliproteins have become commercially available. Dissociation of some of the phycobiliproteins (e.g., A-PC) into subunits with concomitant loss of the fluorescence in diluted conditions may be overcome by chemically cross-linking the subunits (729). A cross-linked A-PC is also commercially available from Molecular Probes Inc.

In the original work of Oi et al. (722) the large size of the proteins was not noticed to cause problems in labeling, but later on steric hindrances have

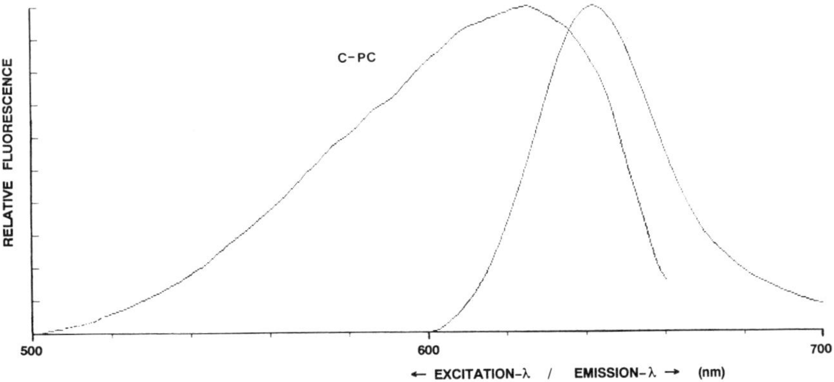

Fig. 7.20. Fluorescence spectra of C-phycocyanin.

been reported (730). In spite of the clear improvement in assay sensitivity achieved when using B-PE instead of fluorescein, the whole expected potential sensitivity improvement has not been achieved in actual FIAs (723), which might reflect the effect of the large size of the label to the assay performance.

The primary, routine, application field of phycoerythrins is in IF and flow cytometry, and several reagent companies have included phycobiliprotein-labeled staining reagents in their assortments. Shapiro used a low-power He-Ne laser for excitation of A-PC–labeled antibodies in IF performed with a flow cytometer (731). An example of a multilabel flow-cytometric application is the four-color staining of B-cell subpopulations, using B-PE and A-PC in addition to fluorescein and Texas Red by Hardy et al. (732), who used an argon-ion laser (488 nm) for excitation of fluorescein and B-PE (respective emissions at 520 and 570 nm), and a dye laser (615 nm) for excitation of Texas Red and A-PC (respective emissions at 620 and 645 nm).

As highly fluorescent compounds, phycobiliproteins are naturally considered potential probes for quantitative FIAs, although actual applications have emerged more slowly. Kronick and Grossman (730) used a B-PE–labeled antibody in an IFMA with microbeads as solid-phases in the detection of human IgG. They obtained a six-fold sensitivity enhancement compared to a respective assay with a fluorescein-labeled antibody. They also reported the problem encountered with the large size of the probe. The same authors have tested B-PE–labeled antibodies as energy acceptors for fluorescein-labeled antigens in a FETI assay of hIgG. Because of its high absorptivity, B-PE is particularly suitable as an energy acceptor to the emission of fluorescein (733), and it has been used, for example, in the assay of digoxin (376). B-PE also has been tested as an energy donor for Texas-Red–labeled antibodies in a sensor-based FETI of phenytoin (71).

In a "particle-concentration-fluorescence immunoassay" (PC-FIA) of Pandex, B-PE is frequently employed as a more efficient fluorescent probe than fluorescein. Using B-PE Francis et al. (734) achieved a four-fold sensitivity enhancement in an IFMA of hIgG. Woods et al. (735) have used B-PE–labeled drugs for controlling drug abuse in racing horses, and Prange et al. (736) have used them for testing for opiates in human urine with a PC-FIA system.

Flow cytometry provides a tool for making quantitative double—or triple—label assays, employing microbeads as solid surfaces. Houghton et al. (533) used both fluorescein and B-PE as labels for simultaneous IFMAs of human IgG and IgM. B-PE–labeled streptavidin was used in a single-label simultaneous assay of two antibodies (65) and in a flow-cytometric FIA of a carcinoembryonic antigen (CEA) (737), in assays based on simultaneous determinations of solid-phase bound fluorescences from two sets of beads differentiated according to their sizes and determined independently from each other.

7.4. ORGANOMETALLIC FLUOROCHROMES

Metallic elements possess many interesting and useful properties which could be exploited in immunological techniques. Those properties became available after the development of appropriate labeling techniques for the covalent coupling of those ions to immunoreagents via stable, bifunctional chelating agents (738). Among the properties utilized (e.g., with antibodies) is radioactivity. For instance, radioactive ^{57}Co functions as a tracer for double-label RIAs as a counterpart for ^{125}I (739) and as a tracer for the B-12 vitamin. α- and β-emitting radionuclides are used as tumor specific *in vivo* radiopharmaceuticals after coupling to anti-tumor antibodies (740, 741). The γ emitters (e.g., ^{111}In and ^{99}Tc) are used as targeted, tumor localization tracers in radioimaging studies and as positron emitters in positron-emission tomography (742–744). Paramagnetic metal ions, especially Gd^{3+}, are routinely applied as contrast-enhancing agents in magnetic-resonance imaging (MRI) (745), and attempts have been made to use them also as tumor targeted image-enhancing reagents (746–748). In addition to the radioactivity, various other properties of metals, such as their chemiluminescence, electroluminescence, phosphorescence, atomic and molecular fluorescence, redox potential, and atomic absorption, are applied for *in vitro* immunoassays (310, 749, 750), and even the term *metalloimmunoassay* has been introduced for an assay based on an antigen labeled with a metal, such as Cr, Ir, Hg, Cu, Pd, Co, Mn, Pt, or Au (310, 751) (Chapter 4.2.4).

Metallic elements, and the complex compounds they form with organic chelating ligands, create a new category of fluorescent probes gaining an increasing number of applications in the immunoassay field. The type of luminescence produced by the chelates depends on the relative position of the excited resonance level of the cation compared to the triplet level of the ligand. Accordingly, the chelates can show either fluorescence, phosphorescence, delayed fluorescence, energy-transfer fluorescence, or charge-transfer fluorescence (Chapter 5.1.4) (752). The use of some metallo-porphyrins as labels in FIAs and PIAs has already been discussed. Other metals of interest are the transition metals Co, Cr, Os, Ir, and Ru, and the lanthanides Eu, Sm, Tb, Dy, and Nd. The reason for the interest those ions—and their chelates—have inspired relates to their exceptional fluorescence properties and especially their unusual fluorescence lifetimes, utilized in time-resolved techniques.

A common problem with the use of metallic ions as labels for *in vitro,* and especially for *in vivo,* assays is their binding to the immunoreagents with a required stability. The stability requirement depends on the cation used and the kinetic stability of its chelates. For example, Ru forms kinetically extremely stable chelates even with considerably simple nitrogen-containing heterocyclic compounds (753), whereas some cations, such as Cu^{2+}, require the most stable macrocyclic complexones before they can be used in *in vivo* imaging studies (743, 754). For *in vitro* assays the stability of the chelates can be stipulated according to the specific requirement of the technology. In any assay the labeled reagents need to be stable for the time required and under the conditions used for the immunoassay.

7.4.1. Lanthanide Chelates

Some lanthanide ions, such as Eu^{3+}, Sm^{3+}, Tb^{3+}, and to a lesser extent Dy^{3+} and Nd^{3+}, exhibit typical fluorescence characterized by the ion, especially when chelated to suitable excitation energy mediating ligands. The fluorescent properties—long Stokes' shift, narrow band-type emission lines, and unusually long fluorescence lifetimes—have made them attractive candidates for FIAs and especially for time-resolved fluorometric techniques, where they actually are gaining rapidly expanding usage.

Lanthanides comprise a $4f^n$ electronic configuration, where the orbitals are largely shielded from the environment and are minimally involved in bonding. The total spreading of λ_{em} by the ligand field splitting is rarely more than a few hundred cm^{-1}, and hence the emission lines are relatively sharp, even in an aqueous solution at room temperature. However, the transitions within the $4f^n$-configuration are electrically dipole forbidden, resulting in a very weak absorption (ε less than 10). Therefore, excitation light absorbing and energy donating ligands are necessary. In the lanthanide series, the relative fluorescence of a particular ion depends on the energy gap between the lowest excited level and the highest ground state manifold level (with the exception of Gd^{3+}, which due to its exceptionally high excited level is efficiently quenched in solutions). (Figure 7.21 shows the main energy levels taking part to absorptions and emissions.) A large energy gap is needed to omit nonradiative processes, because in that case a large quantum of energy would be needed for a nonradiative energy dissipation (755).

The fluorescence decay times of lanthanides primarily depend on the natural lifetime of the lowest excited level, in addition to the competing deactivation processes (756). The major transitions found with those lanthanide ions (in solutions as chelates) and the respective emission lines are shown in Table 7.11.

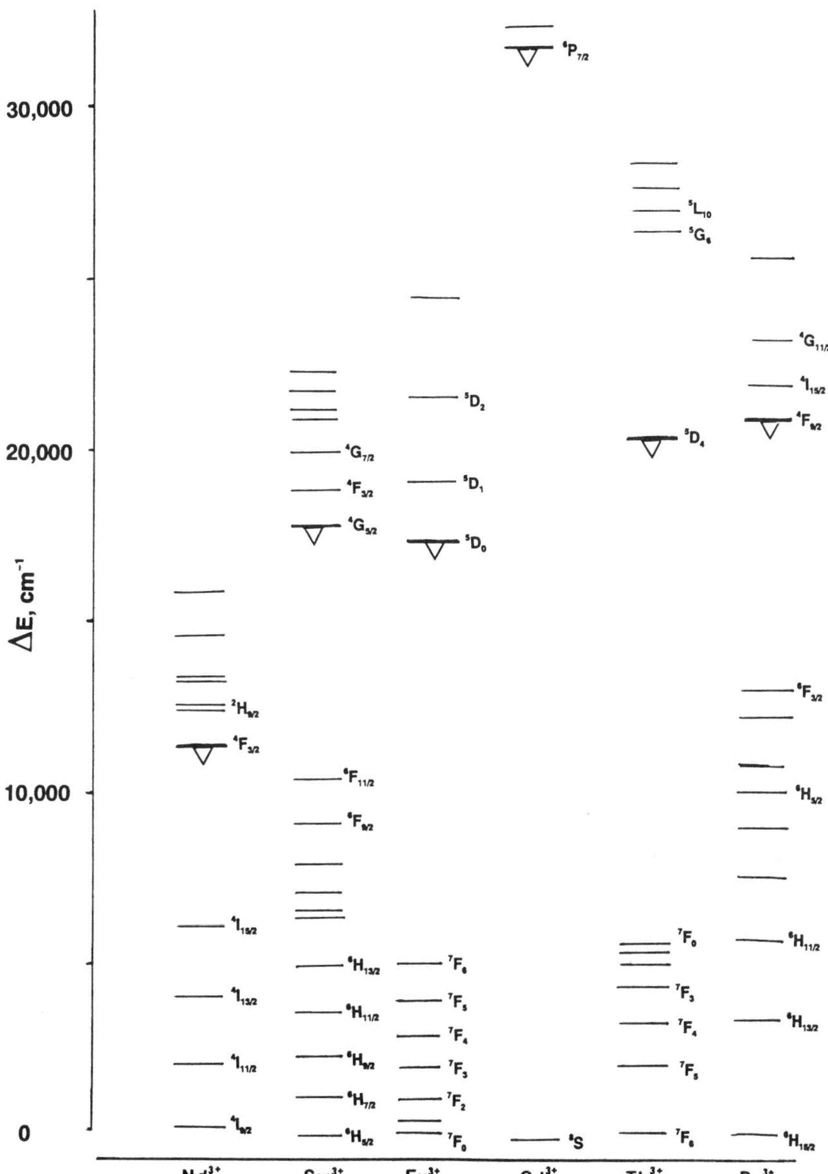

Fig. 7.21. Energy levels of fluorescent tervalent lanthanide ions.

Table 7.11. Emission Lines of Eu^{3+}, Tb^{3+}, Sm^{3+}, and Dy^{3+}

Cation	Transition			Emission
Eu^{3+}	$^5D_0$	→	$^7F_0$	580 nm
			$^7F_1$	590 nm
			$^7F_2$	**613 nm**
			$^7F_3$	650 nm
			$^7F_4$	690 nm
			$^7F_5$	710 nm
Tb^{3+}	$^5D_4$	→	$^7F_6$	490 nm
			$^7F_5$	**545 nm**
			$^7F_4$	590 nm
			$^7F_3$	620 nm
			$^7F_2$	650 nm
Sm^{3+}	$^4G_{5/2}$	→	$^6H_{5/2}$	560 nm
			$^6H_{7/2}$	598 nm
			$^6H_{9/2}$	**643 nm**
			$^6H_{11/2}$	710 nm
Dy^{3+}	$^4F_{9/2}$	→	$^6H_{15/2}$	483 nm
			$^6H_{13/2}$	**575 nm**
			$^6H_{11/2}$	660 nm
Nd^{3+}	$^4F_{2/2}$	→	$^4I_{9/2}$	900 nm
			$^4F_{11/2}$	1060 nm
			$^4F_{2/2}$	1350 nm

The emissions are primarily produced from the lowest excited resonance level of the cations ($^5D_0$ with Eu^{3+}, $^5D_4$ with Tb^{3+}, $^4G_{5/2}$ with Sm^{3+}, $^4F_{9/2}$ with Dy^{3+}, and $^4F_{2/2}$ with Nd^{3+}; Fig. 7.21), and only a minor emission emanating directly from the higher excited level of Eu^{3+} can be recorded from chelates in solution. The major emission lines of the highly fluorescent chelates are formed from a transition called hypersensitive transition and are around 613–615 nm with Eu^{3+}, 545 (and 490) nm with Tb^{3+}, 590 and 643 nm with Sm^{3+}, and at 573 nm with Dy^{3+} (Figs. 7.22–7.25).

Weissman was the first to discover, in 1942 (459), that certain rare-earth chelates emit visible light upon irradiation with UV light, an emission which is characterized by the chelated cation. Whan and Crosby (757) interpreted the mechanism to be intramolecular energy transfer taking place through the ligand triplet state. The requirement for an energy-transfer type of chelate

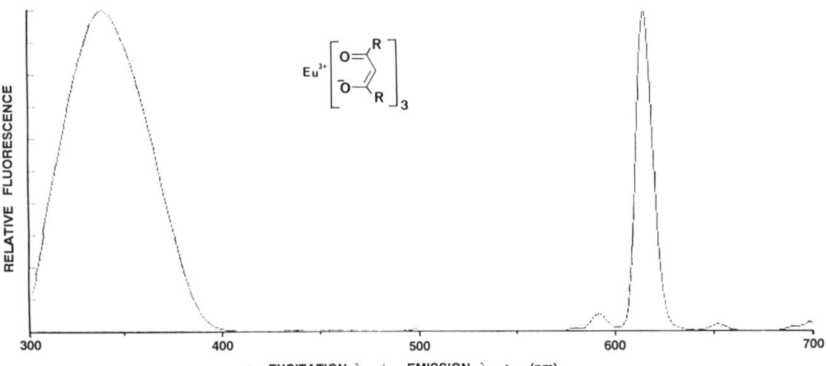

Fig. 7.22. Fluorescence spectra of Eu^{3+} β-diketone (β-NTA) chelate.

fluorescence is that the triplet energy level should be nearly equal but lie above the resonance level of the metal ion in order to facilitate an efficient energy transfer (758).

Lanthanide ions can be classified into three groups according to the fluorescence their chelates produce. Chelates of tervalent ions of La and Gd show molecular fluorescence or phosphorescence, Pr, Nd, Ho, Er, Th, and

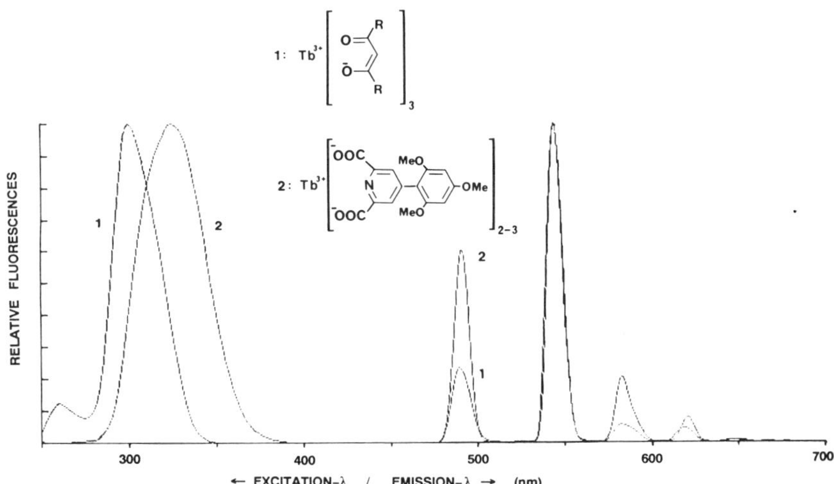

Fig. 7.23. Fluorescence spectra of Tb^{3+} β-diketone (PTA) (1) and trimetoxyphenyl-pyridine-2, 6-dicarboxylic acid (2) chelates.

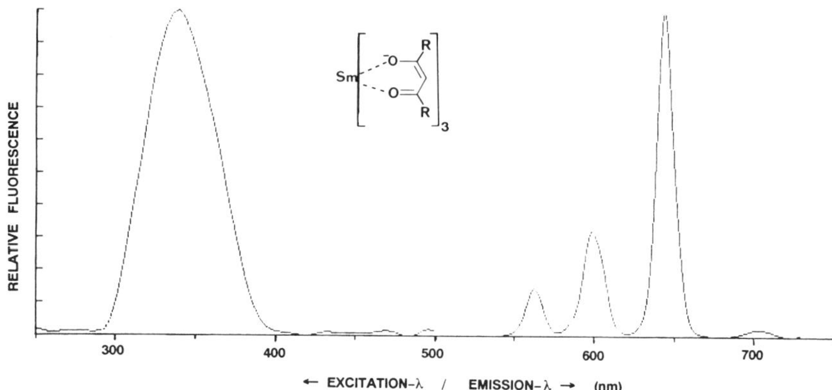

Fig. 7.24. Fluorescence spectra of Sm^{3+} β-diketone (β-NTA) chelate.

Yb form chelates which may possess only weak molecular fluorescence, whereas Eu, Sm, Tb, and Dy can exhibit strong ionic fluorescence when chelated with suitable excitation light absorbing ligands (348). In the last group of ions, energy transfer from the ligand to the chelated ion can be very efficient and may approach 100% (759). Sm^{3+} and Dy^{3+} are less efficient emitters because of the narrow gap in their energy levels between the lowest excited state and highest ground-state vibrational level (Fig. 7.21).

The fluorescence of Eu-chelates is generally quenched in an aqueous solu-

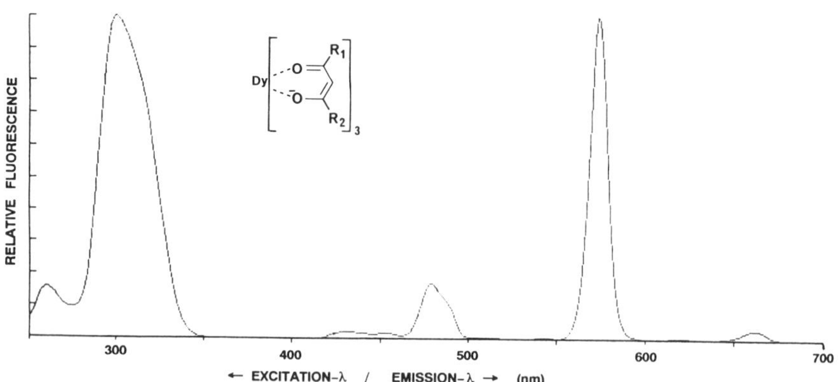

Fig. 7.25. Fluorescence spectra of Dy^{3+} β-diketone (PTA) chelate.

tion. When water molecules are coordinated in the inner sphere of Eu-chelates, the quenching is a result of an efficient, radiationless decay process involving vibronic coupling of Eu $^5D_0$ excited state and OH oscillation. The process is additive in regard to the number of OH oscillators, and hence the fluorescence decay time is inversely related to the number of bound water molecules (760, 761).

In biochemical research, two of the fluorescent lanthanide ions, Eu^{3+} and Tb^{3+}, are applied as Ca^{2+}-antagonistic cations in the study of enzymes and other proteins. The parameters offered by ion fluorescence include the relative fluorescence intensity of the ion, decay time, and energy transfer between the ions and chromophoric groups on proteins or between two bound ions (e.g., from Tb^{3+} to Eu^{3+}). Those parameters can give information about the structure and microenvironment of ion binding sites with various biological compounds and proteins (432, 752, 755, 762–766). Examples of the biological compounds and organelles studied with the use of lanthanide ions are transfer RNA (767), ribosomal RNA (768), DNA and chromatin structure (769), termolysin (770), transferrin (771), calmodulin (using energy transfer between Eu^{3+} and Nd^{3+}) (772), ATP'ase (773), nerve membranes (774), erythrocyte membrane proteins (775), and phospholipids and liposome fusions (776, 777).

In some cases the fluorescence enhancing effect of a biological compound is so high that lanthanides can be used for their fluorometric determination. For example, transferrin can enhance Tb^{3+}-ion fluorescence up to 10^5-fold (771), which forms the basis for fluorometric determination of transferrin with Tb^{3+} as a fluorogenic reagent (778). The value of the technique is diminished, however, by the fact that other proteins can enhance Tb^{3+} fluorescence (779). A therapeutic drug, tetracycline, can specifically enhance Eu^{3+} fluorescence, which forms the basis for the fluorometric determination of tetracyclines with sensitivity at nanomolar concentrations (780). The technique has been evaluated for tetracycline determination in serum samples (781). Wenzel et al. (782) utilized that enhancement in a postcolumn fluorometric detection of tetracyclines in flow-injection analysis.

Fluorescent lanthanide chelates have also been used for fluorometric determinations of the ions from various sources (320, 783), for NMR shift reagents (784), and in searching dyes for lasers (785, 786). Chelating agents are applied for fluorometric determinations of Eu^{3+}, Tb^{3+}, and Sm^{3+} either as such or in combination with polyaminopolycarboxylic acid complexones (mostly EDTA) in the form of mixed-ligand chelates (320, 783). For example, Tb^{3+} has been determined fluorometrically with the use of salicylate or sulfosalicylate (787, 788), with dipicolinic acid (789), and with some aromatic biphenols, such as tiron and dihydroxynaphthalene (790–792), among others.

7.4.2. β-Diketones

β-diketones have achieved the widest applications as fluorescence-enhancing ligands for both Eu^{3+} and Tb^{3+} as well as Sm^{3+} and Dy^{3+}. During the 1960s and 1970s, Eu-β-diketonates were primarily studied for developing fluorescent dyes for lasers (785, 793). Different aromatic β-diketones, especially trifluoro-2,4-butandione derivatives (794) of naphthalene, benzene, furane, and thiophene (Fig. 7.26), are used for fluorometric determinations of Eu^{3+} and Sm^{3+}, primarily after extraction into organic solvents (419, 783, 784, 795–797). Thenoyltrifluoroacetonate chelates of Eu^{3+} have even been used as nonimmunological staining reagents for soil microbes (798–802).

Fluorinated aliphatic β-diketones (Fig. 7.26) can be used for fluorometric determination of Tb^{3+} (346, 803, 804). Because of their higher excited triplet levels, as compared to respective aromatic derivatives, aliphatic β-diketones can be used for simultaneous determination of all four fluorescent lanthanides, Eu^{3+}, Tb^{3+}, Sm^{3+} and Dy^{3+} (347).

For use in immunoassays (aqueous solution), two problems remain to be solved: the solubility of the chelate into water and the avoidance of their quenching caused by water molecules, which tend to fill up the empty coordination sites in the chelates. Ternary chelates composed of one polyaminopolycarboxylic acid and one β-diketone have the solubility required for aqueous applications, and respective chelate structures have also been proposed for FIAs (Chapter 7.4.3). Another system for fluorometric determinations of lanthanides from inorganic samples as well as within immunoassays uses a combination of adduct formation with a synergistic agent and

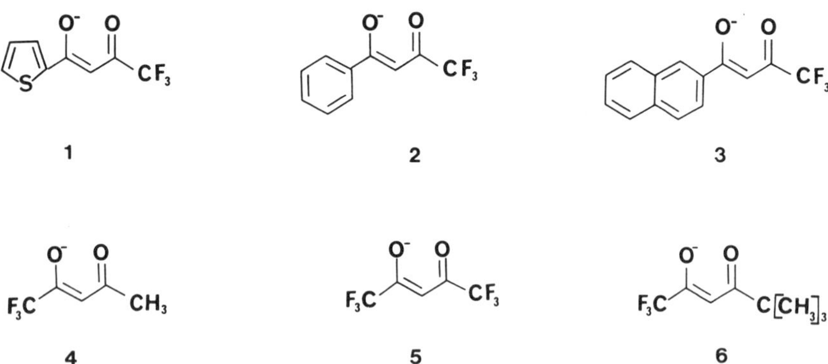

Fig. 7.26. Structures of β-diketones, thenoyltrifluoroacetone (TTA) (1), benzoyltrifluoroacetone (BTA) (2), 2-naphthoyltrifluoroacetone (β-NTA) (3), trifluoroacetylacetone (4), hexafluoroacetylacetone (5) and pivaloyltrifluoroacetone (PTA) (6).

detergent solubilization (346). Various adducts or Lewis bases, such as phosphines, phosphineoxides, or nitrogen heterocycles, have been used to form an "insulating sheet" around the chelates, enhancing the fluorescence by replacing the water molecules in the chelates' inner sphere (805, 806). Brittain has studied the requirement for such adduct formation (807) and has noticed that a strong adduct formation can be accomplished only with highly fluorinated β-diketonato chelates. Solutions developed for fluorometric determinations of lanthanides from aqueous sources (e.g., immunoassays) are comprised of β-diketones, trioctylphosphine oxide as the adduct forming synergistic agent, and a detergent (e.g., Triton X 100) used to form the micelles and to solubilize the chelating components and the formed chelates (346, 797, 803, 808).

The major problem encountered with the development of labeling and detection systems for lanthanides to be used in immunoassays relates to chelate stability and its fluorescence in aqueous conditions. According to the way these problems are solved, published and patented lanthanide chelates utilizing FIAs can be divided into three groups: assays employing a separate fluorescence enhancement step (Chapter 7.4.3), assays using stabilization techniques (Chapter 7.4.4), and assays using *in situ* fluorescent stable chelates (Chapter 7.4.5).

The very first efforts to utilize lanthanide chelates in TR-FIA tried to use the known, fluorescent β-diketone chelates as such as labels. In 1975, Leif et al. suggested the use of Eu-tris β-diketones (hexafluoroacetylacetone, trifluoroacetylacetone, thenoyltrifluoroacetone, or dibenzoylmethane) as fluorescent probes, coupled to antibodies through an adduct forming o-phenanthroline, using its isothiocyanato-derivative as the activated intermediate for conjugation (809, 810). The formed chelates preserved their fluorescences when bound to Sepharose beads, which were used as models for antibodies (811). A similar technique was patented by Wieder and Hidgson in 1977 (812). This patented method is comprised of one β-diketone, which is derivatized in order to couple the tris-β-diketonate chelate onto proteins to form a fluorescent tracer applied in a TR-FIA. He suggested the use of an aminomethyl derivative of thenoyltrifluoroacetone as the linkage forming the β-diketone. Measurement was to take place on dried solid surfaces in order to avoid aqueous quenching (388). An analogous procedure using Nd^{3+} as a near-IR light emitting fluorophore (Table 7.12) has been patented by Kobayashi (426).

An o-phenanthroline derivative containing two β-diketones at positions 2 and 9 was synthesized by Hanson (813). The derivative is a step forward toward more stable and fluorescent chelates. However, none of the systems utilizing β-diketones directly as lanthanide binding reagents have produced any practical applications, simply because the chelates produced do not

Table 7.12. Fluorescent Properties of Lanthanide Chelates

Chelate[a]	Exc. max (nm)	ε (L/M cm)	Em. max (nm)	τ (μs)	Q
Eu ion	393	3	616	110	0.006
Eu-2-NTA$_3$	340	36,000	613	730	0.69
Eu-TTA$_3$	350		613		
Eu-PTA$_3$	295		613	950	
Tb-PTA$_3$	295		545	100	
Tb-EDTA-SSA	300		545		
Tb-TMP-DPA					
Sm-2-NTA$_3$	340	36,000	643	50	0.02
Sm-PTA$_3$	295	31,500	643		
Nd-BTA$_3$	800		900, 1060, 1350		

[a]Abbreviations: 2-NTA = 2-naphthoyltrifluoroacetone; TTA = 2-thenoyltrifluoroacetone; PTA = pivaloyltrifluoroacetone; TMP-DPA = 2′,4′,6′-trimethoxyphenyl-2,6-dipicolinic acid; BTA = benzoyltrifluoroacetone; SSA = sulphosalicylic acid.

fulfill the requirements in regard to stability and aqueous fluorescence. At best the Eu-β-diketones can have chelate formation constants on the order of 10^6, 10^5, and 10^4 (814, 815) for stepwise formation of tris-chelate. For practical applications the lower limit for thermodynamic stability is generally set at 10^{10} (342, 388). In spite of the low formation constant of lanthanide β-diketone chelates, they have rather extensive applications in TR-FIAs, which are based on a separate fluorescence development achieved by a total ligand exchange reaction after the heterogeneous immunoassays have taken place (Chapter 7.4.3).

7.4.3. Fluorescence Enhancement Assays

In fluorescence-enhancement-based FIAs, the chelate used for labeling immunoreagents is totally or partially different from those used for fluorometric determination of the final tracer binding. Two variations have been introduced for the enhancement system: an assay based on a formation of mixed-ligand chelate (*in situ* fluorescent chelate formed after immunoreaction) and an assay based on metal ion dissociation prior to the formation of totally new, fluorescent chelates for fluorometric determination ("dissociation enhanced" TR-FIA).

Ternary chelates—or mixed-ligand chelates—are commonly used in fluorometric determinations of lanthanides from aqueous samples (783). They are formed by using polyamino-polycarboxylates (complexones, e.g., EDTA) as the water soluble, stable chelating agents, and an appropriate bidentate, light absorbing ligand (e.g., β-diketone) as excitation energy collectors and fluorescence enhancers.

The principle for using EDTA derivatives as labeling chelates and β-diketones as enhancing ligands with Eu^{3+} and Tb^{3+} in TR-FIA is patented (816), and the same type of mixed-ligand chelate is used for a homogeneous TR-FIA based on fluorescence quenching of Eu-EDTA–labeled insulin in the presence of β-diketones and an excess of anti-insulin antibodies (817). An analogous system has been patented by Wieder and Wollenberg (818). The patent is based on DTPA-anhydride–labeled thyroxine, chelated with Tb^{3+}, and on the use of sulfosalicylic acid as the fluorescence-enhancing ligand. Wieder has also suggested the use of mixed-ligand chelate formation as a basis for a homogeneous assay using a nitrosotriacetic acid chelate of Tb^{3+} and dipicolinic acid (819).

The drawback of this type of technique relates to the slow formation kinetics of fluorescent mixed-ligand chelates in aqueous solutions. Svetlova et al. (820) have studied chelate formation kinetics in micellar aqueous solution in order to find optimal conditions for this type of assay. In spite of a few approaches, the mixed-ligand enhancement system has not yet gained any wider applications.

The fluorescence-enhancement system, in which the tracer ions are dissociated from the primary labeling reagent prior to formation of a totally new fluorescent chelate for detection purposes, has been developed at Wallac Oy (808, 821) and forms the basis for the commercial DELFIA product line. A rapid dissociation of the Eu ions by use of an acidic solution facilitates the immediate formation of new chelates with β-diketones present in the enhancement solution. The enhancement solution, commercialized by Wallac, contains 2-naphthoyl-trifluoroacetone, TOPO, and Triton X 100 in an acetate buffer of pH 3.2. It is the most frequently utilized enhancing system in the published and commercial TR-FIAs. It produces fluorescent chelates with a relative fluorescence of 24,500 (product $\varepsilon \times Q$), a long Stokes' shift (270 nm), and a decay time of 730 μs (Fig. 7.22, Table 7.12), features which are exploited in time-resolved fluorometry to achieve the sensitivity of 0.05×10^{-12} mol/L in the label detection (475, 808) (Chapter 6.2.3.).

The same solution, based on aromatic β-diketones, is suitable also for detection of Sm^{3+}, even though Sm^{3+} produces a less strong emission than Eu^{3+}, having the product of $\varepsilon \times Q$ only about 700 (822) (Table 7.12). Sm^{3+} labels have also been used in TR-FIAs (823, 824), and Sm^{3+} is well suited as a counterpart to Eu^{3+} in double-label TR-IFMAs, applied, for example, for potato viruses (825). The sharply distinguishable emission lines of the different lanthanides, in addition to their different decay times, makes the lanthanide chelates ideal probes for double- or even triple-label immunoassays, because both spectral resolution (filters) and temporal resolution (time windows) can be combined for their time-resolved fluorometric detection to decrease the spillover between their signals (347, 602, 826).

The aliphatic β-diketone, pivaloyltrifluoroacetone, is used for a fluorometric determination of Tb^{3+}-labeled reagents (346), and the respective enhancement solution is used for double-label TR-IFMAs of serum lutropin and follitropin and for faeces adeno and rotaviruses, using both Eu^{3+} and Tb^{3+} as labels (827, 828). Even though the aliphatic β-diketones (e.g., pivaloyltrifluoroacetone) could be employed for the detection of all four fluorescent lanthanides, its use is restricted by the lower excitation λ, which generally causes higher background for fluorometric measurement and results in lower relative fluorescences (Table 7.12).

Alternative fluorescence-enhancement solutions developed for in-house TR-FIAs primarily contain thenoyltrifluoroacetone as the aromatic fluorinated β-diketone and involve some modifications in concentrations and types of detergents (72, 829, 830). Ekins and Dakubu have patented a modification of the dissociation principle by introducing a two-step enhancement system (831), where Eu^{3+} is first dissociated from the immunoreagents with a strong acid, whereafter a new chelate is formed after the pH rises. This type of enhancement modification can be useful for chelates requiring neutral or alkaline pH for optimal fluorescence, such as 4-trimethoxyphenyl-2,6-dipicolinic acid, used for enhancement of Tb^{3+} (832) (Table 7.12), or tiron, which requires a very alkaline solution for optimal fluorescence (833). Recently it has been found that the fluorescence of Eu- and Sm-β-diketonates can be considerably enhanced by an energy transfer process from nonfluorescent β-diketone chelates of other metals (e.g., Gd^{3+} or Y^{3+}) if present in the same solution at high concentrations (833, 834). It remains to be seen whether this so called "co-fluorescence" enhancement could be utilized in TR-FIAs.

In the fluorescence-enhancement assays, the chelate used for labeling immunoreagents need not be fluorescent as such. Therefore, labeling systems originally developed for *in vivo* use, such as DTPA anhydride or diazo- and p-isothiocyanato derivatives of phenyl-EDTA (Fig. 7.27) (738, 742, 744, 836, 837) can be applied also in TR-FIAs (72, 808, 817, 818, 830, 838). For mixed-ligand formation, the complexone used for labeling needs to allow the binding of one additional bidentate ligand to the chelate to form a fluorescent complex. In the dissociative enhancement technique, the attached ions need to be dissociated from the labeling chelates completely within a short time to facilitate rapid production of stable fluorescence level.

An asymmetric phenyl-DTTA derivative, N^1-p(isothiocyanatobenzyl)-diethylenetriamine-N^1,N^2,N^3,N^3-tetraacetic acid (Fig. 7.27) is the labeling reagent specifically optimized for labeling immunoreagents to be used in *in vitro* assays based on acid dissociation of the chelated lanthanide ions prior

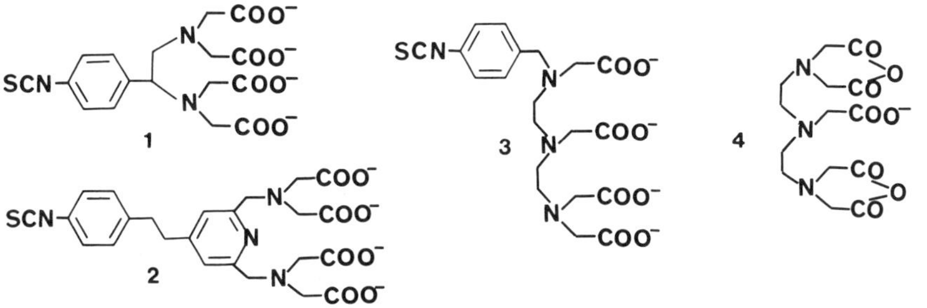

Fig. 7.27. Bifunctional chelating agents used for labeling with lanthanide ions for immunoassays; ITC derivative of phenyl-EDTA (1), ITC-phenyl derivative of pyridine-bis (methylaminodiacetic acid) (2), N_1-p (ITC-benzyl)-diethylenetriaminetetraacetic acid (3), and DTPA anhydride (4).

to the fluorescence enhancement (839, 840). Since its development it has been the labeling reagent in all commercial DELFIA® products (the trademark of Pharmacia-Wallac Oy) and is commercially available from Wallac Oy (Finland), chelated either with Eu^{3+} or Sm^{3+} (Sm^{3+} for double-label assays) (841). For more demanding assay conditions, such as *in vivo* labeling of viable cells with Eu^{3+} in assays of cell-mediated immunology, kinetically or thermodynamically stronger labeling chelates (e.g., DTPA) are needed (842). Also, the direct labeling of DNA-probes with Eu^{3+} to be used in DNA hybridization assays, requires kinetically very stable chelating agents because of the high temperature and the presence of EDTA in the DNA denaturing phase. A pyridine derivative containing bis-imidodiacetic acid groups (Fig. 7.27) is specifically developed for labeling DNA-probes (843, 845). A DTPA anhydride (846) and cyclohexydiaminotetraacetic acid (847) have also been used for DNA labeling in systems employing dissociative fluorescence enhancement.

7.4.4. Chelate Stabilizing Systems

Another technique to overcome the instability and aqueous quenching problems encountered with most of the potentially fluorescent lanthanide chelates is to stabilize the chelates to form *in situ* fluorescent chelates. Two basic techniques have been applied: stabilization of β-diketone chelates by molding them into plastic beads and stabilization of the chelates by using a high excess of lanthanide ions to saturate the fluorogenic ligand (the reverse system to the enhancement assays described above).

Frank and Sundberg have patented an "aqueous stabilized" label system composed of latex beads containing Eu-β-diketonates inside the beads (848, 849). Later Eastman Kodak received new patents to further improve the hydrophilicity of chelate-loaded latex particles by including sugar components to linker arms (850, 851). Similar latex beads, or liposomes, loaded with Eu-chelates, have been patented also by other companies (852–855). Mercolino et al. (856) used a Eu-β-diketone-TOPO chelate as a hydrophobic fluorochrome incorporated into lipid bilayers of liposomes and used it as a label for TR-FIA of hCG.

Another way to stabilize chelates of a moderate stability is to use a high excess of some of the components to saturate either the bound metal (used in the fluorescence-enhancement system with mixed ligands; Chapter 7.4.3) or the bound "fluorogenic" ligand ("reverse enhancement"). Wilmott et al. utilized the enhancing effect of transferrin with Tb-fluorescence in a TR-FIA of gentamicin by saturating the gentamicin-transferrin tracer with an excess of Tb^{3+} (10^{-5} M) (857). An analogous procedure was commercialized later by CyberFluor Inc. (Toronto, Canada). In this system bis-chlorosulfonylphenyl-1,10-phenanthroline-2,9-dicarboxylic acid (BCPDA) (Fig. 7.28) (858–860) is used to label avidin, used in indirect assays, is saturated separately with an excess of Eu^{3+}, and is measured by time-resolved fluorometry from the dried surfaces of white microtitration strips (74, 861, 862). This system was introduced as a part of the FiaGen™ products of CyberFluor (Chapter 8.4.2). Saturation of the ligand with metals derived from samples is avoided by using indirect assay technique and so eliminates the direct contact of BCPDA and the sample.

7.4.5. Stable Fluorescent Chelates

Much effort has been expended to develop and synthesize stable, optimally fluorescent chelates which could be coupled to immunoreagents and used for TR-FIAs. This type of chelate might help simplify TR-FIA techniques, diminish possible contamination problems, and open totally new applications for time-resolved fluorometry. Primarily three types of chelates have been introduced: condensation products of DTPA anhydride with suitable aromatic amines, polyaminopolycarboxylic acid derivatives of pyridines, bi-

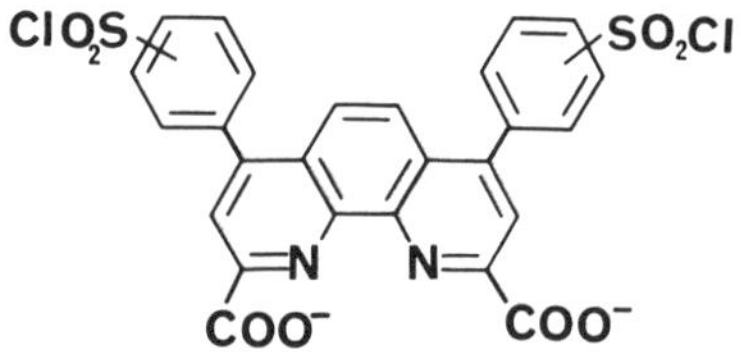

Fig. 7.28. Structure of BCPDA.

pyridines, and terpyridines, and macrocyclic cryptates containing pyridine structures as energy collecting moieties.

The simplest, but also only scarcely fluorescent, stable labels are the same bifunctional complexone derivatives developed for labeling purposes, without any additional absorbing or energy mediating groups. For example, Eu-DTPA has very low absorptivity and thus low relative fluorescence, but it has been used as a fluorescent probe for tissues of animals injected with Eu-DTPA and detected by virtue of a fluorescence microscope (863). Milby et al. used Tb-chelate of diazophenyl-EDTA as a label for TR-FIA of IgG (864, 865). The diazo bond formed with tyrosine residues of antigen is able to absorb excitation (325 nm of a He-Cd laser) and transfer it to the chelated Tb^{3+} with enough efficiency for a "less demanding" assay.

In the first type of synthesized stable fluorescent chelates, the same type of structures are used for fluorometric determinations of Eu^{3+} or Tb^{3+} by using mixed-ligand chelates, with the exception that the bidentate absorbing ligand is covalently coupled to the complexone (e.g., to the DTPA structure). The simplest synthesis consists of the reaction of DTPA dianhydride with aminosalicylic acid (PAS), an amino group of antigen and Tb^{3+} salt, to form a relatively stable and fluorescent conjugate (Fig. 7.29 and Table 7.13), utilized, for instance, for TR-FIAs of albumin (384, 866–869) and testosterone (870). Also, other condensation products of DTPA anhydride and aromatic amines have been tested (384), and actually a cytosine adduct would form fluorescence 2.5 times higher than obtained with DTPA-PAS; however, because of its instability it could not be used for immunoassays (871). A patent application also has been issued regarding the use of DTPA-PAS as a fluorescent probe for time-resolved fluorometry of nucleotides in gel electrophoresis (872).

The majority of stable fluorescent chelates are bis-amino-methyldiacetic acid derivatives of aromatic UV absorbing compounds (often pyridine derivatives) and are primarily found in recent patent publications. The first patent of Eastman Kodak covered aromatic phenol derivatives, such as coumarine-bis (aminomethyltetraacetic acid) (873) (Fig. 7.29) (Table 7.13), but the patent description also included one derivative of 1,10-phenanthroline. In the subsequent patents of the same company, new derivatives were made containing pyridine, bipyridine, terpyridine, or quaterpyridine groups as excitation energy mediators (874, 875). Similar structures, tetraacetic acid derivatives of phenyl-pyridines (Fig. 7.29), are patented also by Travenol-Genetech Diagnostics (876). Various assay principles have been patented based on the use of phenyl-pyridine derivatives, including ligand exchange-based assays, fluorescence quenching assays, enhancement assays, etc. (819). In a TR-FIA of CEA, 4-isothiocyano-2-methoxy-phenyl-pyridine-2′,6′-bis (aminomethyl-diacetic acid) (Fig.7.29) is also used (832). Kankare et al. (877) patented

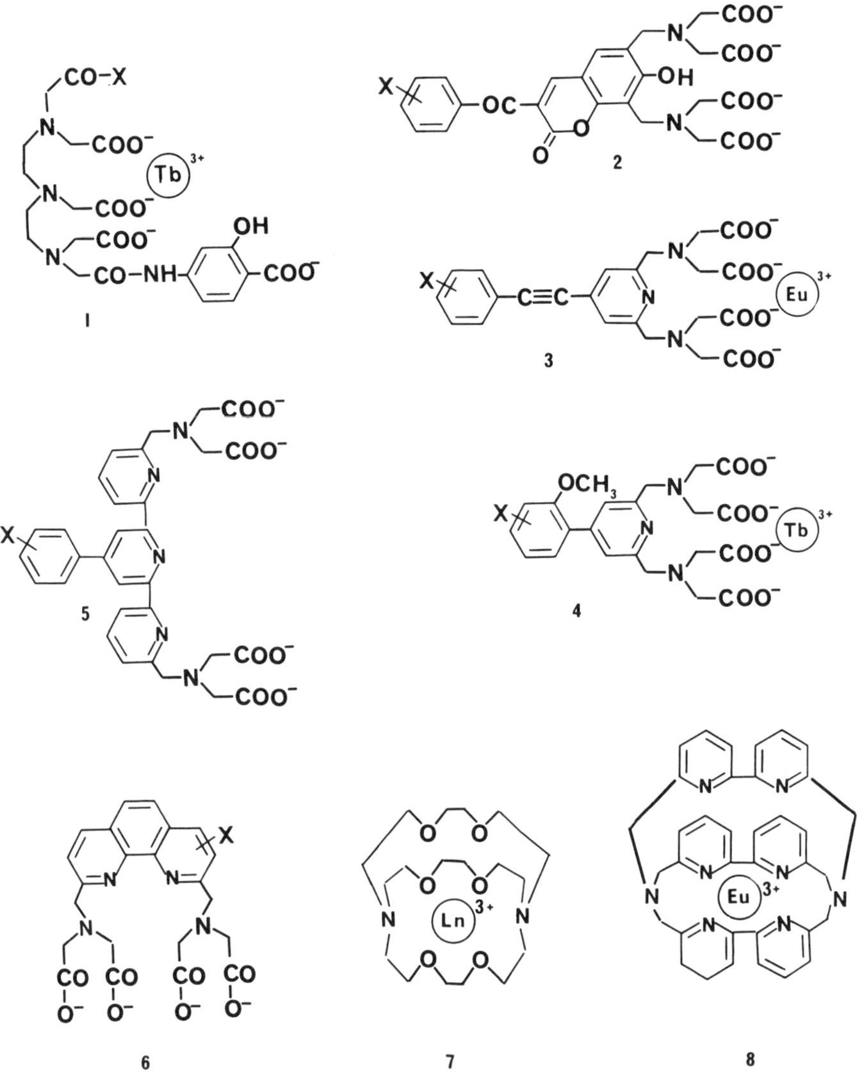

Fig. 7.29. Structures of lanthanide chelates used (or patented) in time-resolved fluoroimmunoassays.

Table 7.13. Fluorescent Properties of Stable Lanthanide Chelates

Ligand[a]	Metal	Exc. max (nm)	ε (L/M cm)	Em. max (nm)	τ (μs)	Q
DTPA-PAS	Tb	312	7,600	545	1550	0.1
DTPA-Cyt.	Tb	305		545	1970	0.1
Coumarin-TA	Eu	396	27,000	614		0.045
Phen-TA	Eu	277		613		0.06
DP-TPDA	Eu	340	13,000	614		0.08
Bipy ⊂ 2.2	Eu	310		613	410	
Phen ⊂ 2.2	Eu	290		614	300	
$Bipy_3$-Crypt	Eu	305	27,000	615	340	0.02
$Bipy_3$-Crypt	Tb	302	29,000	542	330	0.03
W1014	Eu	340		613	550	
W3014	Tb	313		544	1100	

[a]Ligand structures and abbreviations are as mentioned in Fig. 7.28, W1014 and W3014 structures are made by Wallac Oy (351).

structures which are based on pyridine derivatives coupled to a p-substituted phenyl group via an acetylene bridge. Kwiatkowski et al. (878) have published synthetic schemes for introducing stable chelates into oligonucleotide structures. A number of stable fluorescent chelates have been synthesized also by Wallac Oy (351), and a chelate coded W1014 is used in a fluorescence microscopic assay (879) and in a solid-phase TR-IFMA of hCG (880). An environmentally sensitive chelate, W1174, is used for a number of homogeneous TR-FIAs of thyroid and steroid hormones (881, 882) (Chapter 8.4.3).

Cryptates are a group of macrocyclic cage-type chelating agents, which, because of the inherent kinetic stability and the potential fluorescence of their Eu^{3+}, Tb^{3+}, and Ru^{2+} chelates, have recently been extensively studied (883). The basic structure is formed with three polyoxyethylene chains coupled to two nitrogens (Fig. 7.29). Eu^{3+} and Tb^{3+} ⊂ 2.2.2 cryptants have relatively high fluorescence efficiency and show charge-transfer type excitation directly to $^5D_0$ level (884), but energy transfer from UV-absorbing pyridine groups attached to the cryptant structure form a more efficient excitation route (885–887). Cryptates containing a phenanthroline, or one, two, or three bipyridine groups, have recently been synthesized in order to create highly fluorescent Eu-cryptants (Fig. 7.29, Table 7.13). In those cryptants, Tb^{3+} generally produces much weaker emission than Eu^{3+}, due to a partial energy backflow from the metal to the ligand (887).

The use of rare-earth cryptates as fluorescent probes for TR-FIAs has been patented by Mathis and Lehn et al. (888, 889). A cryptant formed of three bipyridines and chelated with Eu^{3+} (Fig. 7.29) was also used in a TR-

IFMA of prolactin, by coupling the amino derivative of the cryptate to antibodies via a heterobifunctional cross-linking agent, SPDP (888, 890). The cryptates have also received attention as potential probes for flow-cytometric detection of DNA hybridization (891).

The kinetic stability of cryptates is their prominent feature. On the other hand, the formation of lanthanide cryptates, where the ion is inside the cavity, needs to be performed in strictly controlled conditions. The positively charged complexes are very sensitive to adduct formation with buffer ions, which may alter the chelate fluorescence (890), and the overall hydrophobicity of unsubstituted bipyridines causes unwanted affinities to serum proteins and surfaces.

Calixarenes are another group of chelating macrocyclic compounds recently introduced as potential chelating ligands for fluorescent lanthanides (892). Still another type of macrocyclic ligand was synthesized by Vallarino (893) for chelation of Eu^{3+} and Tb^{3+}. It was composed of a cyclic Schiff base formed with two ethylenediamines and pyridine-2,6-dialdehydes.

7.4.6. Transition Metal Chelates

Besides lanthanides, some other metals and their complexes have attracted attention as potential luminescent labels in immunoassays. The majority of the published articles and patents deal with Ru^{2+}, but Cr^{3+}, Os^{3+}, and Ir^{3+} have been tested also. When compared to lanthanides, these ions form kinetically more stable chelates. They also produce relatively long decay-time emissions (around 0.1–1 μs) (Table 7.14) exploited in various time-resolved assay principles. The decay times are, however, considerably shorter than those of Eu^{3+} or Tb^{3+} chelates.

Ru-chelates are most intensively studied as photosensitizers for interconversion of light into chemical energy. It forms kinetically inert chelates even with relatively simple nitrogen donors, such as bipyridine and o-phenanthroline. Fluorescence of its chelates is characterized by a long Stokes' shift (Fig. 7.30) and a decay time ranging from 0.1 to 1 μs.

Müller and Schmidt have patented the use of o-phenanthroline for chelation of Ru^{2+} to be used in TR-FIA and exemplified with assays of CEA, hCG, and interferon (894). Bannwarth et al. (895, 896) have utilized an Ru-complex with a derivative of bathophenanthroline, where the carboxyl or sulfonyl groups were used for coupling to DNA. By modifying the measuring conditions and removing dissolved oxygen with sulfite, they increased the decay time of Ru-tris-bathophenanthroline to 7.5 μs, which simplifies TR-fluorometric detection of the complex (897). Davidson and Votier have patented the use of tris-chelates of Cr^{3+}, Os^{3+}, Ir^{3+}, and Ru^{2+} for use in specific binding assays (753). They used a N-hydroxysuccinimide derivative of one

Table 7.14. Fluorescent Properties of Some Transition Metal Complexes

Metal	Ligand	Exc. max (nm)	Em. max (nm)	τ (μs)
Ru	Bipy	475	610–625	0.46
Ru	Phen	470	610–625	0.57
Ir	Bipy	310	495	0.30
Ir	Phen	350	498	0.70
Os	Bipy	480	730	0.13
Os	Phen	480	730	0.13
Cr	Bipy	420	728	0.15
Cr	Phen	420	728	0.17

bipyridine for the coupling reaction, and solid-phase separation on microtitration strips. In the model phase-resolved FIA of TSH the chelate label was released with acid and detected with a phase-resolved fluorometer. An isothiocyanate derivative of o-phenanthroline was used by Thompson and Vallarion to couple a Ru-phen$_3$ chelate to immunoreagents (898). The high affinity of the chelate to DNA was used to concentrate the chelates prior to phase-resolved fluorometric detection. DeCola et al. studied the luminescence and photochemical properties of cage-type complexes formed with Ru-(bipy)$_3$, where chelate stability was further increased by covalent coupling of the bipyridines via a linker group (899).

Ru^{2+} and Os^{3+} show relatively strong electrogenerated chemiluminescence in aqueous solutions, which has been recognized in a number of patent specifications. Weber patented an assay system based on Ru-o-phen as the

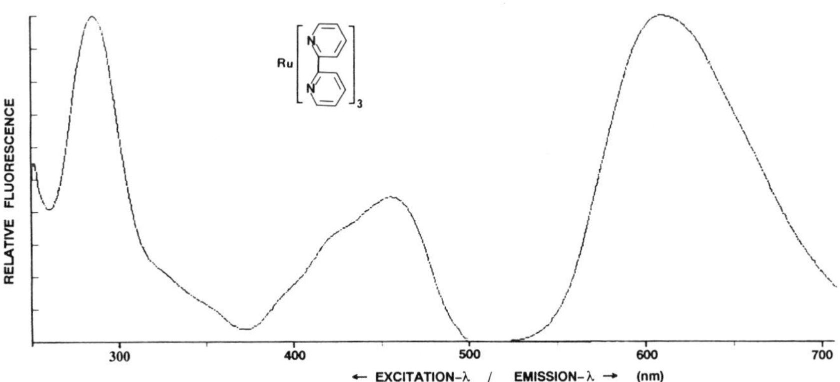

Fig. 7.30. Fluorescence spectra of Ru-tris-bipyridine.

photoelectrochemical label, excited with a laser, quenched by electron transfer to a Co-complex, and determined with an electrode (900). Bard and Whitesides (901) and Massey et al. (902) have issued patent applications on the use of Ru^{2+} or Os^{3+} bipyridine chelates as electroluminescent tracers in immunoassays. An Ru-bipy chelate is also commercialized as "Origen Label" by Igen Inc. (Rockville, MD).

Finally, aluminum, chelated with suitable ligands (such as 8-hydroxyquinoline, Nuclear Fast Red, or purpurin) has been used as a fluorescent staining reagent (903).

7.5. POLYMERIC LABELS

Polymeric labels are one way to increase the detection sensitivity by virtue of increased signal per unit of immunoreagent. With conventional fluorescent probes the benefits of using polymeric labels is hampered, however, by a large decrease in quantum yield as a result of the inner-filter effect (Chapter 5.4.3). Various techniques have been adopted to avoid the quenching. The majority of the polymeric labels have been done with fluorochromes having a long Stokes' shift to avoid spectral overlapping of the excitation and emission. A quantum yield independent spectroscopic technique was introduced by Hirschfeld (364, 436, 904), who used polymeric carriers containing up to 100 fluoresceins. After total bleaching of the probes with powerful laser excitation, the total number of emitted quanta per fluorochrome was shown to be independent of quantum yield, absorption cross section, illumination duration, and illumination intensity. A third method to overcome inner-filter quenching is to use fluorochromes released from immunoreagents prior to detection. Release can be accomplished by enzymatic hydrolysis of the binding arm, acid dissociation (e.g., chelated ions), or detergent lysis of, for example, liposome entrapped fluorochromes.

Polymeric label techniques can be divided into three main groups: immunological polymers, biological or synthetic polymers used as carriers for labels, and liposomes, latex beads, and crystals.

7.5.1. Immunological Complexes

A technique which is widely applied in microscopic staining techniques involves building a complex around the primary immunological recognition reaction. The complex can be formed with avidin-biotin reactions (Chapter 2.7.1), hapten-antihapten reactions (e.g., FITC-anti-FITC), or direct immunoreaction between the label substance and the respective antibodies (e.g., peroxidase-antiperoxidase staining technique). In quantitative immunoassays these techniques are utilized only in a controlled manner, using, for example, avidins, secondary antibodies, or protein A as an additional reagent in indirect assays. Examples of these types of techniques are flow-cytometric IFMA using biotinylated antibodies, phycoerythrine-streptavidin conjugate, biotinylated anti-streptavidin, and a second addition of phycoerythrin-streptavidin conjugate, a method named "super AB complex" (63). Krylova et al. (905) used streptavidin as a linker between a biotinylated antibody and biotinylated polyethyleneimine, tagged with DTPA-Eu labels. Guy et al. (906) formed a complex from phycoerythrin and anti-PE antibodies for flow-cytometric detection of cell surface antigens. An example of an anti-FITC linking system using FITC-labeled antibodies, rabbit-anti-FITC, and FITC-labeled anti-rabbit-IgG is the IF staining of Epstein-Barr viruses ("amplified direct immunofluorescence") described by Schmitz and Kampa (907).

7.5.2. Biological and Synthetical Polymers

Various biological and synthetical polymers have been utilized as carriers for polymeric labels. Primarily these carriers, tagged with a multiplicity of fluorochromes, are used for assays of haptenic molecules, where the simple one-to-one labeling ratio does not provide the required sensitivity. In the simplest systems anti-hapten antibodies are used as carriers for fluorochromes in competitive binding assays (solid-phase assays based on labeled antibodies). Often various additional carrier molecules are used to increase the labeling ratio.

Polylysines of different sizes are most commonly used as readily available polymers containing free amino groups for labeling with fluorochromes. Ekeke and Exley developed FIAs for steroids by coupling polylysine via its terminal carboxy group to the steroid and conjugating the rest of the amines with methylumbelliferyl-3-acetic acid (668–670). Polylysines are also used as carriers for Eu-chelates in labeling steroids (908, 909), prostaglandin (910), a methylated nucleotide (911), and thyroxine (912) used for neonatal screening of T_4 from dried blood samples. Canfi et al. utilized polylysine labeled with DTPA-PAS-Tb for assays of testosterone (870, 871). Manabe et al. used polylysines as carriers for Gd^{3+} to increase the targeted contrast enhancing effect of labeled antibodies in MRI purposes (747).

The use of highly water soluble polymers, such as dextranes, as fluorochromes carriers was patented by Ortho Diagnostics (913). Ranney has patented polychelating agents, formed from dextranes and coupled, for instance, with Gd^{3+}-DTPA, for image and spectral enhancement (914). Gd-DTPA-labeled dextranes are also used for intravascular MR contrast agents in animal studies (915). Hirschfeld used polyethyleneimines as a backbone for a multiplicity of fluoresceins (60–100 FITC/polymer) in his laser excited bleaching technique (364, 436, 904). Krylova et al. (905) also utilized polyethyleneimine as a carrier of Eu^{3+} for TR-FIA. Other polymers used consist of polyacrylic acid (916) and polyvinylamine (845). In DNA labeling the signal improvement by multiple labeling is generally needed (917), and various polymers have been used, including polylysines (846), polyethyleneimines (918), and polyvinylamines (845).

Proteins are also used as fluorochrome carriers. Labeling thyroglobulin with up to 150 chelating ligands, BCPDA, is routinely used in FiaGen TR-FIA products (CyberFluor Inc.), which require higher sensitivities than achieved with streptavidin labeled directly with the ligand (862). Recently Diamandis et al. (919, 920) have introduced still larger complex labels comprised of a mixture of BCPDA-labeled TG and BCPDA-labeled TG-streptavidin conjugate complexed with an excess of Eu^{3+} forming a complex containing up to 480 ligands per unit of streptavidin. Gelatin was used as a carrier for Eu^{3+} in TR-FIA of free thyroxine by Eskola et al. (921).

7.5.3. Liposomes, Latex Beads, and Crystals

Liposomes, microbeads, and microcrystals form the ultimate size of labels applicable in immunoassay. These can incorporate very high numbers of fluorochromes producing a highly amplified signal. On the other hand, their large size can cause steric hindrances and can restrict their applicability.

Liposomes (i.e., vesicles formed of bi- or multiple layer lipid membranes) can be activated with immunoreagents and can incorporate up to 10^5 molecules of small molecular weight compounds. Liposomes have been used as reversible carriers of various compounds—for example, drugs, cytotoxic agents, etc.—subsequently released by the action of antibody-triggered complement lysis, detergent, or cytolysin. Liposomes are prepared from phospholipids and cholesterol by various techniques: mechanical dispersion of dried liposomes in aqueous buffer (922), dispersion of lipids in organic solvent with buffer and subsequent removal of solvent by evaporation, by freeze-drying (923), dehydration and rehydration (924), and sonication (925). Targeting compounds are coupled to the surface of liposomes primarily with covalent reactions (liposome activation). For that purpose suitable phospholipid containing activated groups are incorporated into the membrane. For example, N-hydroxysuccinimide activation of palmitic acid (926), maleimido derivatized phospholipid (927), iodoacetyl activation (928), and a biotin derivative of phosphatidylethanolamine (929) are used for activation. The stability of liposomes is limited, and generally leakage problems are encountered, but reasonably stable lipids can be formed (generally stored frozen) with the appropriate choice of lipids, preparation method, and size.

Liposomes have been used as carriers for immunoassays since the pioneering work of Kinsky et al. (930–932), who has used liposomes for complement-mediated homogeneous immunoassays since 1971. Carboxyfluorescein is the most commonly used fluorochrome encapsulated in liposomes. As a hydrophilic compound, its leakage from liposomes is low, and it is efficiently quenched in concentrated solutions, which makes possible its use in homogeneous assays (Chapter 8.3.5). CF-labeled liposomes are also used in IF, flow cytometry (933–936), and Sep-FIA (929). Other fluorochromes used with liposomes include 4-MU-β-D-galactose (a substrate for β-galactosidase) (937), sulphorhodamine-B (636, 938), aminonaphthalene trisulphonic acid (645), and Eu-chelates (933). Fluorochromes can also be incorporated into lipid bilayers after coupling to lipids (939) or simply by using lipophilic probes, such as water-insoluble Eu-chelates (856).

Monosized polymeric microscopic plastic beads, or latex beads, are quite commonly used in various types of immunoassay as solid-phases or as labels. They are generally prepared by emulsion polymerization and have very narrow size distribution, and so are used as size standards in flow cytometry. If impregnated with fluorescent compounds, these can be used as fluorescent probes in immunoassays.

Dreyer et al. (191, 940, 941) have introduced the use of fluorochrome-labeled immunolatex spheres as markers for scanning electron microscopy, IF, and flow cytometry. Bourel et al. (942) used emulsion polymerized methacrylate particles (0.3 μm) containing ethidium bromide as fluorescent reagents in fluorescence microscopy. A number of commercial companies produce fluorescent particles of varying sizes, surface groups, and fluorescent properties. Particles are available from, for example, Polysciences Inc., (Warrington, PA), Seradyn Inc. (Indianapolis, IN), Covalent Technology Co. (San Jose, CA), and Molecular Probes Inc. Fluoricon particles (Pandex Laboratories) are surface labeled with various dyes and used as standard in flow cytometry.

Higgins et al. (943) used green fluorescent particles (Covaspheres) for an assay of cell surface antigens performed on microtitration plates by measuring the bead fluorescences after suspension in an SDS solution. Mirro et al. (944) utilized Covasphere particles containing rhodamine and fluorescein for an IF test of cell surface antigens. Fluoresbite beads (0.57 μm) are used in the flow-cytometric assay of T-cell receptors, for example (945). Saunders et al. have introduced a nonseparation flow-cytometric immunoassay based on two sets of microbeads (946), with larger (10 μm) beads coated with antibodies and smaller, fluorescent (green) beads of 0.1 μm size (Polysciences Inc.) coated with antigen. The bead-associated fluorescences were determined with a Becton-Dickinson FACS instrument.

Latex beads have also been developed for incorporating a great number of fluorescent Eu-chelates to form "aqueous stabilized" chelate systems for TR-FIA, introduced in a series of patents issued to Eastman Kodak (848–851). The patent of Burdick and Danielson (850) describes a latex bead of discontinuous phases, containing an aqueous phase for chelates. The agglutination of beads in solution is avoided by incorporating hydrophilic surfaces consisting of dextranes, polysaccharides, or polyethyleneglycols (851). Wagner and Baffi have also been issued a series of patents dealing with latex beads or liposomes loaded with Eu-chelates (Chapter 7.4.3) (853–855).

Inorganic crystals are another way to utilize the long lifetime fluorescence of lanthanides in the form of particles. Phosphors are inorganic crystals containing small amounts of other inorganic ions as activators, luminescence centers. The host lattice is usually formed from vanadates, yttrium oxide, metal oxyhalides, halides, phosphates, or silicates. Fluorescent lanthanides (Nd, Eu, Gd, and Tb) are often used as activators. Crystal phosphors can be used both in fluorescence microscopes and as cathodo-luminescent probes excited by electrons in electron microscopes (476). For immunoassays, crystals are ground into small particles (0.1–0.3 μm), coated with suitable polyacids (which creates a negative net charge for the particles), and coated with antibodies. Tanke et al. have used inorganic crystals (e.g., Eu^{3+} doped yttrium oxysulfite and Ag activated ZnS) as fluorophores in the time-resolved fluorescence microscopic IF staining of cell surface antigens (477, 947, 949–950). Crystal phosphors are also used as standards for quantitative microfluorometers (449).

7.6. FLUOROGENIC ENZYME SUBSTRATES

Enzymes are widely applied labels in immunoassays named enzyme immunoassays, EIA (Chapter 4.2.1). Introducing fluorogenic substrates for the measurement of enzyme activities has generally improved the detection sensitivities of the labels, and the resulting enzyme-linked fluorescence immunoassays (ELFIA) are today widely applied in clinical routine and immunological research (Chapter 9), and recently especially in automated systems (Chapter 6.7). Table 4.2 lists detection sensitivities with some generally used substrate systems. Fluorometric detection systems can produce sensitivities decades apart from "conventional" photometric detection. Rotman (250) achieved the ultimate sensitivity of a single molecule detection of β-D-galactosidase using a galactoside derivative of fluorescein (Fig. 7.31). The substrate used by Rotman showed the typical properties required for fluorogenic substrates, where the fluorescence enhancement, combined with spectral shift, results in a very high dynamic range for measurement, 10^5-fold when measured with the wavelength of the product.

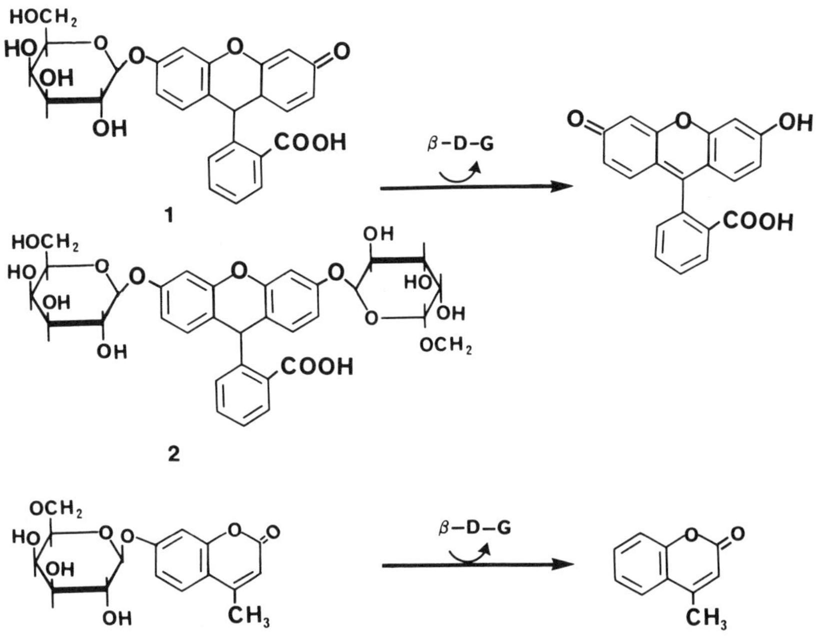

Fig. 7.31. Fluorogenic substrates for β-D-galactosidase.

Fluorogenic substrates have been introduced for most of the enzymes used in EIAs, such as β-D-galactosidase, peroxidase (HRP), phosphatase (alkaline phosphatase), and esterases. The improvement achieved by substituting photometric techniques for fluorometric ones depends on the enzymes and substrates used. Yolken and Stopa (245) achieved 5- to 100-fold improvements in the detection sensitivity of an ALP label when using various fluorogenic substrates (4MU-phosphate, fluorescein-phosphate, flavone-diphosphate) as compared to a photometric substrate, p-nitrophenyl-phosphate. Ishikawa studied fluorogenic substrates with a number of enzymes, and detection improvements vary from 50-fold with HRP to 1,000-fold with alkaline phosphatase (951).

β-D-galactosidase is one of the three most commonly used enzymes in immunoassays. Figure 7.31 shows some fluorogenic substrates used for its determination. The determination of its activity from a single cell was achieved in 1977 by Hösli (952) with the use of a galactoside derivative of umbelliferone. In 1978 (953) he introduced an EIA based on fluorescence detection, named FUMELIA (fluoro-ultra-micro enzyme-labeled immunoassay), which was based on antibodies immobilized into parafilm-membrane microcuvettes, a β-D-galactoside label, and 4-methylumbelliferone-β-D-galactopyranoside (4MUG) as the fluorogenic substrate. Currently 4MUG is a routinely used substrate in a number of ELFIA systems (Chapter 9). Other substrates used with galactosidase include a di-galactosyl derivative of fluorescein, used for digoxin ELFIA measured with the TD_X system (954). Armenta et al. (955) used a macromolecular substrate, dextrane linked with β-galactosylumbelliferone, in a homogeneous ELFIA of ferritin.

β-D-galactoside is also used, as an additional reagent, in SL-FIAs, assays which are based on small molecular weight haptens (e.g., drugs) labeled with enzymatic substrates (Chapter 8.3.2). In SL-FIA the antigens are primarily labeled with 3-carboxyl-umbelliferyl-β-D-galactoside, a label which upon enzymatic hydrolysis (if not bound to respective antibodies) produces a fluorescent antigen-umbelliferone conjugate.

Horseradish peroxidase (HRP) is perhaps the most frequently utilized enzyme in histological and immunological applications and is used frequently in EIAs, ELFIAs and ELLIAs (enzyme linked chemiluminescence immunoassays) as well. Fluorometric determination systems are based on the HRP catalyzed reaction between H_2O_2 and p-hydroxy-phenyl-carboxy acids (Fig. 7.32) (248, 543, 956–958). The condensation product of the reaction has excitation maximum at 326, 315, and 315 nm with propionic acid, acetic acid, and methoxy-acetic acid derivatives of p-phenols, respectively. The respective emission maxima are 410, 414, and 425 nm. Also, tyramine has been used together with H_2O_2 and KCN as a fluorogenic substrate for HRP (959, 960), resulting in a fluorescent product having excitation at 320 nm and emission at 405 nm. The substrates are relatively commonly used in research applications of ELFIA (Chapter 9.2.1). Imasaka et al. (425) used an IR emitting fluorochrome, indocyanine green (exc. at 780 nm), quenched by the product of HRP (H_2O_2), in an ELFIA of insulin. An opposite effect of peroxide to dichlorofluorescin, which is converted into fluorescein, is used for fluorometric detection of several oxidative enzymes (961). The detection of HRP with an "enhanced chemiluminescence" reaction with H_2O_2, luminol, and an enhancer is commercialized as the AmerLite™ system by Amersham International.

A third enzyme commonly used in ELFIA technologies is alkaline phosphatase (ALP). The substrate primarily utilized is methyl-umbelliferyl-phosphate (4MUP) (Fig. 7.33). Yolken and Stopa were the first to use alkaline phosphatase as a label and various substrates including 4MUP for its determination (245). Other substrates subsequently employed include α-naphthyl-phosphate (Fig. 7.33), used, for example, as a substrate for determination of the enzymatic activity of an antigen, prostatic acid phosphatase (PAP) (962). The product, α-hydroxy-naphthalene has its excitation maximum at 340 nm and emission at 415 nm. Lambda Probes Inc. has com-

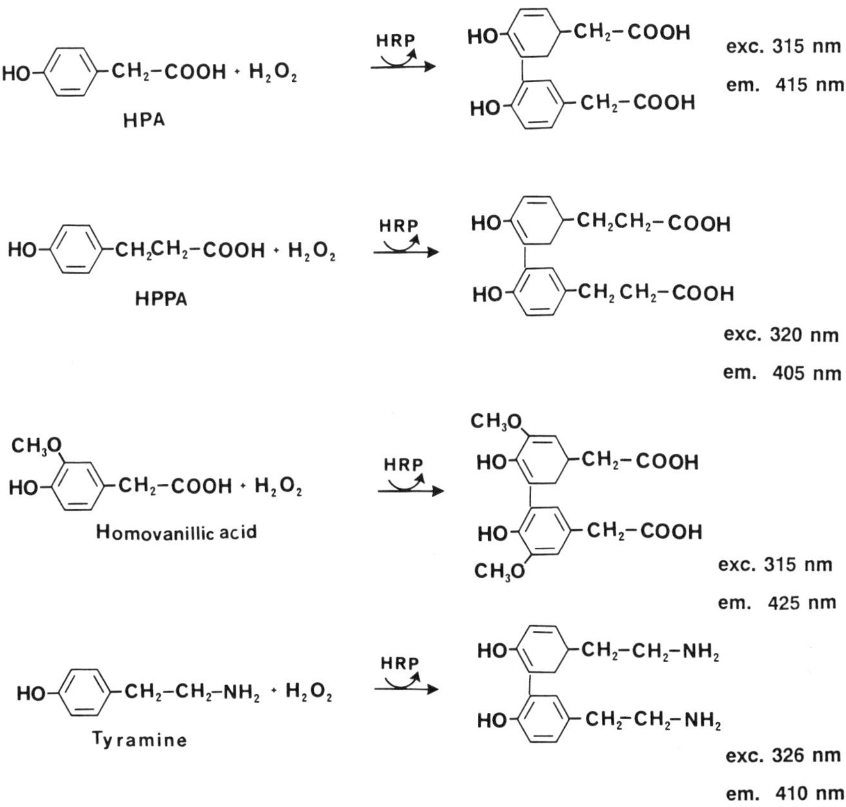

Fig. 7.32. Fluorogenic substrates for HRP.

mercialized a new fluorescent substrate consisting of a phosphoric acid ester of 1-hydroxypyrene-3,6,8-tris(dimethylsulfonamide) (Fig. 7.33), producing a fluorescent hydroxyl derivative (excitation at 495 nm and emission at 555 nm) upon activity of esterases (963). Recently a new commercial fluorogenic substrate, ULTRA-SENS™ has been introduced by JBC Scientific Inc. (San Luis Obispo, CA) (964), which upon hydrolysis catalyzed by ALP produces the fluorescent ULTRA-FLUOR™ product (exc., 430 nm; em., 560 nm). Reportedly the new substrate increases detection sensitivity of ALP beyond that of 4MU. Also, a number of luminogenic substrates have been developed for phosphatases, and those techniques are becoming very popular because of their potential extreme sensitivity. Derivatives of stable dioxetanes have been developed, which upon the hydrolyzing effect of enzymes such as phosphatases, form unstable compounds emitting photons. Alkaline phosphatase triggering of the adamantyl-1,2-dioxetane phosphate substrate is

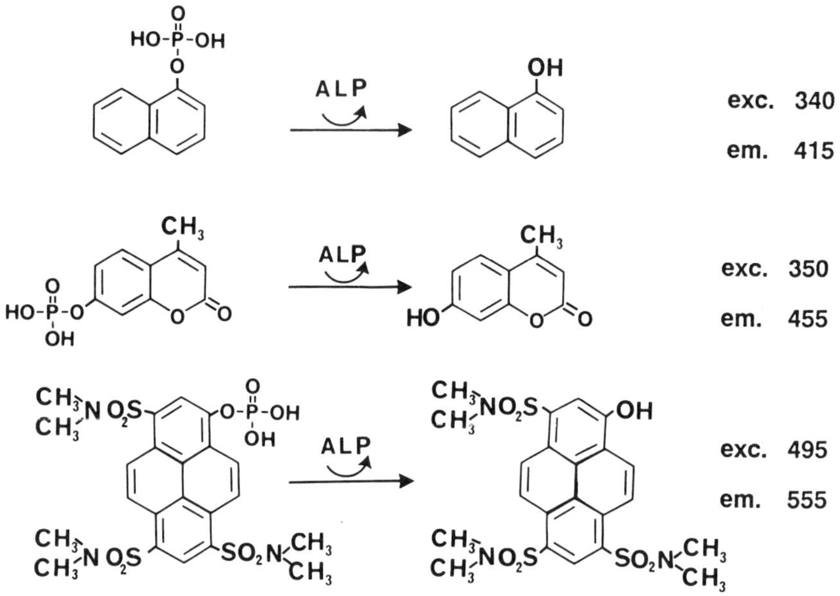

Fig. 7.33. Fluorogenic substrates for ALP.

utilized for chemiluminescence EIAs, for instance (965). Adamantyl-1,2-dioxetane phenyl phosphate is also commercially available as AMPPD™ with an enhancer, "Emerald," from Tropic Inc. (Bedford, MA). Another commercial luminogenic substrate, LumiPhos™ 530 (a trade name of Lumigen Inc., Detroit, MI) produces luminescent Lumigen PPD, 4-methoxy-4-(3-phosphate)-spiro-(1,2-dioxetane-3,2′-adamantane), which is used together with an enhancer for chemiluminescent detection of ALP.

Various esterases are also used in immunoassays as labels (EIA) and as signal modulators (SL-FIA). Umbelliferone, coupled to a small molecular antigen with an ester bond, is used in SL-FIAs based on enzymatic release (competes with antibodies) (966) and surprisingly also in assays based on enzymatic activity of antibodies (967). O'Neal et al. (968) developed a long Stokes' shift (excitation at 337 nm, emission at 480 nm) fluorogenic substrate for esterase by exploiting the excited state proton transfer of hydroxynaphthalene sulfonamide (Fig. 5.14).

Coenzymes, especially NAD(P)H, are also used as fluorogenic substrates in a number of immunoassays, because they can be easily coupled for detection of various enzyme labels, for example, through dehydrogenases. For example, a modified EMIT™ assay has been measured with a fluorometer.

Ishikawa used glucoamylase as a label producing glucose. After coupling with hexokinase and glucose-6-dehydrogenase, the primary enzymatic activity was determined with a fluorometer by measuring the produced NAD(P)H (969).

The application of fluorogenic substrates in IF and flow-cytometric studies requires either precipitating fluorescent products or substrates having such a high affinity to the enzymes that no dissociation happens. An example of such a fluorogenic substrate system comprises 5-chlorotoluene diazonium salt (Fast Red TR) and a substituted naphthol phosphate (AS-MX), used with ALP in a flow-cytometric determination of cell surface antigens on erythrocytes (970).

CHAPTER

8

FLUORESCENCE IMMUNOASSAYS

8.1. CLASSIFICATION OF THE TECHNOLOGIES

Immunological methods are named and classified numerous ways, and currently there is no unified nomenclature covering all assay techniques. The inconsistent terminology used by different authors has created confusion and even misunderstandings. Existing immunoassay techniques are named according to the various features and components used—for example, the type of antibodies, label, detection equipment, separation system, or solid-phase materials used, and so on.

In this chapter fluorescence-based immunoassays are primarily classified according to the label used. Assays comprised of reagents labeled with a fluorescent compound, potentially fluorescent compounds, or a fluorogenic substrate are called fluoroimmunoassays (generic abbreviation FIA). Similarly assays employing phosphorescent compounds as labels are named phosphoroimmunoassays (PIA), assays based on chemi- or electroluminescent labels are termed luminoimmunoassays (LIA), and assays relying on enzymatic labels are called enzyme immunoassays (EIA), analogously to radioimmunoassays (RIA), which utilize radioisotopic labels.

The secondary classification of fluorescence immunoassays is generally made according to the need for a physical separation of the bound fraction of labeled reagent from the unbound fraction prior to the fluorometric detection. Most FIAs are grouped either into separation assays (heterogeneous) or nonseparation assays (homogeneous).

The third level of classification relates to immunological assay performance. Original immunoassays (RIA) were assays comprised of a competition—that is, competitive binding of the labeled antigen and an unknown amount of sample antigen to a limited amount of antibodies—and can thus be named competitive assays or limited-reagent assays. In the context of this chapter, these assays are referred to with the same abbreviations used for general technologies: FIA, LIA, RIA, etc. The term *immunometric assay,* on the other hand, has vague and confusing meanings. The term was originally used for noncompetitive assays performed with ^{125}I-labeled antibodies, where the excess of labeled antibodies was removed by treatment with an excess of solid-phase bound antigen (216, 217). Since then the term *immunometric assay* (IRMA, IFMA) has been used partly for all assays utilizing labeled antibodies and, on the other hand, for assays using a noncompetitive, sandwich technique.

In this chapter, both the competitive and noncompetitive assays are described under the same subtitles even though the type of immunological technology defines the actual assay performance. On the other hand, specified technologies which utilize certain label and certain separation techniques are generally used for both competitive assays of haptenic antigens and noncompetitive assays of larger antigens.

The final level of classification relates to the type of assay technique—for example, the type of homogeneous principle (polarization, quenching, energy transfer, substrate-labeled, etc.)—or the type of solid-phase and separation employed (e.g., magnetic bead separation, microbead filtration, precipitation, etc.). Some of the technologies differ from the other assays to such an extent that they are traditionally classified as separate technologies (e.g., time-resolved immunoassays, immunosensors, etc.).

Which technology is chosen in a particular case depends on the analyte, its size, the required detection sensitivity and dynamic range, the availability of antibodies, labels, and instruments. The simplicity of the technology is also a strong driving force, especially in commercialized technologies, and has led to the exploitation of rapid homogeneous assays for applications which do not require the highest possible sensitivities. When higher sensitivities and wider dynamic ranges are required, heterogeneous assays are generally chosen. The relative merits and drawbacks of homogeneous and heterogeneous assays are summarized in Table 8.1.

Table 8.1. Comparison Between Homogeneous and Heterogeneous Assays

Homogeneous	Heterogeneous
Simple to perform	More complicated assay performance
Easy to automate	Mechanization difficult
Robust procedure	Performance may contain critical steps
Limited sensitivity	Higher sensitivities
Limited dynamic range	Wide dynamic range
Limited menu (small antigens)	General applicability
Sensitive to interferences derived from samples	Less prone to matrix differences

8.2. HETEROGENEOUS FLUORESCENCE IMMUNOASSAYS

Heterogeneous assays are assays based on a physical separation of the fraction of labeled immunoreagent forming the immunocomplex from the free, unreactive fraction prior to the determination of the quantity of marker substance in either of the fractions.

In most techniques the bound fraction of the labeled reagent is measured. When measuring the bound fraction, simultaneous separation and washing of sample constituents eliminates the background interferences derived from samples. This detection does not require the use of tracers with high percentage binding, but can be used even with labeled polyclonal antibodies, where the maximal binding often stays below 1%. The free fraction is nevertheless measured in some competitive assays, and a wide measuring dynamic can result if the zero-level binding of the tracer (B_0) approaches 100%. A lower binding percentage limits the dynamic range of measurement and is hardly practical with reagents with less than 10% maximal binding (e.g., labeled antibodies).

The fluorescence bound to immunocomplexes can be determined directly from the solid surface used; it can be measured from the redissolved precipitate or resuspended beads, or the bound label can be released from immunocomplexes prior to detection. Detergents and alkaline solutions are generally used for releasing labeled reagents from the complexes. This detection can avoid the optical problems encountered when measuring is performed on a certain surface area, and the choice of an appropriate releasing solution can create optimal conditions for the fluorometric determination of the probe used.

Separation systems used in FIAs are to a great extent the same as with other immunoassays: precipitation or chromatographic separation or solid-phase separation with microbeads, balls, or other surfaces (Chapter 3.4). The various heterogeneous assay principles, whether competitive or non-competitive, are classified in this chapter primarily according to the separation system used.

The evolution of heterogeneous FIAs has followed two main lines. One line originated in the development, standardization, and automation of IF tests and has resulted in systems named quantitative IF (QIF), SAFA, and DASS—and later on in routine IFMA techniques. On the other hand, the automation of IF has led to versatile, automated flow-cytometric techniques and to automated imaging systems. The second major trend originated in the desire to develop non-isotopic alternatives to radioisotopic assays. This tendency has resulted in several technologies used primarily in endocrinology, but recently highly sensitive fluorometric immunoassays have been able to replace RIAs and IRMAs in all of their application areas.

8.2.1. Immunofluorescence Tests

Coons's pioneering work in labeling antibodies with fluorescent markers and in detecting antigens with these antibodies has resulted in very wide applications. Immunofluorescence technique has proved to be very advantageous for the rapid and specific determination of antigens in or on biological materials such as tissues or cells, detected with fluorescence microscopes. Most fluorescent antibody staining techniques can be said to be quantitative in a crude, subjective sense, as the fluorescence intensities are expressed as plus symbols, giving a rough idea about the brightness. The first attempts to measure fluorescence emission quantitatively were hampered by unspecific staining, tissue autofluorescence, and the fading of the fluorochromes used.

Today IF is a widely applied semiquantitative technique in serological determinations of anti-microbial antibodies, in the localization of surface antigens, antibodies, complement factors, or immunocomplexes in cells and tissues, in the study of receptors, in determinations of viruses, microbes, and cell populations, in cancer research, and so on (971). Four types of immunological staining are commonly used: direct staining with fluorescent antibodies, indirect staining with fluorescent secondary antibodies, an inhibitory test (control of labeled antibodies), and a complement staining with labeled complement factors or labeled anti-complement antibodies. Numerous commercial test systems are available with slides fixed with microbes or antigens, buffers, and labeled antibodies.

Typical examples of IF applications are the determinations of microbes, such as the detection of chlamydia with a direct fluorescent antibody test (972, 973), the microimmunofluorescence test of chlamydia subtypes (974), the detection of respiratory virus (975), herpes simplex virus (976, 977), rubella virus (978), rotavirus (979), influenza viruses (980), Epstein-Barr virus (907, 981), spirochetes (982), and so on. The IF test is also frequently used in serodiagnosis of microbial and viral infections (by testing circulating antimicrobial antibodies), such as the test for HIV infection (983, 984), antibodies to cytomegalovirus (985), chlamydia (986), and pneumonia (987). Furthermore, it is used for the estimation of various human autoantibodies, such as antibodies against keratin for identification of tumor cells (988) and anti-nuclear antibodies (ANA) (989, 990). IF tests have also been used for detecting steroids in breast cancer cells (991).

8.2.2. Quantitative Immunofluorescence

The major problem in semiquantitative IF tests relates to standardizing reagents and methods and producing quantitative responses. Quantitative microfluorometers have been developed for QIF tests in order to produce results in physical units rather than in subjective plus values (Chapter 6.4). Development of standardized antigen preparations instead of biological tissue sections or cells, on the other hand, has helped to standardize the staining techniques. The resulting QIF technologies do not differ in any respect from FIA or IFMA techniques, except for the terminology used and application field, which to a great extent has been restricted to serological tests for infectious diseases.

The first attempt to standardize IF was introduced in 1963 by Paronetto (183). He suggested the use of cellulose acetate discs for fixing antigens and the detection of the resultant fluorescent spots manually or with a photographic film. Toussaint et al. (184, 272, 273) further developed the technology by using fluorometers for detection of the bound fluorescence directly from the filter surface. Excitation with low intensity light by using neutral filters was employed to avoid photobleaching, and the correction of both the matrix background and the nonspecific binding resulted in a linear relationship between the analyte (antibodies) and the resultant signal. This technique, named SAFA (soluble antigen fluorescent antibody), has since been applied to serodiagnosis of numerous microbial infections: for tuberculosis (184, 992, 993), schistosomiasis (273, 994), *Trypanosoma cruzi* infection (272), histoplasmosis (995), trichinosis (996, 997), rabies (998), *Dirofilaria* infection (999), and adenovirus infection (484).

Micheel et al. later introduced a variation of SAFA technology, which they named SIFA (1000, 1001) and which is based on a nitrocellulose disc solid-phase and uses a microfluorometer for quantitation. Aalberse used principally the same SAFA assay configuration as early as 1973 (185), but he released the bound fluorescein-labeled antibodies from the filter with 0.1 N NaOH and determined the released fluorescence by a fluorometer equipped with a flow cell. This type of SAFA variation has also been used for the diagnosis of hemophilia by quantifying factor VIII-related antigen (1002).

QIF tests are quantitative analogues to IF tests in which the bound fluorescence is quantitated using fluorescence microscopes attached to a photomultiplier tube (508) (Chapter 6.4). In the serological test, either biological materials—fixed cell smears, for instance—or Sepharose beads coupled with antigens (DASS) are used as solid matrixes. In one of the very first QIF applications performed by Goldman in 1960 (270), a microbe, *Entamoeba histolytica,* was measured using a photomicrographic camera. Ueki et al. (520) used slides fixed with human peripheral leukocytes as the antigenic preparation for quantitation of antinuclear antibodies, stained with FITC-labeled anti-human antibodies in the second incubation, and measured with an Olympus microfluorometer. QIF determination can also be performed directly from sample preparations—for example, from urethral or cervical smears used directly as substrates for detection of *Chlamydia trachomatis* (1003).

Microfluorometers are frequently utilized for determining fluorescences bound to beads used as carriers for antigens in the DASS (defined antigen substrate spheres) test system. In the DASS system, introduced by Van Dalen et al. in 1973 (188), microbeads composed of, for instance, Sepharose or agarose are activated with cyanogen bromide, coupled with antigens, and used as defined substrates for QIF (1004). This QIF system is primarily applied to serodiagnosis of anti-microbial antibodies or for measuring total globulin concentrations in serum samples. Knapp et al. (517) have used the beads in a model assay of anti-human and anti-ovalbumin antibodies, and Bloemmen et al. (1005) used the DASS system for evaluating the specificities of labeled antibodies prepared for IF tests. It is used also for measuring total and allergy specific IgEs (186) and anti-collagen antibodies (1006), anti-Fasciola antibodies (1007), serum anti-thyroglobulin antibodies (1009), and immunoglobulin class and subclass levels in murine serum (1010). It is used for the diagnosis of schistosomiasis (189) and for serologic tests of c-type coronavirus (1008) as well. The relatively laborious microfluorometric measurement system is also automated with the ADM (aperture defined microvolume) system, developed for detecting fluorescences from the antigen bearing single beads (513).

8.2.3. Flow-Cytometric Assays

Flow cytometers have been developed for automated analysis of cells, cell surface receptors, and antigens after staining with fluorescent antibodies (Chapter 6.5). The ability to determine cell size by analyzing both forward and side scatterings combined with the use of two lasers and several filters enables the performance of multiparametric analysis of the cells, and cells can even be sorted according to predetermined parameters. The versatility of the instruments also allows for quantitative immunoassays by using microbeads as solid-phases. Two types of multiparametric assays can be carried out in flow cytometers: assays based on two or more microbeads of different sizes and assays based on two or more different fluorescent labels. The possibility of measuring specifically only the bead-associated fluorescence after triggering the detection by scattering also allows for easy construction of the nonseparation assay, where the bead-associated fluorescences are measured with a flow cytometer without any additional washing step.

Flow cytometers are generally used in cellular immunology research, for semiquantitative or qualitative identification of cells, for enumeration of certain types of cells, and for sorting cells. Several parameters can be determined from cells passing through the thin capillary, including the size and shape, DNA content (after staining with DNA-probes), and surface antigens. Examples of the numerous flow-cytometric applications are the single parameter measurement of T-cell receptors (1011), analysis and sorting of antigen specific B-cells (1012), evaluation of gamma-interferon expression in lymphocytes (1013), enumeration of CRI complement receptors in HIV infected donors using phycoerythrin (PE)-labeled streptavidin in a form of complex with biotinylated anti-streptavidin and biotinylated antibodies (63), and quantitation of lymphocyte subsets (1014) and estrogen receptors in biopsy specimens (1015). Fluorescein and rhodamine are used in a two-color staining of IgG and IgM on mouse splenic lymphocytes using a single argon-ion laser excitation (534). In an assay of B-cell maturation, Hardy et al. (64) simultaneously used three fluorescent probes, fluorescein, phycoerythrin, and allophycocyanin. The same authors also have used four fluorochromes (fluorescein, Texas Red, R-phycoerythrin, and allophycocyanin) for simultaneous identification of subpopulations of mouse B-cells using a flow cytometer equipped with two lasers (732). Also, enzymes have been used as labels in flow-cytometric applications by using fluorogenic substrates forming insoluble, precipitated, fluorescent products on the sites of enzyme catalysis (970).

The ability of flow cytometers to specifically determine the bead-associated fluorescences and to perform multiparametric analysis from a single bead has been employed in a number of quantitative IFMA techniques. IFMA assays with fluorescein-labeled antibodies were performed for quantitation of anti-κ light chain antibodies (1016), for screening antibodies in hybridoma supernatant (1017), for detecting immunocomplexes with C1q-coated beads (97), and for detecting anti-gliadin antibodies (536). Viable cells infected with HIV were used as solid-phases in the determination of anti-HIV antibodies (537), and cells infected with herpes simplex viruses in the detection of the microbe antigen (1018). Phycoerythrin-labeled avidin is used for an IFMA of CEA by using two sets of beads coated with antibodies of different affinities in order to widen the dynamic range of the assay (737).

Phycoerythrin is frequently used as a pair for fluorescein in double-staining assays—for example, in an assay of human IgG and IgM (533)—in a system where the microbeads are formed by polymerizing the antigen-coupled monomers during the assay procedure. Size exclusion according to bead size is another technique used for double and triple parametric assays by flow-cytometric detection. McHugh et al. (65) utilized polystyrene beads of 5 and 7 μm sizes, a phycoerythrin-labeled avidin, and a flow cytometer for a simultaneous assay of antibodies against cytomegalovirus and herpes simplex virus. A similar assay design was also introduced for three different candida antigens, using bead sizes of 5, 7, and 9.3 μm (532), and for determination of human IgG and IgM (1019).

The ability to trigger the fluorometric detection with the scattering caused by the beads is employed in a number of nonseparation assays (Chapter 8.3.6). For instance, Lisi et al. (539) have utilized the principle in an assay of human IgG. Saunders et al. (946) used small fluorescent microbeads as labels in a competitive FIA of HRP, using 10 μm beads as solid-phases. In the nonseparation assay, the fluorescence of 5,000 large beads was measured with a flow cytometer without any additional washing steps.

8.2.4. Heterogeneous Assays Based on Precipitation or Gel-Chromatographic Separation

Precipitation of antigen-antibody complexes formed during the immunoreaction, or precipitation of the total globulin fraction including the bound fraction of labeled antigen, was the commonly employed method in early RIAs. Precipitation is also used in a number of competitive FIAs, analogously to respective RIAs. Sometimes precipitation is augmented with the addition of salts (sodium sulfate or half-saturated ammonium sulfate) or polyethyleneglycol (PEG) or by using an excess of secondary antibodies directed against the primary antibodies (DAb-precipitation).

The competitive FIA functions generally with fluorescent antigens. Measurement of fluorescence is accomplished either from the free fraction from the assay supernatant or from the precipitated bound fraction after resuspension in suitable medium. Resuspending or redissolving is generally performed with an alkaline aqueous solution (pH between 10 and 12) such as a 0.1 or 0.2 M NaOH or NaOH-glycerol buffer (668, 1020, 1021) or with a mixture of methanol and NaOH (1022). The alkaline solution rapidly dissociates the formed immunocomplexes and simultaneously creates optimal conditions for fluorescence. The IMMPULSE® system, commercialized by Sclavo Inc. (Sunnyvale, CA), is an FIA which incorporates second-Ab precipitation in competitive assays (Table 8.2), and the bound fluorescence is measured from the solubilized pellet. Table 8.2 contains examples of the competitive Sep-FIAs which are based on separation by precipitation.

Precipitative separation has also been used for some noncompetitive assays, analogously to the use of radioactively labeled antigens in Farr assays, which are primarily used for determinations of serum antibodies. In these assays fluorescently labeled antibodies are used for the determination

Table 8.2. FIAs Based on Precipitation

Precipitation	Analyte	Tracer	Fraction measured	Reference
Salt	Ig	FITC/Ag	Free	276
	Gentamicin	FITC/Ag	Free	1023
	Phenytoin	FITC/Ag	Free	367
	Progesterone	FITC/Ag	Bound	1021
	Progesterone	Phenanthro-imidazole/Ag	Bound	506
PEG	hCG	FITC/Ag	Free	1024
	HSA	Lucifer Yellow/Ag	Free	395
	HSA	DTPA-PAS-Tb/Ag	Bound	384, 871
	Testosterone	DTPA-PAS-Tb/polylys/Ag	Bound	871
	Herbicides	Fluorescein/Ag	Free	1025
	Angiotensin	FITC/Ag	Free	1026
Double-Ab	Cortisol	FITC/Ag	Bound	1027
	Estriol	FITC/Ag	Bound	1028
	Tobramycin	FITC/Ag	Bound	1029, 1030
	Gentamicin	FITC/Ag	Bound	494, 1031
	Phenytoin	FITC/Ag	Free	1032
	Vancomycin	FITC/Ag	Free	1033
	Digoxin	Sulforhod/liposomes/Ag	Bound	636
	Digoxin	FITC/Ag	Bound	1034
	5α-DHT[a]	4-MU-3-A/polylys/Ag	Free	668
	Paraquat	FITC/Ag	Bound	1035
	β-2-microglob.	FITC/Ag	Bound	1022
	Ferritin	FITC/Ag	Bound	614, 1036
	IgE	FITC/Ag	Bound	614, 1037
	AFP	FITC/Ag	Bound	1038
	Albumin	FITC/Ag	Bound	1039

[a]5-alpha-dihydrotestosterone.

of large molecular weight antigens, while labeled antigens are used for the determination of circulating antibodies. The precipitation formation upon immunoreaction is generally augmented with moderate concentrations of salts or PEG. The published noncompetitive precipitation assays are summarized in Table 8.3.

The size difference between the immunocomplexes and the free fractions can also be employed in gel-chromatographic separation. Flow-through fluorescence detectors can be used for monitoring fluorescences from eluted fractions. Katsh et al. (680) used a system in which all small molecular weight antigens bearing free amines were first labeled with fluorescamine; then after the immunoreaction, the antibody-bound fluorescence was determined from the void volume of a Sephadex G 150 column. Agarose gel chromatography was used for fractionation of complexes formed with FITC-labeled antibodies and fungal toxins in a Sep-FIA developed by Warden et al. (504). Hosotsubo et al. (545, 546, 1042) used HPLC for separating hIgG complexes formed with FITC-labeled anti-hIgG in noncompetitive FIAs of serum and cerebrospinal fluid IgGs. Lidofsky et al. utilized HPLC, laser excitation, and flowing droplet detection for a sensitive competitive Sep-FIA of insulin (544).

8.2.5. Fluoroimmunoassays on Beads

Microscopic particles, microbeads, with size distribution between 0.1 μm and 50 μm, are frequently used solid-phase carriers for antibodies or antigens in heterogeneous immunoassays (Chapter 3.4.3). Microbeads have the advantage that they can provide easily adjustable surface areas, which can even be stipulated according to the needs of the particular application. Also, beads can be easily manipulated and processed in bulk amounts (surface treatment, activation, coupling or coating), and in the bead suspension the assay kinetics are rapid due to the short diffusion distances. Four types of techniques are used in handling beads in immunoassays: centrifugation after immunoreac-

Table 8.3. Noncompetitive FIAs Based on Precipitation

Precipitation	Analyte	Tracer	Fraction measured	Reference
Direct	Ig	FITC/Ab	Free	275
Salt augmented	Antibodies	FITC/Ag	Bound	1020
	Factor VIII Ag	FITC/Ag	Bound	1040
	Antinuclear-Ab	FITC/DNA	Bound	1041
PEG augmented	Immunocomplexes	FITC/protein A	Bound	79

tion, filtration from suspension, separation augmented with a magnetic field, and flow-cytometric manipulation and counting.

For immunoassays the important features of beads relate to their surface properties (hydrophilicity, charge, and functional groups), sizes, and densities. The size and density should allow beads to remain in suspension during the immunoreaction (if not mixed continuously). Functional groups can be used for covalent coating, and the surface properties also need to eliminate unwanted bead aggregations. During the development of nonseparation FIAs for soluble antigens, Lisi et. al. (539) found small (1–5 μm) polyacrylamide beads and larger (30–40 μm) dextran beads most suitable in regard to buoyant properties and nonspecific binding properties.

The beads used in immunoassays are composed of, for instance, polysaccharides, such as Sephadex or agarose, which had been used as antigen carriers in the very first FIAs (185, 188). A number of the published Sep-FIAs rely on small polyacrylamide beads, marketed by Bio-Rad Laboratories (ImmunoBeads™), which also have been used in the company's proprietary FIA system (Fluoromatic). The beads have a size of 2–5 μm and a negative surface charge, and they contain functional groups for covalent coupling (549). Most of the currently used microbeads are monodisperse latex beads (e.g., polystyrene) or magnetizable beads. The beads have found extensive applications especially in modern automated batch-type and random-access immunoassay systems (Chapter 6.7).

In Sep-FIAs using bead separation, the immunoassay response is measured by recording the fluorescence either from the free supernatant or from the bound fraction. Measurement of bound fluorescence is performed either from suspended beads, beads on a filter surface or after releasing the fluorescent reagent from beads with suitable solvent. In IFMAs the bound fraction of the tracer is generally measured, and only a few (unsuccessful) attempts have been made to follow the IFMA assay by measuring the unbound fraction of labeled antibodies (1043).

Table 8.4 summarizes some of the Sep-FIAs and IFMAs which rely on microbead solid-phases and centrifugation in separation. Beads such as latex beads and immunobeads are successfully used in both competitive FIAs and noncompetitive IFMAs. On the other hand, FIAs with magnetizable particles were primarily developed for competitive assays, and only a few IFMAs have been tested so far (one of which relied on measurement of the free fraction!) (Table 8.5). On the other hand, magnetic particles have found very wide application in the field of automated ELFIA systems (Chapters 6.7 and 9.2). A magnetic field is used for accelerating bead sedimentation after the immunoreaction, but a rapidly changing magnetic field can also be utilized for mixing beads and keeping those relatively heavy particles in suspension for the time required for the immunoassay to take place.

Table 8.4. Centrifugal Fluorescence Immunoassays on Beads

Solid-Phase	Assay type	Analyte	Bound reagent	Tracer	Fraction measured	Reference
ImmunoBeads	FIA	Thyroxine	Ag	FITC/Ab	Bound	549, 1044, 1045
	FIA	T_3	Ag	FITC/Ab	Bound	1045
	FIA	Cortisol	Ag	FITC/Ab	Bound	1046
	FIA	Deoxycortisol	Ab	FITC/Ag	Free	498
	FIA	Estradiol	Ag	FITC/Ab	Free	430
	FIA	Theophylline				1047
	IFMA	IgG	Ab	FITC/Ab	Bound	493, 1048–1051
	IFMA	IgA	Ab	FITC/Ab	Bound	1052
	IFMA	C-3 component	Ab	FITC/Ab	Bound	1053
	IFMA	C-4 component	Ab	FITC/Ab	Bound	1054
	IFMA	hIgG	Ab	PE/Ab	Bound	730
	IFMA	IgM, albumin	Ab	FITC/Ab	Bound	493, 1051
	IFMA	Blood types		FITC/Ab	Bound	1055
	IFMA	Fibronectin	Ab	FITC/Ab	Bound	1056
Sepharose	FIA	Estradiol	Ag	Umbel./Ab	Free	670
	FIA	Estrogens	Ag	TRITC/Ab	Free	1057
Cellulose	FIA	Phenytoin	Ab	PE/Ag	Free	1058
Styrene	IFMA	AFP	Ab	FITC/Ab	Bound	1059
	IFMA	MAb screen.	Ag	FITC/Ab	Bound	192, 1060
	IFMA	Influenza v.	Ab	FITC/Ab	Bound	495
Microbes	IFMA	Antibodies	Ag	FITC/Ab	Bound	499
	QIF	Streptococ. Ag	Ag	FITC/Ab	Bound	1061
Infected cell	IFMA	HIV-Ab	Ag	FITC/Ab	Bound	500
	FIA	Bovine IgG_2	Ab	FITC/Ag	Bound	1062

Table 8.5. Fluorescence Immunoassays on Magnetic Beads

Analyte	Assay type	Tracer	Fraction measured	Reference
Albumin	FIA	FITC/Ag	Free	196
hIgG	FIA	FITC/Ag	Free	195, 1063
β_1-glycoprot.	FIA	FITC/Ag	Free	1064
Cortisol	FIA	FITC/Ag	Bound	1065
Progesterone	FIA	FITC/Ag	Bound	1021
17-OH-Prog.	FIA	FITC/Ag	Bound	1066
Estradiol	FIA	FITC/Ag	Bound	1067
Thyroxine	FIA	FITC/Ag	Bound	1068, 1069
Bile acids	FIA	FITC/Ag	Bound	1070
Gentamicin	FIA	FITC/Ag	Bound	1071
Phenytoin	FIA	FITC/Ag	Bound	1072
Carbamazepine	FIA	FITC/Ag	Bound	1073
Primidone	FIA	FITC/Ag	Bound	491, 1074
Primaquine	FIA	FITC/Ag	Free	1075, 1076
Theophylline	FIA	FITC/Ag	Bound	14
Quinine	FIA	DTAF/Ag	Bound	1077
Propranolol	FIA	FITC/Ag	Bound	1078
Haloperidol	FIA	FITC/Ag	Bound	1079
Bendazac	FIA	FITC/Ag	Bound	1080
Flecainamide	FIA	FITC/Ag	Bound	1081
Cannabinoids	FIA	FITC/Ag	Bound	1067, 1082
Morphine	FIA	FITC/Ag	Bound	1083
CRP	FIA	FITC/Ag	Bound	1084
	IFMA	FITC/Ab	Bound	1084, 1085
HPL	IFMA	FITC/Ab	Free	1086

The third technique used in FIAs on microbeads is the use of filtration to separate beads from the reaction mixture, to wash them, and even to concentrate the beads on a suitable surface area for measurement. This type of filtration technique is commercialized by Pandex (Pandex Division of Baxter Healthcare Co.) in its particle concentration FIA (PC-FIA), introduced by Jolley et al. (548). The system utilizes small (0.8 μm) latex beads (Epicon particles) covalently coupled with antibodies through surface carboxylic acids. The Pandex system can also use human or microbial cells as solid-phases for screening antibodies against cell surface antigens (Table 8.6). Competitive PC-FIAs generally use B-phycoerythrin–labeled antigens, whereas sandwich assays are performed with fluorescein-labeled antibodies. After immunoreaction, the beads are separated and washed in filter-bottomed plates, and the beads on the filter are measured with a front-surface fluorometer, the Pandex Screen Machine™.

Table 8.6. Filtration of Beads in Fluorescence Immunoassays

System	Assay type	Analyte	Solid-Phase	Tracer	Reference
PC-FIA	FIA	Digoxin	Bead/Ab	PE/Ag	1088
	FIA	Drugs/Horses	Bead/Ab	PE/Ag	735, 1089, 1090
	FIA	Drug of abuse	Bead/Ab	PE/Ag	736
	FIA	Cocaine	Bead/Ab	PE/Ag	1091
	IFMA	Interleukin-4	Bead/Ab	FITC/Ab	1092
	IFMA	α_1-antitrypsin	Bead/Ab	FITC/Ab	1093
	IFMA	Prostaglandin	Bead/Ab		1094
	IFMA	Virus-Ab	Bead/Ab	FITC-Vir	1095
	IFMA	HIV protein	Bead/Ab	FITC/Ab	1096
	IFMA	MAb screening	H.cells	FITC/Ab	198, 1097–1100
	IFMA	Anti A type	Bead/Ag	FITC/Ab	1101
	IFMA	Membrane prot.	Lymphocytes	B-PE/S-avid	1102
	IFMA	IgG subclass	Bead/Ab	FITC/Ab	1103–1106
	IFMA	Anti-TMEV[a]	Bead/Ab	FITC/Ab	1105, 1107
	QIF	Bact.-Ag	Bact. cell	FITC/Ab	1108
	IFMA	Ab screening	*E. coli*	FITC/Ab	1109
Filtrat.	FIA	Estradiol	Sepharose/Ag	RBITC/Ab	430
Filtrat.	IFMA	Preg. zone pr.	Sepharose/Ab	FITC/Ab	1110
	IFMA	Ferritin	Glass bead/Ab		1111

[a]Theiler's murine encephalomyelitis virus.

Beads or cells may also be fixed to a solid matrix, either before or after the primary immunoreaction. For example, the Abbott IM_X system utilizes microparticles captured in glass-fiber cartridges (Chapter 9.2.2). Fixing cells or beads is generally done in qualitative or quantitative IF tests—for instance, in the determination of antibody responses against microbial agents (1087).

8.2.6. Separation with Coated Surfaces

The introduction of antibody-coated tube technology for RIA in 1967 by Catt and Tregear (148) proved to be a crucial point in the evolution of immunoassay technology. Coated tubes, balls, and coated microtitration plates have rapidly gained increasing application as easy and efficient manifolds for immunoreactions and have especially been used for enzyme immunoassays based on either photometric, fluorometric, or luminometric detection (and recently also in some FIAs, such as TR-FIAs) (Chapter 8.4).

In coated tube FIAs (or FIAs with coated microtitration wells) the surface bound fluorescence is most often measured after redissolving it into a specifically optimized measurement solution, and only a few direct tube-surface measuring systems have been developed so far. Elution of the labeled reagent can be accomplished with alkaline aqueous solution, alkaline methanol, or alkaline detergent (e.g., SDS) solution. Alternatively, only the labels are dissociated, as in the assays using liposomes as fluorochrome carriers or in dissociative fluorescence-enhanced time-resolved FIAs (Chapter 8.4.1).

One widely used "conventional" solid-phase FIA system, the IDT FIAX StiQ™ system (International Diagnostic Technology, Santa Clara, CA), is based on a special paddle-shaped dipstick sampler, StiQ™, containing an activated cellulose acetate/nitrate disc (1112). The activated membrane serves to immobilize the antigen for the assay of circulating antibodies and for competitive assays or to immobilize antibodies for noncompetitive assays. Another side of the disc can be used for monitoring the background fluorescence and nonspecific binding of the labeled reagent. A typical assay run involves coating the sampler (or the use of ready coated samplers), incubating it with the sample, washing, incubating with the labeled reagent, washing, and measuring the bound fluorescence with a front-surface fluorometer (IDT FIAX-100 or FIAX 400 fluorometer of Whittaker Bioproducts Inc., Walkersville, MD). The technology has primarily been applied for assays of circulating antibodies, but it has also been tested for some competitive assays (Table 8.7).

Other commercial FIA systems using a solid surface or a three-dimensional matrix include the IMMPULSE™ system, the TRACK XI® Diagnostic System (Microbiological Associates Inc., MD), and a Sep-FIA of the automated random-access system, OPUS of PB Diagnostic System (Table 8.8).

Table 8.7. Applications of the FIAX System

Analyte	Assay	Tracer	Solid reagent	Reference
Immunoglobulins	FIA	FITC-Ab	Ag	1113, 1114
	IFMA	FITC-Ab	Ab	1050, 1115, 1116
CSF-IgG	FIA	FITC-Ab	Ag	1117
CSF-albumin	FIA	FITC-Ab	Ag	1117
IgE	IFMA	FITC-Ab	Ab	1118, 1119
Rheumatoid factor	IFMA	FITC-Ab	IgG	1120–1122
Immunocomplexes	IFMA	FITC-Ab	C1q	94
	IFMA	FITC-Ab	Ab	1123
C-3 component	FIA	FITC-Ab	Ag	1124, 1125
C-4 component	FIA	FITC-Ab	Ag	1124, 1126
C-reactive prot.	IFMA	FITC-Ab	Ab	1121
Factor VIII-Ag	FIA	FITC-Ab	Ag	1127
Anti-actin IgG/IgM	IFMA	FITC-Ab	Ag	1128
Anti-DNA-Ab (ANA)	IFMA	FITC-Ab	Ag	1129–1132
Anti-M_2 Ab	IFMA	FITC-Ab	Ag	1133
Anti-rubella-Ab/IgG	IFMA	FITC-Ab	Ag	1134–1139
Anti-rubella-Ab/IgM	IFMA	FITC-Ab	Ag	1140
Anti-toxoplasma-Ab	IFMA	FITC-Ab	Ag	1141–1146
Anti-cytomegalov.-Ab	IFMA	FITC-Ab	Ag	368, 1147
Anti-measles-Ab	IFMA	FITC-Ab	Ag	1148
Anti-herpes simplex-Ab	IFMA	FITC-Ab	Ag	368, 1147, 1149
Anti-varicella z.-Ab	IFMA	FITC-Ab	Ag	1150
Anti-pasteurella-Ab	IFMA	FITC-Ab	Ag	1151, 1152
Anti-dirofilaria-Ab	IFMA	FITC-Ab	Ag	1153
Anti-candida-Ab	IFMA	FITC-Ab	Ag	1154, 1155
Anti-treponemal-Ab	IFMA	FITC-Ab	Ag	1156
Anti-streptococcus-Ab	IFMA	FITC-Ab	Ag	1157
Anti-borrelia B.-Ab	IFMA	FITC-Ab	Ag	1158, 1159
Anti-legionella-Ab	IFMA	FITC-Ab	Ag	1160
Anti-amoeba-Ab	IFMA	FITC-Ab	Ag	1161
Anti-brucella Ab	IFMA	FITC-Ab	Ag	1162
Tobramycin	FIA	FITC-Ag	Ab	1163–1165

Coated tubes are also used in some analyses utilizing IMMPULSE instrumentation, such as assays of thyroxine, digoxin, and TSH (572, 1166, 1167). A similar technology was applied by other authors using coated tubes or microtitration plates as solid surfaces (Table 8.8). For example, Elliot et al. (938) used digoxin-activated liposomes entrapped with sulforhodamine in an assay, where the bound fraction of tracer was lysed with detergent.

Table 8.8. Solid-Phase Separation FIAs

Analyte	Assay	Tracer	Solid-phase	Reference
Thyroxine	FIA	FITC-Ag	Ab-coated tube	572
	FIA	Coproporph.-Ab	Ag-coated wells	715
Digoxin	FIA	FITC-Ag	Ab-coated tube	1166
	FIA	Coproporph.-Ab	Ag-coated wells	716
TSH	IFMA	FITC-Ab	Ab-coated tube	1167
Histone-Ab	IFMA	FITC-Ab	Ag-coated tube	179
Glucagon-Ab	IFMA	FITC-Ab	Ag-coated tube	1168
HIV-Ab	IFMA	FITC-Ab	Ag-coated well	492
Ferritin	IFMA	FITC-Ab	Ab-coated well	1169
Digoxin	FIA	Liposome/ Rhodam/Ag	Ab-coated tube	938
RIgG	FIA	Coproporph.-Ag	Ab-coated tube	713
Infl.-A	FIA	Coproporph.-Ab	Analyte coating	714
Brucella-Ab	IFMA	FITC-Ab	Ag-Collimmune	551
Hepatitis-Ab	IFMA	FITC-Ab	Ag-Collimmune	1170
Sendai v-Ab	IFMA	FITC-Ab	Ag-Collimmune	1171
CRP	IFMA	FITC-Ab	Ab-PVC matrix	1172
Thyroxine	FIA	Rhodam.-Ag	Ab-coated film	583, 585
Theophylline	FIA	Rhodam.-Ag	Ab-coated film	585, 1173
Phenytoin	FIA	Rhodam.-Ag	Ab-coated film	1174
Carbamazepine	FIA	Rhodam.-Ag	Ab-coated film	1175
Valproic acid	FIA	Rhodam.-Ag	Ab-coated film	1176
Gentamicin	FIA	Rhodam.-Ag	Ab-coated film	1177
AFP	IFMA	FITC-Ab	Ab-coated metal	159
HBsAg	IFMA	FITC-Ab	Ab-coated metal	1178

The TRACK XI® Diagnostic System (Microbiological Associates Inc., Bethesda, MD) is based on a three-dimensional solid matrix containing reagent wells coated with a spongelike rehydrable, swellable structure composed of acrylic resin (Collimmune®), patented by Harte et al. (1179). The matrix contains additional scattering TiO_2 particles and colored phthalocyanine particles, which can specifically scatter the excitation light and are used to decrease background fluorescence. Fluorescences of the company's proprietary fluorochrome (excitation at 420 nm and emission at 570 nm) is measured with a front-surface fluorometer. According to the published articles, the system is primarily used for serological tests of serum antibodies (Table 8.8).

A porous PVC, paper, or cellulose matrix was used in FIA in order to accelerate the immunoreaction with short diffusion distances in a system introduced by Glad (1172), which he named an immunocapillary migration assay.

A way to decrease background interference—especially that caused by scattering during surface measurement—is to use clear polished metal surfaces as solid-phases, surfaces which efficiently reflect the excitation beam. By adjusting the emission collection angle, the effect of scattering can be diminished. Wang et al. (159, 1178, 1180) have utilized this "space-resolved" fluorometric technology in FIAs of alpha-fetoprotein and hepatitis-B surface antigen.

The OPUS system is a fully automated random-access (Chapter 6.7.5) analyzing system employing direct solid-phase competitive FIA for small molecular weight analytes. (Large size analytes and analytes requiring high sensitivity are performed with a fluorometric EIA, ELFIA.) The competitive FIA, "dry chemistry multilayer immunoassay test," is based on three polysaccharide layers coated on a plastic holder. The first layer provides the assay buffer and stabilizers, the reaction layer contains immobilized low affinity antibodies preincubated with fluorescent analyte tracers, and the optical barrier layer absorbs the released tracer. This test principle is used primarily in drug assays (Table 8.8).

8.3. NONSEPARATION FLUOROIMMUNOASSAYS

Nonseparation immunoassays can be defined as immunoassays in which the extent of antibody-antigen reaction can be determined without physical separation of the free fraction from the bound fraction. The term *homogeneous reaction* can be used for any class of chemical reaction that takes place completely in one phase, and accordingly "real" homogeneous FIAs are assays in which the antibody-antigen reaction causes a change in some of the fluorescence properties that makes it possible to monitor the extent of the reaction at any time from the homogeneous reaction mixture. There are a number of nonseparation immunoassays that strictly taken are not homogeneous, such as nephelometric techniques, particle-counting assays, flow-cytometric assays, liposome assays, and various types of "space-resolved" FIAs. In practical terms those assays can be as simple to perform as the real homogeneous assays and are often classified as homogeneous assays because no manual or mechanical separation steps are needed.

The desire for simple homogeneous assays, originally considered impossible with radioisotopic tracers, has been one of the driving forces in developing non-isotopic assay techniques. An easy-to-use assay, which ultimately can be as simple as mixing the sample with a premixed solution of antibody and labeled antigen and measuring the resulting signal, could be easily decentralized for out-patient clinics or bedside tests, into patients' homes, or ultimately utilized in *in vivo* monitoring of analytes with immunosensors.

Homogeneous assays which contain a minimal number of manipulation steps are also easy to automate, and many of the present homogeneous FIAs are automated by using existing clinical chemistry automates (Chapter 6.7.3). Minimizing manipulations also eliminates imprecisions derived from manual steps, and accordingly homogeneous assays, in principle, can produce more precise results. In current homogeneous assays, reactant concentrations are relatively high, and accordingly the assay kinetics are rapid. Rapid results are also needed in some drug assays—in emergency situations, for example.

Despite the simplicity and speed, homogeneous assays also bring along inevitable drawbacks, some of which are summarized in Table 8.1. The most serious limitation is the inferior sensitivity of homogeneous assays and their vulnerability to matrix variations. The presence of endogenous fluors in samples, or highly fluorescent compounds derived, for instance, from medication—even fluorescein is used as a drug (1181)—the high absorptivity of hemolytic and icteric samples, the turbidity and scattering of lipemic samples, and the nonspecific binding characteristics of serum proteins, etc., can interfere with homogeneous assays. Because all the interfering factors of samples are present when the signal is measured, these need to be eliminated. Currently sample interferences are predominately avoided simply by sample dilution, but various sample pretreatments are also frequently applied, such as protein precipitations, analyte extractions, protease treatments, and treatments with various chemicals (Chapter 5.4.5).

The majority of homogeneous assay technologies are well suited only for small molecular weight analytes, haptens, and thus require competitive assay design. That restricts the application of the technology, and competitive assay design itself also restricts the potential sensitivity and dynamic range attainable. Because of these limitations—in addition to the dilution needed to avoid matrix effects as well as the more restricted signal collection—homogeneous assays generally achieve clearly less sensitive analysis than heterogeneous assays. A majority of the technologies can measure analytes present in samples at least at nanomolar concentrations. The assay of serum digoxin, for example, is at the sensitivity borderline for many homogeneous technologies.

The homogeneous assay principle was introduced earlier than the respective heterogeneous principles. As early as 1953 and 1954, Stavitsky et al. (122–124) used erythrocytes activated with insulin in a homogeneous complement lysis assay of insulin. The first fluorescence-based homogeneous immunoassays were developed by Dandliker, who during the 1960s measured antibodies by following the fluorescence polarization changes of fluorescein-labeled antigens upon binding to their antibodies (277, 279, 280). In the early 1970s fluorescence polarization immunoassays (FPIA) were developed for haptenic antigen determinations. That technique fell into disfavor, however, and it was about 20 years before FPIA reached routine clinical laboratories—when Abbott adopted the technology and developed clinical instruments and numerous kits based on FPIA technology.

Today numerous homogeneous assay principles have been introduced. Several technologies are commercialized and have found quite extensive applications in certain areas, especially in measuring drugs (therapeutic drug monitoring, TDM, and tests for illicit drugs).

8.3.1. Fluorescence Polarization Immunoassays

The efficiency of light absorption by a fluorophore is dependent on the angle between the electronic dipole of the exciting light and the absorption oscillators of the molecule. A polarized light will excite only those molecules that have their absorption oscillators parallel to the plane of exciting light. The polarization level of the resultant emission depends on the lifetime of the excited state (τ) and the rotational motion of the molecule. For steady-state measurement polarization is generally expressed by the Perrin equation (Eq. 8.1) (1182).

$$(1/p - 1/3) = (1/p_o - 1/3)(1 + 3\tau/p) \tag{8.1}$$

The rotational relaxation time, p, can be calculated for a spherical molecule according to Equation 8.2.

$$p = 3\,\eta\, v/kT \tag{8.2}$$

Rotational relaxation time is directly proportional to the volume of the molecule (size and shape) and viscosity (η) of the medium.

A large molecule, such as an antibody, has a tumbling time typically around 10 to 100 ns, whereas small molecules, such as haptens, have tumbling times around 0.1 to 1 ns. In steady-state polarization measurement (continuous excitation with polarized light), the resulting polarization of emission depends on the size and shape of the labeled substance and the ratio of rotational relaxation time to the decay time of the fluorochrome. This forms the basis for measuring binary binding reactions—for example, in immunoreaction.

To be practical for an immunoassay, the change in molecular volumes during the immunoreaction needs to be high enough, such as it is during the binding of the haptenic tracer to its antibodies. It gives a practical limit for the size of antigen, which should be below 20,000. The decay time of the fluorophore needs to be longer than the rotational time of the haptenic tracer but shorter than the rotational time of the formed complex. Fluorescein (τ:

4.5 ns) accordingly works very well for normal FPIA, the polarization of which increases drastically upon the binding of the fluorescein-labeled hapten to the respective antibodies.

For large antigens, fluorochromes with somewhat longer decay times have been tested. With proteins the intramolecular tumbling becomes problematic, however, when using steady-state measuring (1183). So far no applications have been made using large binding entities (e.g., microbeads) and long τ probes.

In addition to the size limitations of FPIA, problems arise also from the low affinity nonspecific binding properties of serum proteins, especially that of albumin, which increases the polarization level nonspecifically. To avoid the albumin effect, a simple dilution jump has been used (1184), or various sample pretreatments are required. In the pretreatment solutions either chaotropic ions, proteolytic enzymes, protein precipitating reagents, or solvents are used. The pretreatment of samples is especially needed for analytes that require a high sensitivity that does not allow for high dilutions.

The principle of fluorescence polarization was developed by Perrin in 1926 (1182). About 30 years later, in 1952, the technology was applied in biological systems by Weber (1185). For monitoring immunoreactions, the fluorescence polarization technique has been used since 1961, since the pioneering work of Dandliker et al. (277), who studied the interaction of fluorescein-labeled penicillin (279), ovalbumin (280), and estrone (1186) with their specific binding proteins or receptors. Dandliker has also written a number of review articles about the principle and applications of fluorescence polarization (282, 1184, 1187).

The experimental studies of FPIA during the 1960s and 1970s were conducted with research fluorometers equipped with polarization accessories and have resulted in a limited number of clinical applications (Table 8.9), mainly because of the lack of appropriate instruments for routine assays.

Table 8.9. Early Applications of Fluorescence Polarization in Protein Binding Assays

Analyte	Tracer	Assay type	Reference
Anti-penicillin-Ab	FITC-Penicillin	Direct	279
Estrone receptor	FITC-Estrone	Direct	1186
Anti-ovalbumin-Ab	FITC-Ovalbumin	Direct	280
Anti-Conalbumin-Ab	FITC-Conalbumin	Direct	281
Trypsin	FITC-Casein	Direct	283
Anti-insulin-Ab	FITC-Insulin	Direct	283
hCG	FITC-hCG	Competitive	282, 1188
Fungicides	FITC-Ag	Competitive	1189

Table 8.10. Applications of TD_X

	Analyte	Reference	Evaluation
Antibiotics			
	Gentamicin	1192	1193–1196
	Tobramycin	1192	
	Amikacin	1192	1197
	Streptomycin	1198	
	Netilmicin		1195, 1199
	Isopamicin		1200
	Vancomycin		1201
	Astromicin		1202
Anticonvulsants			
	Phenytoin	365, 1203	1194, 1204, 1205
	Phenobarbital	365, 1203	1194, 1204
	Carbamazepine		1204, 1206, 1207
	Valproic acid		1204, 1208
Antiarrhythmics			
	Quinidine/free		1209, 1210
	Hydroquinidine		1211
	Lidocaine		1212
	Disopyramide/free	1213	
	MEGX	1214	
Other drugs			
	Theophylline	1215, 1216	1194, 1217, 1218
	Digoxin		1194, 1219–1221
	Methyldigoxin	1222	
	Benzodiazepine	1223	1224, 1225
	Flecainamide		1226
	Paracetamol		1227
	Methotrexate		1228
	Cyclosporine	1229–1231	1232–1243
Illicit drugs			
	Morphine	1244	
	Amphetamine	1245	1246
	MHPG	560	
	Barbiturates		1247
	Opiates		1247
	Cocaine metab.	1248	1249–1251
Hormones			
	Thyroxine (T_4)	1252	1253, 1254
	FT_4		1253
	T_3	1255	
	T uptake	1256	
	Cortisol		1257

Table 8.10. Applications of TD_x *(continued)*

	Analyte	Reference	Evaluation
Hormones			
	Free cortisol/U		1258
	Estriol	1259	
	OH-indole acetate	1260	
Proteins and peptides			
	Angiotensin	1261	
	CRP	1262	1263, 1264
	Transferrin		1265

Wider usage of competitive FPIA in clinical routine started during the early 1980s, when Abbott introduced an automated instrument designed for clinical FPIA applications (455, 456, 1190). With instruments of various stages of automation (TD_x, AD_x and IM_x) and over 50 different kits, FPIA has become one of the most used FIA in clinical chemistry (379, 1191). Lately Abbott has been accompanied by other reagent and instrument manufacturers, such as Roche Diagnostics, CANAM Diagnostics, Colony, Sankyo, Innotron of Oregon Inc. (INNOFLUOR™ FPIA), Polymed Co. and Source Scientific Systems (Focus™ FPIA fluorometer).

The reagent pack of TD_x generally contains a pretreatment solution, antiserum, and antigen labeled with a fluorescein derivative. The instrument performs the required dilutions, records the blank value to be substracted, and measures the final polarization level. The technology is used primarily in TDM and screening for illicit drugs, but it is also used for some hormones and even for a few proteins, such as globulins, transferrin, and CRP. Table 8.10 summarizes examples of the articles describing FPIA applications performed on TD_x, AD_x, or the automated IM_x, including the numerous evaluations of the existing kits and other FPIA applications of the TD_x instrument. Some of the assays, such as the assay of cyclosporine, have sparked a great number of evaluations, partly collected in the table.

The research group of Prof. Landon has developed FPIAs since 1976 (1266) and has developed analytical applications for the determination of hormones and drugs. They have been able to simplify the technology further by using a one-step, one-reagent method based on antibodies pre-equilibrated with FITC-labeled antigens. By adjusting the respective affinities so that ligand displacement can take place rapidly, this LIDIA principle provides an extremely simple and rapid analysis. Assays are performed with various research fluorometers, including the Perkin Elmer LS 20 Polarization Fluorometer particularly developed for clinical routine assays (457). FPIA applications performed with homemade reagents are listed in Table 8.11.

Table 8.11. Research Applications of FPIA

	Analyte	Label	Reference
TDM			
	Gentamicin	FITC	1266
	Phenytoin	FITC	372
	Phenytoin	2-Naphthol-sulfonamide	390
	Valproic acid	FITC	1267
	Paracetamol	FITC	487, 1268
	Quinine	FITC	1269
	Theophylline	FITC	489
	Theophylline	Umbelliferyl	672
	Salicylate	FITC	1270
Illicit drugs			
	Opiates	FITC	345
	Amphetamine	FITC	486, 1271
	Methamphetamine	FITC	344, 488
	Benzoylecgonine	FITC	490
	Barbiturates	FITC	1272–1274
	Vanillylmandelate	FITC	1275
	Azidothymidine	FITC	1276
Hormones			
	Cortisol	FITC	370, 373, 1277
	Biopterin	FITC	1278
	Neopterin	FITC	1278
	Deoxycortisol	FITC	1279
	Estradiol	Fluorescein	19
	Estriol	Lucifer Yellow	688
	Testosterone	Lucifer Yellow	688

New manufacturers producing FPIA kits have recently emerged. The kits are intended to be measured either with the existing Abbott TD_X system or with the manufacturer's own instrument, such as the Roche FPIA, developed for the company's Cobas Bio and Cobas Fara chemistry automates. At the moment, alternative products are concentrated in drug monitoring (Table 8.12).

Relatively little effort has been used to develop FPIAs for larger molecules such as proteins. The problems with proteins are related to their large size and their flexibility, as well as the lower sensitivity and more narrow dynamic range obtainable. TD_X has, however, been applied to some proteins, such as globulins, ferritin, and CRP (Table 8.10) and to analytes that do not require high sensitivities.

Table 8.12. Alternative Commercial FPIA Assays

Analyte	Company	Reference
Gentamicin	Roche Diag.	1280
	IBC, Innotron Diag.	1281
Tobramycin	Roche Diag.	1280
	IBC, Innotron Diag.	1281
Vancomycin	Roche Diag.	565
Phenytoin	Roche Diag.	566, 1282
	IBC, Innotron Diag.	1281
Phenobarbital	Roche Diag.	566
	IBC, Innotron Diag.	1281
Carbamazepine	Roche Diag.	566
Theophylline	Roche Diag.	1280, 1283
	CANAM	1281
	IBC, Innotron Diag.	1281
	Colony	1284
Quinidine	Roche Diag.	566, 1282, 1285
Primidone	Roche Diag.	1286
Digoxin	Roche Diag.	1287
Procainamide	Roche Diag.	566, 1282
NAPA	Roche Diag.	566
Dilantin	Roche Diag.	1280

Urios et al. (1188) have made an FPIA for urine hCG using FITC-labeled hCG as the tracer. Reportedly they observed a rather wide dynamic range in the assay—from 0.27 to 64 μg/ml. Yamaguchi et al. (501) were able to measure insulin with a competitive FPIA with a dynamic range from 40 to 600 mU/ml, but only from pure insulin preparations and not from serum samples. A similar insulin FPIA has also been tested by Nithipatikom and McGown (1288), who studied the fluorescence intensity changes, decay-time changes, and polarization changes of FITC-labeled insulin during the immunoreaction. Assays of smaller peptides, such as angiotensin (1261) and neocarzinostatin (454), can be developed more easily.

One approach toward protein FPIAs has been the development of fluorescent probes with longer decay times. Dansyl and umbelliferone derivatives have been tested for FPIA of CK-MB (617). The longer decay-time emitter, dansyl derivative, proved to be too flexible to give an acceptable polarization level. Urios and Cittanova used Lucifer Yellow as a label in a direct assay of IgM (1289). The assay was based on a smaller binding unit, the Fab-fragment of a monoclonal antibody, labeled with the fluorophore and used as a direct reagent for the larger antigen, IgM.

8.3.2. Release Fluoroimmunoassays

Release fluoroimmunoassays are based on labeled antigens rendered nonfluorescent by suitable enzymatically removable groups. Hydrolysis of the bond, typically the ester or glycoside bond at position 7 on the coumarine structure, recovers a fluorescent product. Accordingly the requirements, and to a great extent also the structures, for those labeling reagents are identical to those for fluorogenic substrates (Chapter 7.6).

There are two main variations of release FIA, which appear to be contradictory with each other: antibody-enhanced hydrolysis (employing ester bonds) and a more widely used enzyme hydrolyzed antibody protected FIA called SL-FIA (substrate-labeled FIA) which primarily utilizes glycoside bonded substituents. While the first is based on an enzymelike hydrolytic activity of antibodies, the second uses additional enzymes and the steric hindrance of antibodies inhibiting the action of the enzymes.

In SL-FIA the tracer is an antigen labeled with a fluorogenic substrate. The components of SL-FIA are almost identical to those of ELFIA: an enzyme (esterase or β-galactosidase), a fluorogenic substrate, and an antibody. The actual assay system is, however, opposite that of ELFIA; the substrate and not the enzyme is coupled to the immunoreagent and is used in limited concentrations, while enzymes are in excess. The limited amount of specific antibodies produces the steric hindrance in the bound fraction of the tracer, which inhibits the action of the added enzymes so that only the free fraction contributes to the signal.

SL-FIA was originally developed by Burd et al. (673) in 1977. In their early work they used both umbelliferone-labeled biotin and fluorescein-labeled dinitrophenol as tracers, both labeled through an ester bond. Porcine esterase was used as the hydrolyzing enzyme, but in both cases they noticed increased nonenzymatical hydrolysis caused by avidin and anti-DNP antibodies. All the subsequent applications have been made using β-galactosidase and antigens labeled with umbelliferone, coupled with galactose at position 7 as the substrate (1290, 1291). As compared to ester linkage, the glycoside bond has the benefits of lower serum interference (serum has high esterase activity), more stable linkage and less spontaneous release (lower background), a lack of antibody-induced hydrolysis, and a more stable enzyme (674). Upon hydrolysis the absorptivity of the conjugate is shifted from 343 to 403 nm with simultaneous increase of ε (from 18,000 to 28,000). The overall fluorescence increase is nine- to twelvefold, and, when taking into account the shifted wavelengths, there is practically no background fluorescence with an unhydrolyzed substrate when measured at the wavelength of the product (1290, 1292).

Ames (Ames Division, Miles Laboratories, Elkhart, IN) has commercialized the SL-FIA technique with numerous kits, primarily developed for therapeutic drug monitoring, but also for some proteins. In the early applications various research fluorometers were used prior to the development of the company's filter fluorometer, Fluorostat™, specifically designed for SL-FIA. Table 8.13 lists the published applications of SL-FIA and some of the kit evaluations of Ames TD_A assays.

A rapid dry-reagent strip procedure has also been developed with use of the SL-FIA principle, based on reagents dried on a filter paper (1310). The antibody and tracer are either precomplexed (LIDIA) or precomplexing is avoided by adding tracer to the paper in organic solvent (576). This assay format results in very simple and rapid analysis; for instance, the final fluorescence is measured after three minutes of incubation after the addition of 35 μl of the diluted sample (1324).

As a simple homogeneous assay, SL-FIA has also been automated with existing chemistry automates. The Technicon II AutoAnalyzer is used for SL-FIA of theophylline (569), the Kontron SFM 25 for automation of theophylline and valproic acid tests (503), the Cobas Bio centrifugal analyzer for

Table 8.13. Applications of TD_A SL-FIA

Analyte	Reference	Evaluation
Tobramycin	1293, 1294	1295, 1296
Gentamicin	674, 1293, 1297	1295, 1298
Kanamycin	1293	
Amikacin	1293, 1299	
Netilmicin	1293, 1300	1199
Sisomycin	1293	
Phenytoin	1292, 1293	1301-1304
Phenobarbital	1293, 1305	1301, 1302
Primidone	1293, 1306	1302, 1307
Carbamazepine	485	1302, 1307, 1308
Theophylline	1293, 1309, 1310	1302, 1311-1313
Quinidine		1301
Procainamide		1314
Disopyramide		1315
Valproic acid	1316	1317
Dibecacin	1318	
Caffeine	1319	
Ethosuximide		1320
Human albumin	1321	
hIgG	1322	
hIgM	1323	

automation of theophylline, phenytoin, and phenobarbital assays (568), and the MULTISTAT III analyzer for phenytoin, phenobarbital, carbamazepine, and theophylline assays (1325).

In addition to the commercially exploited Ames SL-FIA, some publications describe variations of the technology without further applications. Li and Burd (695) tested FMN as a fluorogenic substrate coupled to theophylline via an AMP linker, which allows the use of pyrophosphatase as the releasing enzyme. Dean et al. (1326) have developed a double-label SL-FIA procedure based on β-galactosyl-coumarin–labeled phenobarbital and 4-methylcoumarin-phosphodiester–labeled phenytoin. With the use of two enzymes, β-galactosidase and phosphodiesterase, both released labels can be measured from the same solution with appropriate filters. O'Neal et al. (968) used acetoxynaphthalene sulfonamide as a long Stokes' shift probe for labeling phenytoin and porcine esterase as the releasing enzyme in the SL-FIA. In this assay serum endogeneous esterase activity was eliminated by destroying it prior to assay.

Since the discovery of the enzymelike activity of antibodies and avidin by Burd et al. (673) during the early work on SL-FIA with ester bonds, antibody augmented esterase activity was also evaluated in release FIAs by Kohen et al. 17-α-hydroxyprogesterone was conjugated with an ester bond to umbelliferone (967), and testosterone was linked to umbelliferone with a thioether bond (1327), for an antibody-enhanced hydrolysis assay of the haptens. Ester-bond hydrolyzing activity was also noticed with a monoclonal antibody against DNP, where the hydrolysis was more stoichiometric than actually catalytic due to the slow dissociation of the hydrolysis product, DNP (1328). Kohen et al. (966) have also labeled estriol with NAD to be detected with an enzymatic-cycling reaction by fluorometric measurement of formed NADPH.

8.3.3. Fluorescence-Quenching and Enhancement Immunoassays

Homogeneous fluorescence-quenching and fluorescence-enhancement immunoassays are straightforward applications of the fact that most fluorescent probes are sensitive to their environment reflected in their fluorescent properties. Changes in their environment, such as a change in polarity, when labeled haptenic antigen is bound to antibodies, a change in dielectric strength, hydrogen bonding, pH, rotational freedom, viscosity, the vicinity of energy donating or accepting groups, quenching atoms or absorbing groups, etc., produces changes in some of their fluorescent properties, in wavelengths, quantum yield or decay times—changes which allow for immunoreaction monitoring directly from the homogeneous reaction mixture.

Despite a number of published articles—and even the existence of one kit in the past—these direct enhancement or quenching assays have not become widely used. The effect is relatively uncommon, sometimes unpredictable, and usually dependent on the antibody batch used. The technology has been further standardized by employing antibodies directed against the fluorophores used as additional signal modulating components. This indirect quenching FIA attracted much attention in the 1970s and early 1980s, resulting in a number of patents (1329–1332), but has not produced further applications so far. Still another way to improve the signal modulation is to apply quenching or energy accepting groups in other components of immunoreaction (see FETI, Chapter 8.3.4).

Two principles have been used for fluorescence-enhancement immunoassays: an assay based on a polarity sensitive fluorescent probe and an assay based on antibody alleviated heavy atom quenching within an antigen-fluor conjugate. A typical environmentally sensitive fluorescent probe, such as a dansyl derivative and ANS, exhibits remarkable fluorescence enhancement upon binding to protein surfaces or antibodies. The principle has been used to study antigen-antibody reaction kinetics with use of a dansyl group as the antigenic hapten (1333). Rezaei-Poor Kardost et al. (641, 642) used 1-naphthylamine-5-sulfonic acid–labeled nucleotides as tracers for a homogeneous assay of antinuclear antibodies. In the test antibody binding was manifested by 12- to 35-fold increase in the fluorescence quantum yield. Liburdy used N-(3-pyrene) maleimide–labeled anti-hIgG antibodies, the fluorescence of which was increased upon binding to hIgG as a result of a proposed pH change in the microenvironment (652, 653). Handley et al. (682) tested the suitability of MDPF and fluorescamine-labeled thyroxine for an enhancement FIA and achieved a steeper standard response with MDPF.

Even though fluorescein is generally quenched when bound to antibodies, an enhancement effect also has been reported with fluorescein-labeled estradiol (19), although the enhancement was not strong enough to be used for an actual immunoassay. Another example of enhancement FIA with a fluorescein-labeled hapten is the assay of thyroxine (1334). In this assay fluorescein is quenched by the four iodine atoms in T_4, and the quenching is partly alleviated upon binding of the tracer to anti-thyroxine antibodies.

Various fluorescence-quenching immunoassays have found somewhat wider applications, mainly because they employ the generally used fluorescein as the labeling reagent for haptenic antigens and methods have been further standardized by using indirect quenching assays.

A fluorescein-labeled gentamicin was the first tracer found to undergo fluorescence quenching upon binding to anti-gentamicin antibodies by Shaw et al. in 1977 (1335), and the respective assay is also patented by Smith (1336). The obtained fluorescence quenching is relatively small, however, when compared to background fluorescence of sample constituents, and the assay requires recording of the blank values for each sample separately.

Dilution of samples is also necessary to avoid the inner-filter effect. Gentamicin FQIA was commercialized by Technicon Instruments Ltd. (London, UK) and also automated using the Technicon AutoAnalyser (366). The FQIA of gentamicin was also available as a commercial kit (371, 1337, 1338).

The FQIA principle is applied to some other haptenic antigens, such as cortisol (369), netilmicin (1339), and cortisol with use of 17α-hydroxy-4,6,8 (14)-pregnatriene-3,20-dione as the fluorescent tracer undergoing quenching upon immunoreaction (1340).

The indirect quenching FIA (IQ-FIA) calls for the use of antibodies directed against the label (generally fluorescein), used as an additional signal modulating reagent, which makes the principle more generally applicable and suitable for larger (primarily only) antigens. Fluorescein is an efficient immunogenic hapten (594) against which antisera of high titer and affinity can be prepared easily (1341). The fluorescence of fluorescein is almost completely quenched (up to about 90%) upon binding to anti-fluorescein antibodies as a result of the vicinity of tryptophan and tyrosine amino acid residues near the antigen-binding sites (612, 1340–1342). As a result of the comparable high affinity of anti-fluorescein antibodies, indirect quenching FIAs are generally performed by sequential addition; the first reaction between analyte and specific antibodies is allowed to proceed to completion prior to the addition of anti-fluorescein for modulating the fluorescence of only the free-labeled antigen, not sterically protected. Regardless of the rather efficient quenching, in practical applications the intrinsic fluorescence of samples makes a significant contribution to the total signal, so background monitoring and correction is also needed in indirect quenching FIAs.

According to the authors of published papers, different names have been introduced for the same assay principle. Ullman called the assay *double-receptor FIA* because the assay consists of two receptor bindings simultaneously (1330). Smith et al. (1343) and Nargessi and Landon (1344) have named the technology *indirect quenching FIA* to emphasize its distinction from direct FQIA. Zuk et al. (1345) called his assay *fluorescence-protection immunoassay,* because the analyte-specific antibodies protect the FITC-labeled antigen from quenching by anti-fluorescein antibodies. A variation of the technology, "alternative binding FIA" describes the alternative binding of labeled antigen either to anti-analyte antibodies or to anti-fluorescein antibodies, which are coupled together to improve the steric exclusion (1343, 1346).

Nargessi, Landon, and Smith have developed indirect quenching FIAs for serum proteins albumin, IgG, and human placental lactogen (1344, 1347, 1348). Ullman et al. have described the use of fluorescein- and dansyl-labeled albumin, insulin, and morphine as tracers for indirect FQIA in a patent description (1330) and also used the principle in an assay of IgG (1345) and cardiolipin (1349). Even though indirect quenching FIA does not work as such for haptenic molecules, two variations have been developed for small antigens. Anti-analyte and anti-fluorescein antibodies coupled together to a complex are used in a competitive alternative-binding assay for thyroxine (1346). Yoshida has patented a principle composed of a support matrix where haptenic antigens were coupled and which functions as a spacer between antigen and fluorescein (1329). A rather similar principle was later used in an assay of phenytoin (644) with a polylysine as the carrier.

8.3.4. Fluorescence Energy-Transfer Immunoassays

Fluorescence energy (excitation) transfer immunoassays (FETI) make use of two labels coupled to immunoreagents, at least one of which is fluorescent while the other is an energy accepting or quenching group. The assay is based on the energy transfer between these two groups, if brought to close proximity as a result of an immunoreaction. Dipole-dipole energy transfer is dependent, among the others, on the degree of overlapping of the emission of the donor with the absorption of the acceptor, and on the sixth power of the distance between the two groups (Chapter 5.3). In practice this requirement means that energy can be transferred efficiently within a distance of about 10 nm and very inefficiently at greater separation distances.

FETI was first described by Ullman et al. in 1976 (552). The first assay used a fluorescein-labeled morphine as the energy donor for rhodamine-labeled antibodies. To maximize the quenching of fluorescence of the labeled morphine, antibodies were labeled with up to 15 rhodamine per IgG. Poor solubility of rhodamine, however, restricts the labeling level of antibodies. The technology was further developed by the Syva Co. (1350) and marketed with the company's automated Syva Advantage fluorometer. Considerable effort has been used to find suitable energy donor-acceptor pairs for FETI (621, 622, 1351). The 4′,5′-dimethoxy derivative of fluorescein has shown optimal spectral characteristics for an energy acceptor, good spectral overlapping with fluorescein, and practically no fluorescence of its own. Because of its negligible fluorescence, the background resulting from direct excitation of the acceptor probe is omitted. Subsequently, many FETI applications have been made using different fluorescein derivatives (carboxyfluorescein, FITC, DTAF, or various methoxy- and chloro-substituted fluoresceins) as the primary donor fluorochromes and dimethoxyfluorescein as the nonfluorescent acceptor (Table 8.14).

Besides fluorescein and rhodamine, a number of alternative labels have also been tested in the energy-transfer-based homogeneous FIAs (Table 8.14), including phycoerythrin (PE), pyrene, Texas Red, Lucifer Yellow, quinacrine, eosin, fluorescamine (FL), squaric acid, and gallocyanine.

Table 8.14. Fluorescence Energy Transfer Immunoassays[a]

Analyte	Donor	Acceptor	Reference
Morphine	FITC-Ag	TRITC-Ab	552
	FITC-Ag	Dimethoxy-fluor-Ab	1352
hIgG	FITC-Ag	TRITC-Ab	552
	PE-Ag	Pyrene-Ab	650
	FITC-Ag	PE-Ab	730
	PE-Ag	Texas Red-Ab	730
	Fluor-Ag	Dimethoxy-fluor-Ab	1353
hIgA	Fluor-Ag	TRITC-Ab	618, 1354
hIgM	Fluor-Ag	TRITC-Ab	1354, 1355
Light chains	FITC-Ag	TRITC-Ab	1356
C-3-comp.	FITC-Ag	TRITC-Ab	1357
CRP	FITC-Ag	TRITC-Ab	1358
Transferrin	FITC-Ag	Dimethoxy-fluor-Ab	1359
Retinol-BP	FITC-Ag	Dimethoxy-fluor-Ab	1360
Albumin	FITC-Ag	TRITC-Ab	542, 1361
	Lucifer Y.-Ag	RBITC-Ab	689
	FITC-Ag	Eosin-Ab	683
	Quinacrine-Ag	Eosin-Ab	683
Prealbumin	FITC-Ag	Dimethoxy-fluor-Ab	1362
TBG	FITC-Ag	TRITC-Ab	619
Thyroxine	FITC-Ag	TRITC-Ab	1363
T uptake	FITC-Ag	TRITC-Ab	1363
Cortisol	FITC-Ag	Dimethoxy-fluor-Ab	1364
Digoxin	PE-Ag	Fluor.-Ab	376
	Squaric.-Ag	Gallocyanine-Ab	696
Phenytoin	PE-Ag	Texas Red-Ab	71, 1365
Nortriptyline	FL-Ag	FITC-Ab	681

[a]Abbreviations: Fluor = fluorescein derivative other than FITC; FL = fluorescamine.

Black charcoal particles have also been tested as efficient "eclipsing" components (622, 1366). The heavy atom quenching caused by iodine is utilized to form a nonfluorescent energy acceptor for fluorescein (1367). Luedtke et al. (1368) used dansyl and N-fluorescyl derivatives as the donor-acceptor pair for a study of the distance between the antigen-binding sites within an antibody. Energy transfer between antigen-binding sites was evaluated also by using fluorescein- and rhodamine-labeled thyroxines, but the quenching level obtained (6.5%) was not sufficient for any practical immunoassay (1369). Morrison has utilized a time-resolved fluorometric detection of the energy transfer between the short decay-time acceptor (PE) and the long decay donor (pyrene derivative) to improve the signal-noise ratio by avoiding direct background of short duration (650). Wieder and Hale have patented an energy-transfer-based time-resolved FIA principle based on Ln-chelate labels and exemplified with an assay of theophylline (1370). Fluorescent Ln-chelate–labeled antigens are quenched by a suitable emission absorptive organic fluorochrome or suitable quenching heavy metal. Chelates were also used as labels in the patent of Stavrianopoulos et al. (81) describing an energy-transfer type of assay based on the use of a complement (C1q).

Also, luminogenic substances, such as derivatives of isoluminol, have been used as energy donors for FITC-labeled antibodies in developing energy-transfer immunoassays (601). In the assays, the primary energy is produced by a chemical reaction, and the assay is accordingly classified as a lumino-immunoassay, even though the final emission is produced by fluorescein.

8.3.5. Liposome Immunoassays

Liposomes have gained applications in many areas of the medical and biological sciences. They are used as carriers for small and large compounds, for the targeted delivery of drugs, for encapsulating various compounds, for stabilizing unstable compounds, and also for encapsulating signal producing compounds for immunoassays. Kinsky et al. (930–932) were the first to show that liposomes incorporating immunoreagents on their surface could be used as label carriers in immunoassays and that the liposomes taking part in immunoreaction and having immunocomplexes on their surfaces can be disrupted by the action of complement binding, resulting in the release of the encapsulated label. All types of marker substances have since then been entrapped in liposomes, including enzymes (1371, 1372), enzyme substrates (930, 1373), dyes (1374, 1375), electron spin labels (1376), radioactive tracers (1377), and fluorophores (646, 1378).

In fluorescence immunoassays, liposomes serve two purposes: to function as carriers for the plurality of labels to amplify the signal (see Chapter 7.5.3), and to offer a way to construct sensitive nonseparation FIAs, which, unlike most homogeneous assay principles, also work with large antigens. Heterogeneous liposome assays are generally based on liposome lysis and the release of the label with concomitant fluorescence enhancement, but in some applications the liposomes are measured without lysing. Homogeneous liposome assays are primarily based on the liposome-lysing effect of complement binding using a suitable animal serum as the source of the complement, but cytolysins such as mellitin also can be used as the lysing component—after coupling to a haptenic antigen, for instance (1250, 1379).

Liposomes are unilamellar or multilamellar vesicles of very different sizes corresponding to the procedures used for their production. They are made from mixtures of phospholipids, cholesterol, and fatty acids. Large unilamellar liposomes can be formed by, for example, reverse-phase evaporation (628, 1380), and their size distribution can be further adjusted by extrusion through membranes. Other methods used include sonification (925), microemulsification (1381), mechanical dispersion (922, 924), and freeze drying (923). Covalent and noncovalent activation of liposomes with immunoreagents, as well as the fluorescent probes used for encapsulation, are briefly descried in Chapter 7.5.3. The stability of liposomes (leaking of the marker) is generally problematic both for their use and storage. Liposome stability can be affected by choosing the right components, preparation method, and sizes (1381). Reduction with DTT has been found to stabilize formed liposomes (1382). Also, the hydrophilicity of encapsulated fluorescent probes is an important factor in determining the leakage rate. Weinstein et al. (1383) reported a half-time of 5 minutes for fluorescein-loaded liposomes at +5 °C, compared to a half-time of a few weeks with the more hydrophilic carboxyfluorescein. Fiechtner et al. (1384) synthesized a series of more hydrophilic fluorescein derivatives in order to further increase liposome stabilities and to form practical reagents for routine or even commercial liposome immunoassays. To avoid the metal ion quenching noticed with metal chelating polycarboxylic acid derivatives (1385), they used hydroxyalkyl-substituted fluorescein derivatives.

The applications of liposomes in FIAs are listed in Table 8.15. Most liposome immunoassays are homogeneous complement-mediated liposome-lysis FIAs, also called microcapsule immunoassays (MCIA) (1382), but a few solid-phase Sep-FIAs and IFMAs have been developed using liposomes as label carriers.

Despite the fact that liposomes have the potential to solve two of the major problems with homogeneous FIAs—the problem of signal and sensitivity and the problem of universal suitability, (especially for large antigens)—they have not yet gained wider acceptance. Also, commercial systems are, so far, restricted to a few visual test systems, such as the Q Test of Becton Dickinson, which is based on rhodamine sulfate loaded liposomes and visual detection of the formed color (1399). The problems may be related to the preparation of liposomes, their stability, the leaking of encapsulated fluorochromes, and the incomplete action of the complement (a single antigen-antibody reaction is not always enough to trigger complement binding).

8.3.6. Other Nonseparation Fluorescence Immunoassays

In addition to the above described technologies, a number of additional nonseparation FIA techniques have been developed which are either "real" homogeneous assays or solid-phase separation assays, where the detection is performed preferentially either from the free or bound fraction.

Table 8.15. Liposome Immunoassays[a]

Analyte	Technique	Label	Reference
Mycotoxin T-2	Complement lysis	CF	1386
Anti-streptolysin O	Complement lysis	CF	1387
Anti-mycobact. Ab	Complement lysis	Calcein	505, 1388
Hepatitis BsAg	Complement lysis	CF	1389
Anti-hIgG	Complement lysis	CF	1390
CRP	Complement lysis	CF	1391
Ferritin	Complement lysis	CF	1382, 1392
AFP	Complement lysis	CF	1393
α_2-plasmin inhibitor	Complement lysis	CF	1394
CEA	Complement lysis	CF	1395
Erythrocyte lipid Ag	Complement lysis	Aminonaphthalene-trisulfonate	646
Ganglioside GM2	Complement lysis	CF	1378
Cell phenotyping	IF	CF	934
Membrane proteins	QIF	FITC-PS.	939
Cell surface Ag	IF	CF	1396
Phenytoin	Complement lysis	CF	1397
Theophylline	Complement lysis	Calcein	628
	Sep-FIA	CF	1398
Digoxin	Sep-FIA	Sulforhodamine	636
	Complement lysis	CFTMA	1384

[a]Abbreviations: CFTMA = carboxyfluorescein-trimethylol-amide; PS = phosphatidylserine

Halfman has patented a "real" homogeneous assay, which he named solvent perturbation FIA. It is based on an additional reagent in the reaction mixture, which modulates the signal of the labeled haptenic antigen, if not bound to the antibodies (396). Various detergents have been tested as the quenchers for fluorochromes, and SDS is especially efficient as a signal modulator of fluorescein-labeled gentamicin (397) and amphetamines (1400). Effects of the micelle-forming detergents and cyclodextrines on the fluorescence level and decay time of fluorescein-labeled phenytoin have been measured by a phase-resolved fluorometer (398). An analogous procedure has been used with Eu-chelate–labeled haptenic antigens (1401). In the competitive assay the chelate label was either bound to albumin, which is present in the assay buffer in excess and enhances the chelate fluorescence, or labeled antigen is bound to respective antibodies and fluorescence is quenched. The principle is further applied for TR-FIA of serum thyroxine (881) and urine estrone-3-glucuronide (882).

In addition to fluorescence intensity, fluorescence decay time also can change during immunoreaction. McGown (389) measured both the fluorescence intensity change and decay-time change of fluorescein-labeled phenobarbital and Texas Red-labeled albumin upon immunoreaction using phase-resolved fluorometry. The observed decay-time changes from 4.04 to 3.94 ns and 4.07 to 3.98 ns, respectively, were reportedly enough for a quantitative assay. Soini et al. (1402) have patented a general technique utilizing decay-time differences in a homogeneous TR-FIA exemplified with an assay of insulin. The fluorescent properties of lanthanide chelates have also led to a patent describing several postulated ways to construct homogeneous assays, including the formation of mixed-ligand chelates in immunoreaction, ligand exchange during reaction, intraligand quenching, and different energy transfer routes (1370).

The majority of published nonseparation FIAs could also be called "space-resolved" FIAs, because these are generally normal Sep-FIAs or IFMAs on solid-phases, and only the fluorometric determination of either of the fractions makes a difference between bound and free. A number of these assays is based on microbeads as solid-phases. In the flow-cytometric FIAs, only the bead-associated fluorescence is detected by triggering the detection with scattering caused by beads migrating through the capillary (Chapter 8.2.3). Examples of nonseparation flow-cytometric assays are the assay of hIgG (539) and the assay of peroxidase (946). Particle-associated fluorescence can also be determined by analyzing signal fluctuations and distinguishing slowly fluctuating bead-associated fluorescence from the rapidly fluctuating background of freely diffusing reagents. Fluctuation analysis was used in 1977 for measuring stained virions by Hirschfeld (436). Elings et al. introduced fluorescence fluctuation immunoassays for gentamicin (1403, 1404) and hIgG (429) by exciting the samples with an argon-ion laser and using beads from Bio-Rad Immunofluor reagent kits.

Mansouri and Schultz (82) introduced an immunosensor for measuring glucose with a specific protein binding assay, which is based on a fiberoptic and a reaction cuvette attached to the distal end of the fiber. Both excitation and emission collection were predominately accomplished from the free fluorescent dextrane in solution. An analogous technology was described in a patent received by Kankare et al. (877) employed for assays of albumin and globulins by using a fluorescent Eu-chelate label and measuring primarily only the free fraction of the tracers. Labsystems Oy has patented a similar assay principle utilizing magnetic particles as the solid-phase, pulled to the sides of cuvettes with a magnetic field before measuring the free fraction of tracer from the solution (1405).

An evanescent wave is a commonly used method for the excitation of only those fluorescent molecules that are near the reflecting surface (see Chapter 6.1.3). Kronick and Little used the technology for an immunoassay of morphine performed on quartz slides (439, 440). Evanescent wave excitation is frequently used in waveguide immunosensors (Chapter 8.5) using optical fibers containing a coated area near the distal end of fiber. With the evanescent wave, only the tracer bound to surfaces is excited and its emission collected.

By using solutions that strongly absorb the excitation, it is also possible to create conditions in which only the surface-bound fluorochromes are excited and measured. This principle is patented by Labsystems Oy, using conventional fluorochromes (1406), and by Becton Dickinson using Eu-chelate loaded liposomes or latex particles as labels (853, 1407).

8.4. TIME-RESOLVED FLUOROMETRIC IMMUNOASSAYS

Time-resolved fluorometry, or time-resolved photoluminescence in general, is an instrumental design to collect emission at a certain time interval after the pulsed excitation and to improve the detection sensitivity by means of a temporal rejection of background. A majority of the assays require specialized technologies, such as handling lanthanide chelates, which is a very distinctive technique compared with handling of organic fluors in "conventional" FIAs. Therefore all time-resolved photoluminescence techniques, including competitive and noncompetitive time-resolved fluorometric immunoassays, phase-resolved fluorescence immunoassays, and phosphorescence immunoassays, are described here as a separate section.

The reason for using time-resolved fluorometry in immunoassays originates in the realization that the sensitivity of the "conventional" fluorometric method is seriously restricted by the high background interference inevitably present in any routine analysis. Despite the fact that fluorometric detection of fluorescent compounds can have the utmost sensitivity, reaching a single molecule detection level in specific conditions (337–340), fluorometric detection in routine conditions is limited to nano- or micromolar concentrations, and the sensitivity is highly dependent on the background level present (342, 388). Before direct fluorometric methods can impose a real challenge to radioisotopic techniques, background elimination is absolutely needed, and various techniques have been developed to discriminate background interference (Chapter 5.4.5). Time-resolved fluorometry provides an ideal way to distinguish a specific signal from nonspecific background, provided that the signals differ substantially from each other in their decay times. Background elimination by time resolution was introduced in 1942 by Weissman (459) in a phosphorometric analysis, and during the 1960s Winefordner further developed time-resolved instruments by using pulsed light and gated detection (385, 386). The evolution of time-resolved techniques and instrumentation has been reviewed by Soini and Lövgren (464), and some features of instrument development are also described in Chapter 6.2.6.

To be practical for immunoassays, time-resolved techniques require fluorescent probes having decay times clearly longer than the average background noise, which accrues from scattering ($\tau = 0$), the background fluorescence of sample and reagent constituents ($\tau \approx$ 1–10 ns) and the background luminescence of solid materials, such as plastic disposables, filters, and lenses (τ ranging from microseconds to milliseconds). Therefore, development of fluorescent probes with long decay times has played an important role in the successful use of time-resolved fluorometry. The development of long fluorescence decay-time probes composed of lanthanide chelates has actually opened the possibility of improving detection sensitivities considerably by employing time resolution (Chapter 7.4), and time-resolved fluorometric immunoassays with chelate labels have resulted in sensitivities equal to or even exceeding those achieved with radioisotopic labels, making fluoroimmunoassays real alternatives to radioimmunoassays.

Recently several review articles have been written about time-resolved fluorometric immunoassays (74, 253, 347, 351, 464, 826, 1408–1413). From time-resolved fluoroimmunoassays especially two technologies utilizing europium chelate labels have gained wide applications and are commercialized with the product names DELFIA® (Wallac) and FiaGen™ (CyberFluor Inc.). Other chelate systems have found fewer applications so far, as is also the case with assays based on organic photoluminescent probes, phase-resolved fluoroimmunoassays (PR-FIA), and phosphoroimmunoassays (PIA).

8.4.1. Dissociative Enhanced Time-Resolved Fluorometric Immunoassays

Fluorescence enhancement assays—that is, assays comprised of immunoreagents labeled with practically nonfluorescent but stable lanthanide chelates and relying on a separate fluorescence-enhancement step performed after the immunoreaction—were actually the first practical lanthanide-chelate-based time-resolved fluoroimmunoassays (1414, 1415). The two ways to perform the fluorescence enhancement, either by forming mixed-ligand chelates or by dissociating the ions prior to the formation of new fluorescent chelates, are described in Chapter 7.4.3. Dissociative enhancement has proved to be a more rapid and practical approach, because this technique allows independent and separate optimization of the labeling of, for example, antibodies with lanthanide ions (839, 840) and of conditions for the fluorometric detection of the ions (347, 808, 821). This technique is available commercially under the trade name DELFIA® and has been used with a great number of analytes.

The DELFIA assay principle is particularly well suited for solid-phase-based two-site immunofluorometric assays, where it has found its widest and most successful applications. Originally polystyrene tubes or polystyrene balls were used as solid-phases, but later all applications have been made using surfaces of microtitration strip wells as solid-phase manifolds. Table 8.16 lists both the research applications and articles describing commercial products and their clinical evaluations. A majority of the techniques rely on a two-site assay approach with two monoclonal antibodies, one on the surface and the other labeled with Eu^{3+}, but polyclonal antibodies are frequently used as well. Some of the published applications employ labeled avidins, secondary antibodies, or protein A as universal reagents in indirect assays.

Minor modifications of the technique relate to labeling reagents and constituents of the enhancement solution and are described in more detail in Chapter 7.4.3. A two-step enhancement, dissociating the ions with acid prior to the adjustment of pH to form optimally fluorescent chelates, was tested both with Eu- and Tb-labeled antibodies using β-diketones for the enhancement of Eu^{3+} and a dipicolinic acid derivative for the enhancement of Tb^{3+} (832). A similar approach was used by Xu et al. (1564) with Tb-labeled albumin and tiron as the fluorescence-enhancing ligand. Baxter Travenol has patented a variation of the enhancement technique called interligand metal transfer assay (1565), in which fluorescence enhancement is accomplished with an excess of trimethoxyphenyl-pyridine-2,6-dicarboxylic acid (without acid dissociation) exemplified with assays for thyroid hormone determinations.

Eu-labeled antibodies were originally used for competitive TR-FIAs of haptenic molecules after immmobilizing the haptenic antigens to solid-phases via carrier protein conjugates. The same assay performance can be achieved by immobilizing antibodies and labeling the carrier protein instead, but in both cases problems can arise from the fact that a critical component of the competition is immobilized, and its leaking causes severely decreased binding percentages. Therefore, the newer applications are primarily constructed by using an excess of secondary antibodies (e.g., anti-mouse IgG for monoclonal antibodies) on the solid-phase and both critical components, primary antibodies and tracer in solution.

Table 8.17 lists the applications of competitive DELFIA-type techniques primarily used for haptenic antigens but also for some larger antigens. Relatively few of the applications rely on a tracer conjugated with a single chelate.

Table 8.16. Time-Resolved Immunofluorometric Assays Based on Dissociative Fluorescence Enhancement[a]

Analyte	Tracer	Reference	Evaluation
Thyrotropin (TSH)	Eu-MAb	1410–1411	573, 1416–1438
TSH neonatal	Eu-MAb		1439–1445
TSH	Eu-Streptav.	73	
hCG	Eu-MAb	838, 1446–1451	573, 1452–1458
βhCG	Eu-MAb	1459–1461	
Follitropin (FSH)	Eu-MAb	823, 1462	573, 1463–1466
	Sm-MAb	823	
	Eu-streptav.	72	
(monkeys)	Eu-MAb		1467
Lutropin (LH)	Eu-MAb	1462, 1468, 1469	573, 1464, 1470–1473
	Eu-streptav.	1474	
Prolactin (PL)	Eu-MAb	1475	573, 1430, 1464
Alpha-fetoprot (AFP)	Eu-MAb	1476	1441, 1477–1480
	Sm-MAb	824	
Insulin	Eu-MAb	1481, 1482	
Proinsulin	Eu-MAb	1483	
ACTH	Eu-MAb	1484	
Growth hormone (hGH)	Eu-Ab	1485	
	Eu-streptav.	1486, 1487	
α_1-Interferon	Eu-Ab	1488	
Nerve growth fact. (NGF)	Eu-Ab	1489	
Epidermal GF (EGF)	Eu-MAb	1490–1492	
Lactoferrin	Eu-Ab	1493	
Placental prot. 5	Eu-Ab	1494	
Placental prot. 14	Eu-Ab	1495	

Table 8.16. Time-Resolved Immunofluorometric Assays Based on Dissociative Fluorescence Enhancement[a] *(continued)*

Analyte	Tracer	Reference	Evaluation
Somatomedin BP	Eu-Ab	1496	
Sex hormone BG (SHBG)	Eu-MAb	1497	1498–1500
Myoglobin	Eu-MAb	1501	
Ferritin	Eu-Ab		1502
Phospholipase A_2	Eu-MAb	1503–1509	
Trypsinogen-1/2	Eu-MAb	1510	
Cysteine proteinase inhibitors	Eu-Ab	1511, 1512	
CRP	Eu-Ab	1513	
β_2-microglobulin	Eu-Ab	1514	
Thyroglobulin	Eu-MAb	1515	
CEA	Eu-MAb	832	
CA-50	Eu-MAb		1516–1519
CA-125	Eu-MAb	1520, 1521	
CA-242	Eu-MAb	1522, 1523	
PSA	Eu-MAb/Ab	1524, 1525	
IRT	Eu-MAb	1526	
RIgG	Eu-Ab	808, 1414	
IgG (Ab)	Eu-Protein A	80	
IgE	Eu-MAb	1527	
MIgG	Eu-polym-biot.	905	
MAb screening	Eu-Ag	1528	
Myelin basic prot.	Eu-Ab	1529	
Anti-insulin Ab	Eu-insulin	1530, 1531	
Anti-thyroglob. IgG	Eu-TG-DNP	1532	
Anti-rubella, IgG	Eu-anti-hIgG	1415, 1533	

Table 8.16. Time-Resolved Immunofluorometric Assays Based on Dissociative Fluorescence Enhancement[a] *(continued)*

Analyte	Tracer	Reference	Evaluation
Anti-tetanus, IgG	Eu-anti-hIgG	1534	
Anti-HIV, IgG	Eu-anti-hIgG	1535	
	Eu-HIV peptide	1536	
Anti-Schistosoma	Eu-anti-hIgG	1537	
Anti-Campylobact.	Eu-anti-hIgG	1538	
Anti-Amoeba IgG	Eu-anti-hIgG	1539	
HBsAg	Eu-Ab	1540, 1541	
Rubella Ag	Eu-MAb	1542	
Adenovirus Ag	Eu-anti-RIgG	1543, 1544	
	Eu-Ab	1545–1547	
Rotavirus Ag	Eu-anti-RIgG	1543, 1544	
	Eu-Ab	1545	
Influenza viruses	Eu-Ab/MAb	1543, 1544, 1548–1555	
RSV	Eu-Ab	1556, 1557	
Astrovirus	Eu-Ab	1558	
Schistosoma Ag	Eu-Ab	1559	
Plant viruses	Eu-Ab	1560–1563	
Estradiol	Eu-anti-idiotype	100	

[a]Abbreviations: BP = binding protein; DNP = dinitrophenyl; TG = thyroglobulin.

Table 8.17. Competitive TR-FIAs with Dissociative Fluorescence Enhancement

Analyte	Solid-phase	Tracer	Reference/Evaluation
Total T_4	Albumin-Ag	Eu-Ab	1566
	Second.-Ab	Eu-Ag	573, 1464
T_4 Screening	Second.-Ab	Eu-Ag	1567
	Second.-Ab	Eu-gelatin-Ag	1567
Free T_4	Second.-Ab	Eu-Albumin-Ag	1464, 1568
	Second.-Ab	Eu-gelatin-Ag	921, 1569
T_3	Second.-Ab	Eu-Ag	573, 1464
Cortisol	Albumin-Ag	Eu-Ab	53, 573
Estradiol	Thyrogl.-Ag	Eu-Ab	908
	Albumin-Ag	Eu-streptav.	1487
	Second.-Ab	Eu-Ag	1570
Progesterone	Thyrogl.-Ag	Eu-Ab	908
	Second.-Ab	Eu-Ag	1570, 1571
	Ab	Eu-HRP-Ag	1572
	Albumin-Ag	Eu-prot. A	1573–1575
17-α-OH-prog. screen.	Second.-Ab	Eu-Ag	909, 1576
	Second.-Ab	Eu-polym.-Ag	909, 916
Testosterone	Albumin-Ag	Eu-Ab	1577, 1578
Prostaglandin F2α	Ab	Eu-polylys.-Ag	1579, 1580
5-methyl-deoxy-cytid.	Second.-Ab	Eu-polylys.-Ag	911
	Thyrogl.-Ag	Eu-Ab	1581
Adipokinetic hormone	Thyrogl.-Ag	Eu-Ab	1582
Digoxin	Albumin-Ag	Eu-Ab	156, 1583, 1584
Aflatoxin	Albumin-Ag	Eu-Ab	830
Azidothymidine (AZT)	Albumin-Ag	Eu-second.-Ab	1585
Acrivastine	Thyrogl.-Ag	Eu-second.-Ab	1586
Albumin	Ab	Tb-Ab	1564
TBG	Second.-Ab	Eu-Ag	1587

The improvement of signal level has been attained by labeling either antibodies, carrier proteins, or antigen-conjugated polymers with several chelate groups.

The DELFIA technology has nicely demonstrated the benefits of time-resolved fluorometry in producing high detection sensitivity through background elimination. Because in this technology the chelates used for labeling antibodies are different from those used for fluorometric detection, those phases (labeling and detection) can be optimized separately. This is an especially crucial point when labeling antibodies, where it is of utmost importance to maintain the immunological and natural properties of the antibodies in order to obtain high specific binding and minimal nonspecific binding. Therefore, the labeling reagent used in DELFIA applications is a nonaromatic, highly hydrophilic, and negatively charged Eu-chelate of isothiocyanate derivative of diethylenetriaminetetraacetic acid (839, 840) which is practically nonfluorescent. After the immunoreactions and ion dissociation, new, optimally fluorescent chelates are formed with a quantum yield of 70% (Chapter 7.4.3). The detection sensitivity of that chelate with time-resolved fluorometry is around 1×10^{-17} mols/200 μL (475). In DELFIA immunometric assays which employ high affinity monoclonal antibodies, the dynamic range and assay sensitivities can be much higher than with the respective immunoradiometric assays (1448). According to clinical evaluations of commercial immunoassays kits for TSH, the DELFIA kit has proved to be one of the most sensitive methods available (1416–1438).

An additional feature of DELFIA technology is its suitability for double- or even triple-label assays, a suitability made possible by the characteristic fluorescent properties of the different lanthanide chelates (Chapter 7.4). By choosing the type of β-diketone in the enhancement solution, either the pair Eu^{3+} and Sm^{3+} (822–825) or Eu^{3+} and Tb^{3+} (346, 827, 828) can be used as labels and measured simultaneously, or one after the other, from the same enhancement solution (Chapter 11.1).

8.4.2. Time-Resolved Fluoroimmunoassays with Stabilized Lanthanide Chelates

As described in Chapter 7.4, the chelate systems developed for TR-fluorometric immunoassays can be classified into three groups: enhancement systems, systems using stabilized chelates, and systems employing stable fluorescent chelates. In the enhancement system described above, the major problems encountered with lanthanide chelates—namely, stability and fluorescence in aqueous solutions—are split into two phases. Stability problems are solved by using stable chelates for labeling, and, after ion dissociation, ligand excess conditions to ensure chelation of all ions. Avoiding of aqueous quenching is accomplished by addition of synergistic agents and micelle-forming detergents, to extrude water molecules from chelates and to form optimal conditions for fluorescence. The second way to avoid the stability and quenching problems is to stabilize the inherently unstable fluorescent chelates to form *in situ* fluorescent chelate systems.

One way to stabilize fluorescent β-diketone chelates is to incorporate them into liposome membranes (856) or into latex particles (848–855). Despite the fact that such fluorescent beads containing a plurality of highly fluorescent Eu-chelates are extremely fluorescent, these have not so far been applied in practical immunoassays or even in fluorescence microscopic studies for cell-surface antigens.

Another technique to form *in situ* fluorescent chelates is to couple the enhancing ligand to some of the immunocomponents and saturate the ligand with a high excess of fluorescent lanthanide ions. Wilmott et al. (857) were the first to use a fluorogenic chelating ligand as a marker for antigen. They labeled gentamicin with transferrin, which in the presence of an excess of Tb^{3+} greatly enhances Tb^{3+} fluorescence, and used the system for a TR-FIA of gentamicin. Since the introduction of a derivative of bathophenanthroline, 4,7-bis(chlorosulfophenyl)-1,10-phenanthroline-2,9-dicarboxylic acid (BCPDA) by Evangelista and Pollak (858–860) and the development of procedures for labeling proteins with the ligand and for saturating conjugates with Eu^{3+} (861, 862), this Eu^{3+} fluorescence-enhancing ligand has been extensively used for labeling immunoreagents (primarily streptavidin) and for TR-fluorometric immunoassays by a research group led by Elefterios Diamandis at CyberFluor Inc. (Toronto, Canada). The TR-FIAs based on this ligand and the TR fluorometer developed for immunoassays are available commercially as FiaGen™ products by CyberFluor.

In this system, immunoreagents are generally not labeled directly with the ligand due to the problems arising from metal ions being in the samples (they can saturate the ligand), but all the assays work with biotin-labeled antibodies, and BCPDA is conjugated to streptavidin, which is incubated with the formed complexes in the wells as a separate step, in an assay buffer containing an excess of Eu^{3+} (74). Aqueous quenching is omitted by removing all water from the reaction vessel prior to TR-fluorometric measurement of the dried surfaces of the white microtitration strips used.

All the early applications relied on BCPDA-labeled streptavidin (Table 8.18), but for some assays the signal level is improved by using a "biological polymer," thyroglobulin coupled with streptavidin and conjugated with high number of ligands. With thyroglobulin as a carrier the protein labeling level is increased from 14 to 150 and the respective detection limit of the conjugate lowered sevenfold (1588, 1589). By incubating a streptavidin-thyroglobulin-BCPDA complex with an additional amount of BCPDA-

Table 8.18. Time-Resolved Immunofluorometric Assays with the CyberFluor System

Analyte	Tracer	Reference
TSH	Streptav.-TG-BCPDA	1591, 1592
TSH screening	Streptav.-TG-BCPDA	1593
TBG	Streptav.-BCPDA	1594, 1595
FSH	Streptav.-TG-BCPDA	1596, 1597
LH	Streptav.-BCPDA	1598–1600
	Streptav.-TG-BCPDA	1601, 1602
hCG	Streptav.-BCPDA	1603, 1604
	Streptav.-TG-BCPDA	861, 1588
Prolactin	Streptav.-BCPDA	1605, 1606
	Streptav.-TG-BCPDA	1606
AFP	Streptav.-BCPDA	1607, 1608
	Streptav.-TG-BCPDA	1590
hGH	Streptav.-BCPDA	1609
CEA	Streptav.-TG-BCPDA	1610, 1611
Ferritin	Streptav.-BCPDA	1612, 1613
CK-MB	Streptav.-TG-BCPDA	1614, 1615
Isoamylase	Streptav.-BCPDA	1616–1618
Adenovirus	Streptav.-BCPDA	1619
Anti-rubella IgG	Streptav.-BCPDA	1620
Anti-rubella IgM	Streptav.-BCPDA	1620, 1621
Albumin	Streptav.-BCPDA	1622

labeled thyroglobulin and with a controlled excess of Eu^{3+}, a macromolecular aggregate can be formed which contains up to about 480 ligands per streptavidin (919, 1590). This complex is used in TR-FIAs to further increase the signal level and the assay sensitivity.

Applications of the technology have been published largely, so far, only by the R & D group at CyberFluor. Noncompetitive applications are listed in Table 8.18. All assays except that of rubella antibodies are based on antibody coated wells, biotinylated antibodies, and various forms of BCPDA-labeled streptavidins (streptav.). The anti-rubella IgG assay is based on antigen coated wells and biotinylated anti-human IgG, whereas the anti-rubella IgM test is an IgM-capture assay based on an added rubella antigen and biotinylated anti-rubella antibodies.

Competitive assays of CyberFluor are generally based on the surface immobilized haptenic antigens, biotinylated mono- or polyclonal antibodies, and BCPDA-labeled streptavidin or streptavidin-thyroglobulin (TG) conjugates. The published applications are summarized in Table 8.19. Some minor modifications of the technology also have been tested. In the cortisol assay (1631), anti-cortisol was directly immobilized on wells, and competition

Table 8.19. Time-Resolved Fluoroimmunoassays with BCPDA-Labeled Streptavidins

Analyte	Solid-phase	Tracer	Reference
Tot. T_4	Bovine glob.-Ag	Streptav.-BCPDA	1623, 1624
Free T_4	Prot.-Ag	Streptav.-TG-BCPDA	1625
T_3 uptake	Prot.-Ag	Streptav.-BCPDA	1626, 1627
Cortisol	Albumin-Ag	Ab-BSA-BCPDA	1628
	TG-Ag	Streptav.-BCPDA	1629, 1630
	Ab	Biotin-TG-BCPDA	1631
17-OHP	TG-Ag	Streptav.-TG-BCPDA	1632
Digoxin	TG-Ag	Streptav.-BCPDA	1633, 1634

of the sample analyte took place with cortisol coupled to streptavidin. The bound streptavidin was determined with biotinylated and BCPDA-labeled thyroglobulin. Another modification of the cortisol assay used antibodies which were labeled through coupling to BCPDA-labeled albumin, forming a more direct competitive assay approach compared to the use of labeled streptavidin (1628).

As stated by the authors, this technique has the advantage of being insensitive to contamination of reagents with extraneous Eu^{3+}, which can be regarded as a potential risk for the enhancement-based systems. On the other hand, the use of these chelates requires extra steps for streptavidin and Eu^{3+} incubations and for drying the surface prior to measurement. High-sensitivity assays also require rather complicated polymeric label systems. However, very high sensitivities have been achieved; by using limited surface areas for coating, small volumes for the assay, and a polymeric label (480 ligands per streptavidin), a sensitivity of 30,000 molecules of AFP in the sample volume has reportedly been achieved (1590).

The technology is relatively new and has so far resulted in a limited number of clinical evaluations. The clinical potential of the technique remains to be seen.

8.4.3. Time-Resolved Fluoroimmunoassays with Stable Fluorescent Chelates

The development and synthesis of thermodynamically and/or kinetically stable and optimally fluorescent chelates has long been the goal of some intensive research and has resulted in a number of postulated structures (Chapter 7.4.5). The reason for the high interest relates to the potential advantages those chelates would offer: avoiding the problems of the above described techniques, producing potentially higher sensitivities, and opening totally new applications for time-resolved specific binding assays, such as homogeneous assays and *in situ* stainings (IF, QIF, DNA hybridizations) and so on. Despite the extensive work, a very limited number of practical approaches has been published so far (Table 8.20), and the postulated structures and applications can be found primarily in patent descriptions (753, 873–877, 888, 889, 894).

The simplest stable chelate used for TR-FIA is the Tb-chelate of diazophenyl-EDTA (864, 865), a chelating ligand originally developed for labeling proteins with radioactive metals (744) and subsequently used as a nonfluorescent Eu-chelator in enhancement-based TR-FIAs. Another straightforward synthesis is to couple light absorbing and fluorescence-enhancing ligand to DTPA-anhydride (384, 867). Most of the other synthesized stable and fluorescent chelates are derivatives of pyridine, bipyridine, terpyridine, or phenanthroline containing two iminodiacetic acid groups or cryptate structure to ascertain chelate stability and containing fluorescent lanthanides or ruthenium as the light emitting ion (Chapter 7.4.5 and 7.4.6). These chelates have been used for separation-based time-resolved FIAs and IFMAs, homogeneous TR-FIAs, IF tests, and DNA hybridization assays (Table 8.20)

Time-resolved FIAs based on lanthanide cryptates composed of one, two, or three bipyridines or o-phenanthrolines (Chapter 7.4.5) were introduced by FluoCis (Oris Industries, France) (1638, 1639). The intention has been to construct simple homogeneous TR-FIAs, but so far only a model TR-IFMA of prolactin has been described (888, 890).

Table 8.20. Time-Resolved Fluoroimmunoassays with Stable Fluorescent Chelates[a]

Analyte	Technique	Tracer	Reference
IgG	Sep-FIA	Tb-diazophenyl-EDTA	864
Ag	Sep-FIA	Eu-diazophenyl-EDTA	865
Albumin	Sep-FIA	Tb-DTPA-PAS	384, 867, 869
Testosterone	Sep-FIA	Tb-DTPA-PAS	870, 871
Prolactin	IFMA	Eu-cryptate	888, 890
CEA	IFMA	Tb-phenylpyridine-TA	832
hCG	IFMA	Eu-W1014	880
Cell surf. Ag	IF	Eu-W1014	1635
Myosin	IF	Eu-W1014	879
T_4	Homogeneous	Eu-W1174	881
Estrone-3-glucuronide	Homogeneous	Eu-W1174	882, 1636, 1637
Theophylline	Homogeneous	Tb-phenylpyridine-TA	1565

[a]Abbreviations used: PAS = para-aminosalicylic acid; TA = tetraacetic acid; W1014 and W1174 (chelates coded by Wallac).

Stable fluorescent chelates also have created interest as potential probes for time-resolved fluorescence microscopic studies. Tanke et al. have successfully used inorganic crystals composed of Eu-doped phosphors (Chapter 7.5.3) as probes for IF (947–950). Due to their large size, crystals are suitable only for staining cell surface antigens, and therefore simple small chelates would be preferred. Problems with the current chelates relate to their lower fluorescence intensity and photostability. However, some IF applications with fluorescent chelates have emerged (879, 1635).

One problem encountered with those stable and fluorescent chelates is the relatively low fluorescence intensity obtained so far. Another is derived from the aromatic nature of the light absorbing group in the ligands, which tends to increase the nonspecific binding properties of labeled reagents, noticed, for instance, with o-phenanthroline derivatives (210). It is obvious, however, that when those problems are solved, these chelates will find extensive applications in different fields of immunological techniques.

8.4.4. Phosphorescence and Phase-Resolved Fluorescence Immunoassays

Phosphorescence, delayed fluorescence, and phase-resolved fluorometry have also been used to take advantage of the time behavior of photoluminescent probes to improve the performance of respective photoluminescence immunoassays. Phosphoroimmunoassays (PIA) are instrumentally equal to TR-FIAs with chelates, but PIAs utilize the long lifetime emission produced by phosphorescent probes, such as erythrosin, eosin, or metallo-porphyrins. Those compounds exhibit relatively strong RTP in optimized conditions, in deaerated solutions, solid surfaces, or micelles (1640) (Chapter 5.5). Sidki and Smith have issued a patent application describing a PIA using erythrosin as the phosphorescent label and preventing the quenching by dissolved oxygen by removing it with sulfite, bisulfite, or metasulfite (1641). Eosin also produces delayed-type fluorescence (Chapter 5.1.3) which can be used analogously to phosphorescence (1644). Despite the fact that phosphorescence could provide high sensitivities, the applications have been primarily developed for analytes requiring only moderate sensitivity (Table 8.21). Recently, however, new phosphorescent probes composed of metallo-porphyrins have been introduced by Savitsky et al. (717). The very high phosphorescence intensity of Pd-coproporhyrin might make it possible to extend the applications of PIA into sandwich-type assays of peptides and proteins, analytes requiring high assay sensitivities.

Phase-resolved fluorometry is another technology to determine the decay times of various fluorescent compounds (Chapter 6.2.3). The technology and its applications have been reviewed extensively by Lakowicz (478) and

Table 8.21. Phosphorescence and Phase-Resolved Fluorescence Immunoassays

Analyte	Technique	Tracer	Reference
Primidone	PIA magnetic sep.	Erythrosin	1641, 1642
Carbamazepine	PIA homogeneous	Erythrosin	1643
IgG	Delayed FIA	Eosin	1644
Anti-insulin	PIA sandwich	Pd-coproporphyrin	717
Phenobarbital	PR-FIA homog.	Fluorescein	389, 1645
Lactoferrin	PR-FIA FETI	FITC-TRITC	1646
Albumin	PR-FIA homog.	Texas Red	639
Benzo[α]pyrene	PR-FIA sensor	—	1647
TSH	PR-FIA sandwich	Ir-bipyr.	753

McGown (389). With phase-resolved fluorometry, decay times and decay-time differences even within a time frame of subnanoseconds can be determined, which has been the basis for most homogeneous PR-FIA applications (Table 8.21). The phase-resolved principle also can be used for elimination of background noise—for example, by employing selective phase nulling. However, all the present PR-FIA applications have been tested with analytes present in samples at relatively high concentrations, and it is still uncertain whether phase-resolved fluorometry can provide new prospects for practical quantitative fluorescence immunoassays.

8.5. FLUOROIMMUNOSENSORS

Sensors are devices developed for monitoring analytes continuously from the solutions studied. They can be flow-through analyzing systems or remote sensors. The final goal set for the immunosensor is to carry out *in situ* monitoring of analytes in biological fluids, the same way as, for example, pH can now be followed with pH sensors. Sensors as real future immunoassay systems would enable continuous monitoring of the essential compounds in for instance, emergency situations, in blood analysis at bedside, and in doctors' offices, outpatient clinics, patients' homes, etc. Photoluminescence is utilized as the measured signal in numerous sensor principles; for example, pH can be monitored with pH-sensitive fluorescent probes such as derivatives of coumarin or pyrenes, and oxygen can be monitored by the quenching it causes for the phosphorescence of porphyrins or fluorescence of polycyclic hydrocarbons. Electrolytes, carbon dioxide, and ammonia also can be determined with fluorescence indicators attached to a fiber sensor (1648).

Due to the prospects immunosensors have, there is extensive work going on to develop immunosensors utilizing various immunoassay technologies and labels. Immunoassays are not, however, intrinsically very suitable for sensors due to the indirect signal production, slow kinetics, and difficult standardization of immunoassays. For sensors the immunoassay needs to be robust and simple, standardization and quality control need to be performed internally, and for multi-use the technology should be homogeneous, reversible, or easily regenerated. Rapid regeneration and signal production require rapid association, but also rapid dissociation rates, especially in the ligand-displacement-based homogeneous assays. In that respect assays that do not require any added labels would be preferred, if they could produce strong enough responses.

Systems used in the development of immunosensors have been based on, for example, transmembrane potential (1649), electrodes (1650), loaded liposomes (1651), and enzymes with various detection principles (1652), including fluorometry (1653). Most of the developed immunosensors are optical immunosensors (1654–1657) based on technologies such as Langmuir-Blodgett film technology, ellipsometry (surface plasmon resonance measures thickness and refractive indices of thin film) (1658), electroluminescence (655, 1659), and internal reflection spectrometry based on attenuated total reflection (ATR) and total internal reflection (TIRF).

Total internal reflection (evanescent wave) is frequently used in the development of fluorescence immunosensors (443, 1660–1662). Evanescent wave excitation on a quartz plate was used in 1975 by Kronick and Little (439) in an immunoassay of morphine. Sutherland et al. (1663, 1664) have applied both planar quartz plates and optical fibers as waveguides in the determination of methotrexate by employing the decreased transmission as a result of the binding of the hapten to immobilized antibodies, and in the determination of IgG by the enhanced emission at 520 nm as a result of sandwich formation with FITC-labeled antibodies.

Three types of waveguides have been introduced and used in fluoroimmunosensors: disposable thin film cuvettes containing waveguides, quartz fiber waveguides, and planar waveguides with bulk excitation. The emission produced can be detected either conventionally at a 90° angle (Fig. 8.1a), in line by measuring the tunnelled fluorescence (c), or from back-generated tunnelled emission (b). According to the theory of reciprocity, only the evanescently excited fluorescence will be back coupled into the fiber and will propagate in the waveguide (1665). Accordingly, on-line detection or detection of back-generated emission from the fiber produces higher sensitivities.

A capillary fill device is an optical fluoroimmunosensor developed at Serono (Serono Diagnostics) (1666). It is based on two glass plates, one silanized and covalently coupled with antibodies or antigens and one containing the dried fluorescent reagents. Within the thin capillary rapid binding kinetics result in an equilibrium within 1 minute. The surfaces are bulk illu-

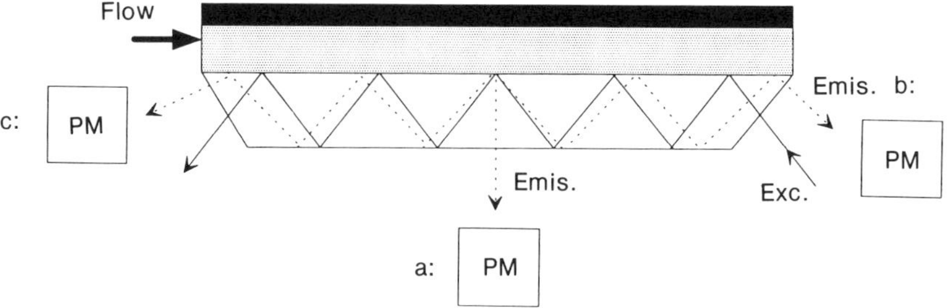

Fig. 8.1. Detection principles in a flow cuvette excited with evanescent wave. Detection from side (a), in line (c), or from back-generated tunnelled emission (b).

minated from the sides, and the evanescent wave emission is separated from the emission produced from unbound reagents by the angle they propagate in the waveguide. The system is used, for example, to detect hIgG (1666) and anti-rubella antibodies (1667).

Fiber waveguides, coated covalently with antibodies by their distal end (Fig. 8.2), are especially suitable for remote sensors. The coating of optical fibers is generally performed covalently using cross-linking reactions with silanized surfaces (177, 1668). Tronberg et al. used a fiber sensor for a competitive FIA of rabbit IgG using FITC-labeled anti-RIgG (1668), and Andrade et al. (1669) used a remote semicontinuous fiber immunosensor to detect blood coagulation proteins. Regeneration of the sensor was performed with a chaotropic ion (KSCN), which, however, has a tendency to destroy surface bound antibodies, especially if they are immobilized noncovalently.

Another way to utilize fiberoptics in remote sensors is to use dialyzing membrane closed cuvettes at the distal end of the fiber (Fig. 8.3). Fluoroimmunoassays within the membrane are preferably homogeneous or assays based on *in situ* spatial separation. Anderson and Miller (71) employed a FETI principle with B-PE–labeled phenytoin as a large molecular weight energy donor and Texas-Red–labeled avidin, with biotinylated anti-phenytoin antibodies, as the energy acceptor. Phycoerythrin functions as a fluorescent probe, an energy donor, and a large carrier to keep the tracer inside the sac. In this system ligand displacement and reaching new equilibrium required about 5–20 minutes. A similar approach has been used in a specific protein binding assay for glucose, using rhodamine-labeled concanavalin A and fluorescein-labeled dextrane (1670). A "space-resolved" spatial separation principle has been used in a glucose sensor developed by Mansouri and Schultz (82) using immobilized concanavalin A on a surface not excited by fiber and fluorescein-labeled dextrane, which is released from the surface by competition with sample glucose. In that system response time was 5–7 minutes.

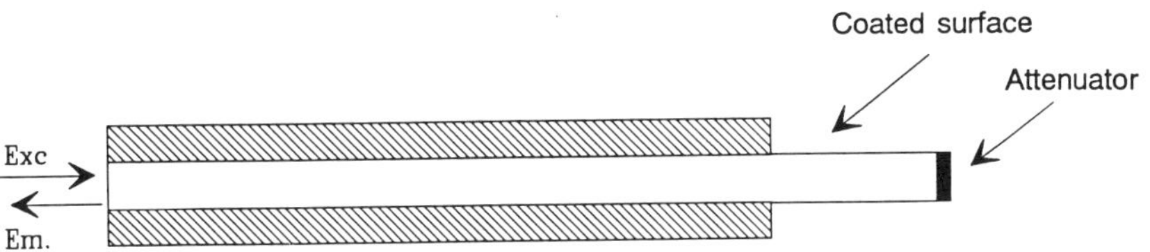

Fig. 8.2. Diagram of a fiberoptic waveguide sensor.

An ideal fluoroimmunosensor should give response as a change in fluorescence without the need to add labeled reagent to the sample. For example, the use of unlabeled FIA by employing the intrinsic fluorescence of tryptophan residues on proteins has been suggested (1671). This principle is working only in a few special cases, however. Benzo[α]pyrene can be monitored with fiberoptic sensors coated with anti-benzopyrene antibodies just by measuring the increased emission (656, 1672). Detection sensitivity and specificity can be further increased by employing phase-resolved detection for the long decay-time emission of pyrene (1647). Reck et al. (1673) have developed an optode based on a flow cuvette with dialysis membrane closed TBG, the intrinsic fluorescence of which is quenched upon binding of diffused thyroxine. Problems with TBG binding relate also to the slow formation and dissociation kinetics making the detector response timely.

Bright et al. (643) used a fiberoptic sensor coated with a Fab-fragment of anti-albumin antibodies labeled with dansyl-chloride. Concentrations of albumin in samples were monitored directly by the increase in fluorescence the bound albumin caused to the dansyl-labeled Fab.

Despite the extensive work carried out by some active groups, fluoroimmunosensors have not yet gained wide practical applications. Problems might be related to the slow kinetics of antibody-antigen interactions, the

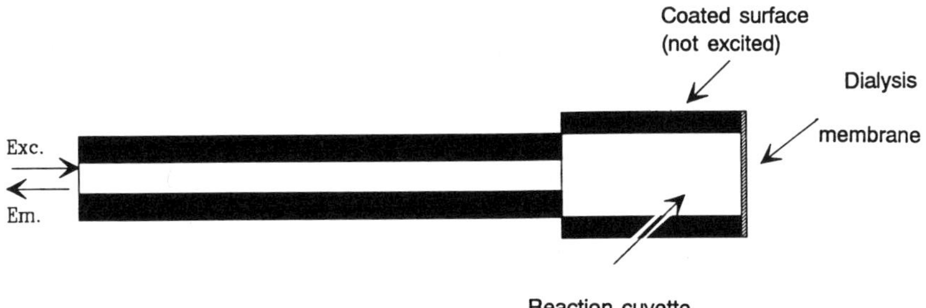

Fig. 8.3. Diagram of a dialysis membrane closed cuvette at the end of fiber sensor.

biocompatibility of materials used (1674), the difficult regeneration of sensors, and the high background level, affected especially by scattering. Also, the addition of labeled reagents to samples with sensors needs to be arranged —for example, by using continuous or pulsed pumping from a reagent reservoir (1669). Because of the high background it would be obvious that time-resolved fluorometry with fiber sensors should be used to increase the sensitivity. Petrea et al. (1656) have tested the use of Eu-labeled antibodies with fibers by using the enhancement principle, but the successful use of chelates would require the use of stable fluorescent chelate labels.

CHAPTER

9

FLUOROMETRIC ENZYME IMMUNOASSAYS

Fluorometric enzyme immunoassays (ELFIA) are assays based on enzyme-labeled immunoreagents and the fluorometric determination of the enzyme-catalyzed reaction. They are typical EIAs and differ from "conventional" photometric EIAs only in respect to the substrates and instruments used. With fluorometric substrates the detection sensitivities of enzymes can be increased by several orders of magnitude (see Chapter 7.6 and Table 4.2). Even though the increased detection sensitivity is not directly transferable to actual immunoassays, where the ultimate sensitivity is determined as much by the nature of antigen-antibody interaction as by the detection sensitivity of the label (1675), ELFIA technologies represent one of the most sensitive immunoassay technologies today. Fluorometric detection also widens the dynamic range of assays as compared to photometric reading, which is practically restricted to an absorption range from more than 0.001 to less than 2 absorption units. Both fluorometric and luminometric substrates are gaining increasing application in EIAs, and it seems to be a general tendency, especially with commercial automated systems (Chapter 6.7), to move from chromogenic substrates to fluorogenic or luminogenic substrates.

At the moment enzymes are the most widely used non-isotopic labels in the immunoassay field (Chapter 4.2.1), and the total application field of EIA is enormous. The use of fluorogenic substrates and fluorometric determination in EIA is only one feature of the technology, and accordingly this overview concentrates only on the specific points of ELFIA.

Fluorogenic substrates were used for the determination of enzyme activities as early as 1977 (952). In 1978 umbelliferone galactoside was used as a substrate for β-D-galactosidase determination in EIAs described by Hösli et al. (953) and by Ishikawa and Kato (1676), and in 1979 umbelliferone phosphate was used as a substrate for alkaline phosphatase (ALP) by Yolken and Stopa (245).

9.1. ENZYMES AS LABELS

Enzymes are proteins catalytically converting substrate molecules into products. The high turnover number of enzyme catalyzed reactions is the basis of the high amplification producing the high detection sensitivity. In addition to the high turnover number, enzymes used as labels need to have very good stability also to enable long-term storage of labeled reagents. In addition, the enzymes used as labels should be insensitive to interfering compounds (activators, inhibitors, or substrates) present in samples and, on the other hand, samples should have very low respective catalytic activity. For convenient detection, suitable substrates are also needed. Enzyme molecules also should remain intact and active after covalent coupling to immunoreagents. The enzyme protein as such should have the lowest nonspecific binding characteristic possible, and the coupling reaction should not interfere with either the activity of the enzyme or the affinity of the antibody. High detection sensitivity of the enzyme itself does not generally guarantee high sensitivity in the immunoassay, because the sensitivity of immunoassays tends to be nonspecific binding (NSB) restricted.

The most frequently used enzymes in immunoassays are peroxidases (horseradish, HRP), phosphatases (alkaline phosphatase, ALP), and β-D-galactosidase (βDG) (1677). During the 1980s HRP was used in a majority of EIAs (1678), but the advent of automated immunoassay systems seems to favor the use of ALP as the label and 4-MUP as the substrate (Chapter 6.7). Other enzymes used include glucose-6-phosphate dehydrogenase (1679) and glucoamylase (969), which, along with numerous other enzymes, can be measured fluorometrically by coupling to NAD(P)H-producing enzymes.

The labeling of antibodies with enzymes is traditionally performed with various cross-linking reagents, such as glutardialdehyde or carbodiimides, with simultaneous production of all kinds of cross-linked side products. One very simple labeling procedure, used especially with HRP, is to use the carbohydrate moiety of antibodies, form reactive aldehydes with periodate oxidation, and couple the aldehyde with the amines of HRP present in high excess. Another way to avoid unwanted reactions is to apply heterobifunctional reagents, used especially with the SH group in the hinge region of Fab′ (209, 497, 958, 1680–1682). Quite a number of the research applications of ELFIA rely on enzyme-labeled Fab′-fragments (Table 9.1).

Most ELFIA techniques are based on solid-phase separation, and only a few nonseparation homogeneous ELFIAs have been introduced. As solid-phases the same materials are applied as in immunoassays in general (Chapter 3.4). Polystyrene balls have been used in numerous ELFIA, as well as various microbeads, such as Sepharose particles (Table 9.1). Silicone rubber pieces (1676, 1680) and nitrocellulose membranes (1683) are solid-phases more rarely applied in other immunoassay types. Currently microtitration plates are becoming a standard solid-phase in all EIAs, partly because there are numerous photometric and fluorometric plate readers commercially available (Chapter 6.6.1). In totally automated random access systems, a tendency

Table 9.1. Applications of ELFIA for Proteins

Analyte	Tracer	Solid-phase	Substrate	Reference
Insulin	HRP-Ab	Sepharose	Tyramine,H_2O_2	959, 1684
	HRP-Ab	Disc	HPA,H_2O_2	543, 1685
	HRP-Fab′	Ps-ball	HPPA,H_2O_2	152, 958
hGH	HRP-Fab′	Ps-ball	HPPA,H_2O_2	209, 497, 1686
TSH	HRP-Fab′	Sepharose	Tyramine,H_2O_2	959
	βDG-Ab	Ps-ball	4MUG	1681
Ferritin	βDG-Fab′	Ps-ball	4MUG	1687
	βDG-Fab′	Silicone	4MUG	1680
β_2-microglob.	HRP-Fab′	Beads	HPPA,H_2O_2	1688
PAP	HRP-Fab′	Sepharose	α-naphthyl-P	962
β-interleukin	HRP-Fab′	Ps-ball	HPPA,H_2O_2	1689
	βDG-S-avid.	μ-plate	4MUG	1690
IL-receptor	βDG-S-avid.	μ-plate	4MUG	70
Myoglobin	HRP-Fab′	Ps-ball	HPPA,H_2O_2	1691
EGF (rat)	HRP-Fab′	Beads	HPPA,H_2O_2	1692
Neural. GF	βDG-Ab/Fab′	μ-plate	4MUG	75, 1693
Compl. compon. C-3, C-5	βDG-Ab	μ-plate	4MUG	1694

prevails toward the use of microbead solid-phases, separated by filtration or by a magnetic field.

In ELFIA, as well as in conventional FIAs, the performance of the instruments is generally not critical for the assay performance, due to relatively high background fluorescence and the existence of NSB background. In some assays sensitivities are increased by exploiting "high performance" fluorometers. Lidofsky et al. (543) applied laser fluorometry with flowing droplet detection in insulin ELFIA by measuring the HRP-produced fluorescent product from hydroxyphenylacetic acid (HPA). The ultimate sensitivity of one enzyme molecule detection has been achieved with a microfluorometer using β-D-galactosidase and a β-D-galactopyranoside derivative of deoxyfluorescein as the substrate (250). Hösli et al. have reported the development of ultramicroscale ELFIA using a miniaturized cuvette (953). Schneckenburger and Unsöld (469) utilized time-resolved fluorometric determination of 4-MU for high sensitivity measurement of βDG.

9.2. APPLICATIONS OF ELFIA

Most applications of fluorometric enzyme immunoassays are two-site immunometric assays. Relatively few research applications of ELFIA have been developed, and the most important application of ELFIA will be in automated immunoassay systems (Chapter 7.6).

The batch-analyzing systems Pharmacia CAP™ and 3M Diagnostic FluoroFAST™ were primarily developed for allergy testing. Automated systems from Americal Dade (Stratus) and Abbott (IM_x) are intended for wider clinical use, and those systems have resulted in a great number of applications and clinical evaluations. Quite a number of totally automated random-access analyzing systems have been introduced, which very often rely on ALP as a label and 4MUP as the fluorogenic substrate. Product menus are to be finalized for those systems and only a limited number of manufacturer-made applications in the form of abstracts are available at the moment.

9.2.1. Research Applications of ELFIA

The research applications of ELFIA have to a great extent been developed in Japan—for example by the research group of Professor Ishikawa—and perhaps as a result analytes measured reflect those analytes frequently determined in Japan, such as insulin and growth hormone. The immunometric ELFIA applications developed for peptides and proteins are summarized in

Table 9.1, serological, microbiological, and allergic applications in Table 9.2, and assays of haptenic molecules (competitive ELFIAs) in Table 9.3.

At present most applications of ELFIA for proteins, peptides, and haptenic molecules are developed in research laboratories and are based on HRP or galactosidase as labels and many different types of solid-phases. Virological, microbiological, and allergy test applications are primarily based on phosphatase as the labels in addition to a few assays using galactosidase, and most assays use microtitration plates or strips as the solid-phases. In allergy testing the reason is that the tests are primarily commercial tests (3M Diagnostic Systems FluoroFAST and Allergenetics FAST), and probably during the commercialization of batch-type ELFIA systems, applications of the microtitration plate format will increase.

Despite the facts that homogeneous, photometric EIAs are relatively abundant and various homogeneous principles have been invented, including Syva's EMIT, prosthetic group labeling, enzyme channelling immunoassays,

Table 9.2. Serological, Microbiological, and Allergy Tests with ELFIA

Analyte	Tracer	Solid-phase	Substrate	Reference
HBsAg	βDG-Ab	μ-plate	4MUG	167
Anti-HBc IgM	HRP-Ab		HPA,H_2O_2	1695
Infl. A virus	βDG-Ab	Tube	4MUG	1696
Rotavirus	ALP-Ab	μ-plate	4MUP	245
Newcastle virus	ALP-Ab	Membrane	4MUP	1683
Arbovirus	ALP-sec.Ab	μ-plate	4MUP	1697
Feline. leuk. virus	ALP-Ab		4MUP	1698
Chlamydia	ALP-Ab	μ-plate	4MUP	1699
Salmonella	βDG-Ab	μ-plate	4MUG	1700
Anti-viral-Ab	βDG-Ab	μ-plate	4MUG	168
Anti-Borrelia Ab	ALP-Ab	μ-plate	4MUP	1701
Anti-Coxiella Ab	ALP-Ab	μ-plate	4MUP	1702
Monocl. screening	ALP-Ab	H. cells	4MUP	1703
Anti-estrogen Ab	ALP-Ab	μ-plate	4MUP	1704
Anti-nuclear Ab	ALP-Ab	μ-plate	4MUP	1705
	HRP-Ab	Tube	HPA,H_2O_2	1706
	ALP-Ab	Nylon ball	4MUP	166
IgE tot.	ALP-Ab	μ-plate	4MUP	1707
Allergy-spec. IgE	ALP-Ab	μ-plate	4MUP	1707–1710
Anti-mite IgE	βDG-Ab	μ-plate	4MUG	1711
Anti-pollen IgE	βDG-Ab	μ-plate	4MUG	1712
Rhinitis	ALP-Ab	μ-plate	4MUP	1713

Table 9.3. Competitive ELFIA Applications[a]

Analyte	Tracer	Solid-phase	Substrate	Reference
Gentamicin	βDG-Ag	Ab	4MUG	1714
Cytokinins	ALP-Ab	Ag	4MUP	1715
Digoxin	βDG-Ab	Beads-Ag	Gal-F	954
Neocarzinostatin	HRP-Ag	Sepharose-Ab	Tyramine,H_2O_2	960
Cotinine	ALP-biot.	μ-plate-Ag	4MUP	1716
Testosterone	HRP-Ag	Cellul.-Ab	HPA,H_2O_2	1717
Estradiol	HRP-Ag	Beads	Homovanil. H_2O_2	956
17-OH-Prog.	HRP-Ag	Bead-doubl. Ab	HPPA,H_2O_2	18, 1718
21-deoxy-cort.	HRP-Ag	Bead-Ab	HPPA,H_2O_2	1719
Aldosterone	HRP-Ag	Tube	HPA,H_2O_2	912
Pregnanediol-glucuronide	G6P-DHG-Ag	Cellul.-Ab	G6P, NAD	1720
Insulin	Glucoamyl. Ag	Sephadex-Ab	Amylose/NAD	969

[a]Abbreviations: G6P = glucose-6-phosphate dehydrogenase; Gal-F = galactosyl-fluorescein.

enzyme-enhanced immunoassays, and enzyme-labeled liposome assays (1721, 1722), homogeneous ELFIAs are not widely applied. Some homogeneous photometric EIAs can be converted to homogeneous ELFIAs by using coupled enzymatic reactions and fluorometric determination of formed NAD(P)H (1723), applied, for instance, in Syva's EMIT assays using the company's Syva Advance™ fluorometer (1724). Armenta et al. used a fluorogenic macromolecular substrate, dextrane coupled with β-galactosylumbelliferones, to construct homogeneous ELFIA for serum ferritin (955).

9.2.2. Batch-Analyzing ELFIA Systems

Commercial ELFIA systems are primarily developed for totally automated systems and less frequently for systems employing semiautomated or manual technologies. The FAST™ system of 3M Diagnostic is based on microtitration plates, immobilized allergens, ALP-labeled anti-hIgE, 4MUP substrate, and the FluoroFAST plate reader (1707–1709, 1713, 1725–1727). The allergy-analyzing system of Pharmacia Diagnostics, the Pharmacia CAP system, is based on a spongelike matrix, βDG as the label, and 4MUG as substrate (1728).

The first totally automated batch-analyzing system, the Stratus system (American Dade Division, Baxter Health Care, Miami, FL), uses glass fiber filter solid-phase cartridges for immobilizing the caching antibodies (1729, 1730). After the immunoreaction has taken place on the filter with ALP-labeled reagent, the added fluorogenic substrate solution (4MUP) functions simultaneously as a washing solution, and the fluorescent product diffuses from the center of the filter toward the edges ("radial partition"). The fluorescence of the formed product is measured kinetically from the center of the fiber filter with a front-surface fluorometer (571). Table 9.4 summarizes applications of the technology and some clinical evaluations of existing products.

Another widely used automated batch-analyzing system based on ELFIA technology is the Abbott IM_X. The system, called a microparticle capture enzyme immunoassay (MEIA), is based on microbead solid-phases using a glass fiber filter matrix for immobilizing the beads (410). Similarly to Stratus, this system also is based on ALP as a label and 4MUP as a substrate. The fluorescent product is measured with a front-surface fluorometer from the filter surface attached to a specific filter cartridge. Table 9.5 lists some of the applications of IM_X and their clinical evaluations.

9.2.3. Random-Access ELFIA Automates

At the moment several totally automated random-access immunoassay sys-

Table 9.4. ELFIA on Glass Fiber

Analyte	Tracer	Solid-phase	Substrate	Reference	Evaluation
TSH	ALP-Fab′	Ab	4MUP	1731	1732–1734
hCG	ALP-Ab	Ab	4MUP	1735, 1736	1737–1740
LH	ALP-Fab′	Ab	4MUP	1741	
FSH	ALP-Fab′	Ab	4MUP	1742	
Prolactin	ALP-Ab	Ab	4MUP	1743	
CK-MB	ALP-Ab	Ab	4MUP		1744
Ferritin	ALP-Ab	Ab	4MUP	1745	1746, 1747
Tot. IgE	ALP-Fab′	Ab	4MUP		1748
HBsAg	βDG-Ab	Ab	4MUG	1749	
HBsAg	βDG-S-avid	Ab	4MUG	69	
Tot. T_4	ALP-Ag	Ab	4MUP		1750
Free T_4	ALP-Ag	Ab	4MUP		1751
T_3	ALP-Ag	Ab	4MUP	1752	
Cortisol	ALP-Ag	Ab	4MUP		1737
Digoxin	ALP-Ag	Ab	4MUP	1730	
Vancomycin	ALP-Ag	Ab	4MUP	1753	
Procainamide	ALP-Ag	Ab	4MUP	1754, 1755	

tems have been introduced (Chapter 6.7.5), and the number of applications for the systems has been reported in posters and abstracts. Surprisingly, many of the systems introduced employ fluorometric EIA as the immunoassay system. The OPUS system of PB-Diagnostics employs two measuring systems and utilizes ELFIA for large analytes, very similarly to the Stratus ELFIA. The ELFIA is performed on glass-fiber paper attached to a unit dose cartridge and is based on ALP as the label and 4MUP as the substrate. Washing is performed as in the Stratus system, with the substrate solution (capillary flow washing), and fluorescence is followed kinetically. Applications introduced so far include assays of HBsAg (587), HIV antibodies (1787), hCG (1788), CEA (1789), and digoxin (1790).

The AIA 600 and 1200 of TOSOH Co. are basically the same as the earlier introduced Photon ELITE of Hybritech. This system is based on magnetic-particle separation, ALP as the enzyme, and 4MUP as the substrate. An application announced in 1990 relates to measurement of PAP and PSA (1791), β_2-microglobulin, ferritin and prolactin (1792), and TSH, T_4, and T_3 (1793). The automatic system of Kallestad is based on a specific dry reagent delivery module which contains the assay specific solid-phase, ALP-labeled immunoreagents (antigen or antibody), and 4MUP as the substrate. The abstracts presented at the AACC meeting in 1990 include a two-site assay of hCG (1794), a competitive assay of cortisol using double-antibody

Table 9.5. ELFIA with MEIA-IM_x System

Analyte	Tracer	Solid-phase	Reference	Evaluation
hCG	ALP-Ab	Ab	1756	1757, 1758
FSH	ALP-Ab	Ab	1759, 1760	1761
LH	ALP-Ab	Ab	1762	1761
PL	ALP-Ab	Ab	1763	
AFP	ALP-Ab	Ab	1764–1766	
Ferritin	ALP-Ab	Ab	1767	1768
β_2-microglob.	ALP-Ab	Ab	1769	
CK-MB	ALP-Ab	Ab	1770	
CEA	ALP-Ab	Ab	1771	
PSA	ALP-Ab	Ab	1772	
CEA	ALP-Ab	Ab	1773	
HBsAg	ALP-Ab	Ab	1774	
HBsAg	ALP-anti-biot	Ab (+biot-Ab)	1775, 1776	
Anti-HBc, IgM	ALP-Ab	Ab	1777	
Anti-HB-A, IgM	ALP-Ag	Ab	1778	
Anti-HBc	ALP-Ab	Ag (competit.)	1779	
Anti-HIV	ALP-Ab	Ag	1780	
Anti-Toxopl. IgG	ALP-Ab	Ag		1781
Anti-rubella	ALP-Ab	Ag		1781
Tot. T_4	ALP-Ag	Ab		1782
T uptake	ALP-Ag	Ab		1782
Tot. T_3	ALP-Ag	Ab		1783
Free T_3	ALP-Ag	Ab	1784	
Prog.	ALP-Ag	Ab	1785	
B_{12} vit.	ALP-Ag	Binding prot.	1786	

solid-phase (1795), an assay of free T_4 with back titration (1796) and direct competitive assays of digoxin (1797) and theophylline (1798). A system named Pulse FIA is under development by Beckman. That too is based on ELFIA, with ALP as a label and 4MUP as the substrate. Noller has introduced a list of applications performed with the system (1799), including assays, hormones, drugs, peptides, viruses, and microbes.

VISTA is based on DuPont's chromium dioxide magnetic particles and uses ALP as the label and 4MUP as the substrate for fluorometric detection. Chromium-dioxide-magnetic-particle-based ELFIAs were presented at the 1988 AACC meeting for a number of analytes (Table 9.6).

At the moment ELFIA technique is commonly used in companies developing automated immunoassay systems. The demands for the immunoassay applied in automated systems are very high; the reagents need to be very stable, and the produced response must be unchanged to allow the use of

Table 9.6. ELFIA with Chromium Dioxide Magnetic Particles

Analyte	Tracer	Solid-phase	Reference
TSH	ALP-Ab	Ab	1800
hCG	ALP-Ab	Ab	1801
FSH	ALP-Ab	Ab	1802
AFP	ALP-Ab	Ab	1803
CEA	ALP-Ab	Ab	1804
Ferritin	ALP-Ab	Ab	1805
β_2-microglob.	ALP-Ab	Ab	1806
HBsAg	ALP-Ab	Ab	1807
Anti-HBsAg	ALP-Ag	Ag	1808
Anti-HBc	ALP-Ab	Ag (competit.)	1809
Anti-HAV, IgM	ALP-Ab (+HAV)	S-avid (+B-anti-hIgM)	1810
Anti-HIV	ALP-Ab	Ag	1811
Tot. T_4	ALP-Ag	S-avid.	1812
T uptake	ALP-Ag	S-avid.	1812
T_3	ALP-Ag	S-avid.	1813
Free T_4	ALP-Ag	S-avid.	1814
Cortisol	ALP-Ab	Ag	1815

standard curves from memory. High sensitivities are also needed, and there is a high demand to develop assays that are as rapid as possible. Fluorometric detection improves the sensitivity, and microparticle solid-phases are generally used to provide sufficient capacity and rapid diffusion.

CHAPTER

10

OTHER SPECIFIC BINDING ASSAYS USING FLUORESCENCE

Even though antibodies are the most widely used and most important specific binding reagents in the clinical analysis of biologically important compounds, numerous other specific binding reactions are employed for certain types of assays. The uses of thyroxine-binding globulin for the assay of T_4, of intrinsic factor for the assay of B_{12}, of protein A for the analysis of IgG, of lectins for monitoring glycosylated groups on proteins, and of a biotin-avidin pair for the amplification signal for various immunological applications are briefly described in Chapter 2.7. Different types of assays, in respect to technical performance and application field, also can be made using receptors on cell surfaces (or solubilized receptors), DNA- or RNA-probes, or certain intact viable cells of the immunological system. The most important alternative, or complementary, system to immunoassays will be DNA hybridization assays using labeled DNA-probes. If current hybridization technology can be simplified—for instance, to use fluorescent probes instead of radioisotopes—DNA hybridization assays will become an important tool in clinical laboratories for the diagnosis of viruses and microbes, for early identification of cancer cells through the determination of oncogenes, and for identification of genes and mutations leading to inherited disorders.

10.1. RECEPTOR ASSAYS

Receptor proteins and receptor containing cells are determined and enumerated routinely using fluorescent antibodies and IF or flow-cytometric methods (63). Receptors commonly measured include the TSH receptor (1816), insulin receptors (1817), and prolactin and growth hormone receptors (1818) in addition to estradiol receptors (1819). Actual quantitative determinations of receptor amounts or their affinities from cell surfaces or tissue homogenates are not generally done with fluorometric techniques but rather with radioactive tracers. Assays such as estrogen receptor determinations on breast cancer tumors are frequently done with ^{3}H-labeled steroids (1820–1823). A few studies have, however, been conducted for using fluorescently labeled ligands for the determination of respective receptors.

Many of the technologies developed for the quantitation of soluble antigens could be transferred to the quantitation of soluble receptors, provided that the sensitivity obtained would be sufficient. Dandliker et al. (1824, 1825) used fluorescein-labeled estradiol, GH, and prolactin for homogeneous determinations of cellular receptors based on the fluorescence polarization increase upon the binding of the tracer to the receptor. In addition to fluorescein (1826–1828), dansyl- and NBD-derivatized steroids also have been synthesized and tested for receptor assays (1829), but these needed to be extracted into organic solvent before the specific fluorescence could be distinguished from cell autofluorescence (685). A fluorescent estrogen receptor reagent is also commercialized with the trade name FLUORO-CEP® by Wampole Laboratories (Cranbury, NJ). Rhodamine-labeled T_3 was tested in a microscopic assay of cellular binding protein (1826), but its value was diminished by the partial aggregation it undergoes.

Background fluorescence—for example, the autofluorescence of cells, if intact cells are used for assays—causes the same problem for receptor assays as it causes for normal fluorescence immunoassays. Sensitivity can be improved by using polymeric labels; for instance, fluorescent microbeads (Fluoresbrite beads, Polyscience, Inc.) are applied in a flow-cytometric determination of IgE receptors on T-cells (945).

10.2. CELL-MEDIATED IMMUNOLOGICAL ASSAYS

Cells of the immunological system can also be used as reagents in immunological tests, or as analytes determined with cell-mediated immunological tests. For those assays, viable cells need to be labeled with signal-producing compounds—or the cell components (such as the cellular enzymes) are used as labels leaking out from the cells when cells die. One such cell-mediated cytotoxicity assay is the test of natural killer cell activity (NK cells), routinely performed using ^{51}Cr-labeled target cells and measuring the chromium release during the killing process (1830). Chromium labeling of cells was originally developed for an assay for lysing nucleated cells introduced by Goodman in 1961 (1831) and later extended to other cytolytic cell-mediated reactions (1830, 1832). Due to the radioactivity of ^{51}Cr, there has been a strong tendency to develop alternative non-radioisotopic technologies to replace the chromium release assay.

The requirements for cell labeling are that the label and the labeling procedure not be toxic for the cells, that spontaneous release of the label be minimal, that the labeling procedure and assay of the release be simple and robust, and that the labeling not cause any morphological change to the target cells possibly recognized by the effector cells. Alternative labels introduced include the intrinsic enzymes of cells such as ALP (1833), lactate dehydrogenase (1834), or various chemiluminescent detection systems (1835, 1836).

Carboxyfluorescein, as a diester derivative, is the most commonly used fluorogenic compound for labeling viable cells. As a nonpolar hydrophobic compound, diester easily penetrates the cell membrane, and in viable cells the ester bonds are rapidly hydrolyzed by the action of cell esterases. The resulting hydrophilic CF stays inside the cell and cells become fluorescent (fluorochromasia) (625). CF-labeled target cells are used for NK cell cytotoxicity tests—for example, by the enumeration of viable fluorescent cells with a flow cytometer after the action of NK cells (1837). Schols et al. (1838) used CF-labeled T_4 lymphocytes for an assay of the anti-HIV activity of antiviral drugs. The assay was based on the inhibition of the cytopathic effect of HIV by the drug.

Alternative fluorescent probes used for the purpose are Hoechst dye No. 33342, a DNA fluorochrome used to label target cells for T-cell cytotoxicity assays (1839), green emitting PKH-1, which binds to cytoplasm membranes, and propidium iodide, which stains nonviable cells (1840). New derivatives of carboxyfluorescein also have been introduced, such as an acetoxymethylester of 2′7′-bis(carboxyethyl)-5,6-carboxyfluorescein, which reportedly has lower spontaneous leakage through cell membranes (1841). It is also commercially available from Molecular Probes, Inc. and is suited for cytotoxicity tests (627, 1840). Ethidium bromide, generally used for labeling nucleotides in cells, was proposed for antibody-mediated cytotoxicity assays in 1975 (1842).

Labeling target cells with Eu-DTPA is successfully used for the assay of NK-cell activity by the determination of the released Eu-chelates after dissociative fluorescence enhancement with time-resolved fluorometry (842, 1843–1845). In this system the target cells are labeled with a hydrophilic Eu-chelate after partial disintegration of the cell membrane with dextrane sulfate and correction of the damage with glucose and Ca^{2+} after incubation with Eu-DTPA to keep the cells alive.

10.3. DNA HYBRIDIZATION ASSAYS

Recombinant DNA technology is predicted to have a major impact on future clinical diagnosis. Its importance is obvious in areas where traditional immunological techniques for one reason or other are not satisfactory, such as the identification of genetic disorders at an early foetal stage of development (muscular dystrophy, familial hypercholesterolemia and cystic fibrosis), early detection and identification of cancers (oncogenes), detection of microbes (salmonella) and viruses—even at the latent phase in host DNA—and identification of DNA samples in forensic medicine. In microbiology DNA-probe techniques are becoming important complements to immunoassays for the identification of microbes in cases where conventional microbiological and immunological methods are not applicable—for example, when the microbe is difficult to grow, the antigenicity is poorly known, or the microbe is in latent phase.

In a conventional hybridization assay, nucleic acids are immobilized on a filter and detected using a complementary DNA-probe labeled with a radioactive nucleus, generally ^{32}P. This technique requires, however, laborious sample pretreatment and fixation, and the hybridization is slow. In a sandwich hybridization, two DNA-probes complementary to adjacent positions of the sample sequence are utilized the same way as two antibodies in two-site sandwich immunoassays, by immobilizing one and using the other as labeled reagent (1846). Another modification of the technology is named affinity-based collection hybridization (ABC), which enables the primary hybridization to take place in solution (1847). In this technique one probe is affinity labeled with a hapten or biotin to ensure the subsequent collection of formed hybrids on the solid surface, and the other probe is labeled with the marker.

10.3.1. Alternative Labels for Nucleotides

Today radioactive isotopes (^{32}P, ^{125}I, ^{35}S, or ^{3}H) are the labels primarily used in hybridization assays, and their binding is determined with β counters or autoradiography. As with immunoassays, in hybridization assays a general tendency is to develop non-radioisotopic detection systems. The drawbacks of radioisotopes involve the legal, emotional, health, and disposal problems related to the handling, use, and storage of radioactive materials. Also, the detection, if performed with autoradiography, is laborious, semi-quantitative, and time consuming. Detection can be achieved with automated counters, but these produce a somewhat lower detection sensitivity. The problems inherent with isotopic techniques have also effectively prevented the distribution of the technology for routine clinical use. The advantage of radioisotopes relates to their robust use and high sensitivity, which has been difficult to exceed with non-radioactive labels in practical assay conditions.

A number of different non-radioactive labels have been developed for nucleic acid probes—for use in virus diagnosis, for instance (1848). Various enzymes are used as labels through the use of indirect labeling by haptenized probes. In *in situ* hybridization, fluorogenic substrates that produce insoluble fluorescent deposits are used. Also, the "enhanced luminescence" detection of the HRP catalyzed chemiluminescence of luminol (1849) and ALP triggered dioxetane luminescence, enhanced with micelles and energy transfer with fluorescent compounds (598) are used. Chemiluminescence-based hybridization assays with acridinium-ester-labeled DNA-probes have also been introduced (1850). Fluorescent probes offer an easy and direct method of detection, used especially for *in situ* hybridization and DNA sequencing, even though the sensitivity obtained with organic fluorochromes and conventional fluorometers is less than with radioisotopic tracers or enzymes (1851, 1852).

Polymerase chain reaction (PCR), a technology able to multiply the target DNA up to 10^6-fold by repeated cycles of denaturation of the template, primer annealing, and extensions (1853), has made it possible to exploit even less sensitive detection techniques for hybridization assays.

10.3.2. Labeling of Polynucleotides

Polynucleotides are generally labeled at multiple internal sites or by either the 3′ or 5′ terminus. The marker substances are coupled either directly to nucleotides (e.g., ^{32}P) or, more often, indirectly using biotin or haptens, and streptavidin or anti-hapten antibodies as carriers of labels.

Biotinylation of DNA-probes has become one of the most frequently used labeling technologies. Polynucleotides can be biotinylated enzymatically, chemically (photobiotin), chemically after transamination of cytidines, or by biotinylation of intercalating compounds, such as psoralen (1854). Enzymatic nick-translation with bio-11-dUTP (1855) is a routinely used method for labeling polynucleotides. Chemical biotinylation of intact DNA also can be made directly with highly reactive biotin derivatives, such as an azido derivative of biotin (photobiotin) (1856, 1857), a diazo derivative of biotin (1858), a hydrazide derivative of biotin with glutaraldehyde (1859), or after incorporation of amino-derivatized nucleotides (e.g., allylamine UTP) into RNA (1860). For biotinylation or other derivatization, reactive amino groups can be introduced into polynucleotides by a transamination reaction—for example, by a bisulfite catalyzed reaction with diamines (1861). In addition to the amino groups sulfhydryl groups also have been introduced to the 5′ terminus to be coupled with SH-reactive fluorochromes (1862). Psoralen has been used for labeling DNA with Eu^{3+} by coupling a polylysine to a psoralen SH-group and incorporating DTTA groups to polylysine with DTPA anhydride (846).

Other affinity pairs also are utilized for indirect labeling of DNA-probes. Azido-DNP is used as a photoactive labeling reagent analogously to the use of photobiotin, which can produce labeling levels of 7–23 DNP/1000 bases (1863). Aminoacetylfluorene was used as a linking hapten for fluorescent antibodies through mouse anti-acetylfluorene in a study of three-color fluorescence in *in situ* hybridization (1863). FITC can also be used as a hapten for *in situ* hybridization by using rabbit-anti-FITC and FITC-labeled anti-rabbit IgG (1864).

Terminal L-deoxyribonucleotidyl transferase and polynucleotide phosphorylase are applied to add polyriboadenylic acids (8000 AMP groups) to the 3′ terminal end of the probe (1865), detected after the hydrolysis to ATP with a bioluminescence reaction with pyruvate kinase and luciferase. ATP detection, however, encountered practical problems with the high background. With a similar technology Trainor and Jensen (1866) prepared polyfluorescein-labeled DNA-probes. Other techniques to prepare polymeric labels for nucleotide probes function with macromolecules conjugated with a plurality of labels and coupled to the probes. Fluorescein-labeled polyethyleneimine was coupled to a DNA-probe with glutardialdehyde and used for quantitation of mRNA on T- and B-lymphocytes (918). Ylikoski et al. (917) have issued a patent application for a polymeric label technology for introducing multiple Eu-chelates to a DNA-probe to be used in time-resolved fluorometric hybridization assays.

10.3.3. Labeling of Oligonucleotides

Oligonucleotide probes have recently attracted attention as probes for nucleic acid hybridization assays, because their use involves an easier labeling procedure and the hybridization assay can be done at a lower temperature and in a shorter time (1867). On the other hand, it is difficult to obtain the same sensitivities with oligonucleotides due to the lower amount of label oligonucleotides can incorporate.

Various technologies have been developed for labeling oligonucleotides. Many of them have been developed to be used as primers in DNA sequencing studies and are performed with automated DNA synthesizers using phosphoramidate activated building blocks. Labeling at the 5′ terminal end can be performed after producing an aliphatic amino group to the 5′ end. Smith et al. (1868) studied the labeling of amino terminal oligonucleotides with a number of fluorescent probes, including FITC, Texas Red, TRITC, and NBD chloride. Schubert et al. (1869) labeled oligonucleotides at the 5′ terminal end with biotin or fluorescein. Biotin also can be incorporated into an oligonucleotide directly with a synthesizer using a phosphoramidate-activated biotin derivative (1870).

For hybridization assays, improvements in sensitivity can be achieved by using polymeric labeling procedures. Singh et al. (1851) made poly-fluor-labeled probes by synthesizing adenine-modified oligonucleotides labeled with dansyl groups. By choosing a suitable linker and spacer arm, both total fluorescence and quantum yield reportedly can be enhanced with suitable polymeric labels. Kwiatkowski et al. (878) have described different routes to label oligonucleotides either with a nonfluorescent Eu-chelate (for a dissociative fluorescence-enhancement assay) or with a fluorescent Eu-chelate (for *in situ* hybridizations) using diaminohexane-modified deoxycytidines to yield 20–30 Eu^{3+} per oligonucleotide. These probes have been used to detect HIV-1 nucleic acid by ABC hybridization assay after PCR using time-resolved fluorometry (1871). Sund et al. (845) utilized polyvinylamines and polyacrylates coupled to a synthetic oligonucleotide with a cross-linking reagent as linear carriers for a multiplicity of Eu-chelates.

Ruthenium is a nonlanthanide metal which also has a relatively long fluorescence decay time and has been used as a probe in time-resolved fluorometric assays (Chapter 7.4.1). Bannwarth et al. prepared fluorescent DNA-probes by coupling Ru-tris-bathophenanthroline to the 5′ terminal end, modified with 5′-amino-5′-deoxythymidine (895, 896) through a carboxylic group on the phenyl ring.

Bauman et al. (1872) described the synthesis of 3′-terminus–labeled RNA-probes for *in situ* hybridization studies. FITC and TRITC were first coupled to hydrazine to yield thiosemicarbazides, subsequently coupled to a periodate oxidized ribose ring in RNA.

10.3.4. *In Situ* Hybridization

Fluorometric DNA-probe techniques can be divided into qualitative microscopic *in situ* staining techniques and quantitative hybridization assays of analytes, similarly to the classification of fluorescent-antibody techniques into immunofluorescence and immunofluorometric assays. In *in situ* hybridization, nucleotide probes labeled with organic fluorescent probes are used for staining specified DNA or RNA sequences, microbes, or genes, and the detection is performed with a fluorescence microscope, microfluorometer, image cytofluorometer, or flow cytometer.

Examples of the applications of *in situ* hybridization are determinations of adenoviruses with TRITC-labeled RNA-probes (634), detection of HIV-related RNA and DNA in infected lymphocytes with haptenized probes, an anti-hapten antibody, and a FITC-labeled secondary antibody (519), detection of DNA sequences by indirect staining with FITC-labeled RNA, rabbit-anti-FITC, and FITC-labeled anti-rabbit IgG (1864), and localization of RNA with a biotinylated probe and TRITC-labeled avidin (1873).

Dual- and triple-label staining techniques are possible also with fluorescent nucleotide probes, similar to the use of fluorescent antibodies in double- or triple-label IF staining. Bakkus et al. (1874) used FITC-labeled streptavidin and TRITC-labeled antibodies with haptenized RNA-probes for the detection of oncogene expression. Nederlof et al. (1875) developed methods for multiparameter analysis using three different fluorescent probes, FITC,

TRITC, and AMCA, with biotinylated and haptenized probes and with a probe labeled with mercury and an SH-group containing a TNP derivative.

Even though sensitivity is not a major problem in *in situ* hybridization studies, more sensitive label systems have been developed for qualitative assays. Valet and Oser suggested the use of Eu-cryptates as probes determined with TR fluorometry with a flow-cytometric application (891). More sensitive response also can be obtained by using enzymes as labels with fluorometric or luminometric substrates.

10.3.5. Quantitative Hybridization Assays

In quantitative hybridization assays there is a need for high sensitivity, and therefore the use of conventional fluorescent probes is limited to low-sensitivity detection applications—or applications utilizing PCR prior to actual hybridization. The high sensitivity required has also limited the usage of non-isotopic detection systems, due to the relatively high sensitivity obtained with ^{32}P. Urdea et al. (1876) recently compared some fluorescent probes (fluorescein, Texas Red, and sulforhodamine) with isoluminol, ALP (with chromogenic substrates), and HRP with chromogenic and luminogenic detection in oligonucleotide labeling. The probes were compared in a sandwich hybridization assay with a ^{32}P-labeled probe. The fluorescent probes and luminol yielded about 2,000–10,000-fold, ALP 200-fold, and HRP 2-fold less sensitive assays than ^{32}P.

Non-radioisotopic labels used in quantitative hybridization assays include enzymatic labels, detected with fluorometric or luminometric substrates, and various chelates detected with time-resolved fluorometry.

Coutlée et al. (1877, 1878) developed an assay for DNA detection by using biotinylated RNA-probes, biotin binding solid-phase, and monoclonal antibodies against RNA-DNA hybrids, labeled with βDG and determined with a fluorogenic substrate. The system was applied for measurement of HIV DNA after PCR. Nagata et al. (1879) used βDG-labeled avidin in dot-blot hybridization on surfaces of microtitration plate wells with the use of biotinylated probes and achieved a detection level down to picogram amounts of DNA. Alkaline phosphatase is another enzyme frequently used for hybridization assays, especially because of the extreme sensitivity of the chemiluminescence detection method of ALP using dioxetane-phosphate substrate systems (598, 1880). ALP with 4MUP as the fluorogenic substrate was also used, for example, for the detection of phage DNA by Murakami et al. (1881).

Time-resolved fluorometry is the other non-radioisotopic technology sensitive enough for hybridization assays. Applications have been developed primarily by using the dissociative fluorescence-enhancement principle, which employs nonfluorescent Eu-chelate labels. Some studies have been carried out also with stable fluorescent Eu-chelates and fluorescent Ru-chelates. Syvänen et al. (1882) used Eu-labeled anti-mouse IgG for detecting hybrids formed with sample DNA and a 7-iodoacetylaminofluorene haptenized DNA-probe, after incubating with mouse antibodies against the hapten. Eu-labeled streptavidin is used with biotinylated DNA-probes for the dot-blot hybridization assay for adenovirus type 2, for example, (1883) and in the sandwich hybridization assay of *E. coli* plasmin (1884).

In indirect hybridization assays the chelates originally optimized for *in vitro* immunoassays can also be used to label, for instance, streptavidin for detection with dissociative fluorescence enhancement (Chapter 7.4.3). A label attached directly to a DNA-probe has to have very high kinetic chelate stability to resist the dissociation of metals at the temperature and EDTA concentration used in hybridization conditions, and therefore the chelate optimized for DNA labeling is different from that used for immunoassays (843). Oser et al. (846) used psoralen conjugated to polylysine for coupling with chelating groups formed with a DTPA-anhydride reaction and chelated with Eu^{3+}. The probe was used in filter hybridization for hepatitis B virus detection. The DTTA-amide chelate used, however, was found unstable during hybridization. A more stable Eu-chelate composed of a pyridine-bis (methyliminodiacetic acid) derivative (843, 878) was used for labeling a DNA-probe with nick-translation and random priming, using chelate-labeled dCTP (1885). With a labeling level of 3.5 Eu/100 bases, a detection sensitivity of 10^5 targets was achieved. DNA-probes labeled with Eu-chelates after transamination of DNA were used for detecting adenovirus DNA on a spot hybridization assay on a nitrocellulose filter (1886), detection of papilloma virus type 16 with a sandwich hybridization (1887) and with ABC hybridization on microtitration strips (1888). Oligonucleotide probes labeled with Eu-chelates have been used for detecting HIV-1 viruses (1871) and human T-lymphocytic virus II (HTLV) (1889) performed after a PCR multiplication.

Kwiatkowski et al. (878) have described the synthesis of an oligomeric DNA-probe labeled with a stable and fluorescent Eu-chelate suitable for *in situ* hybridizations. Saavedra and Picozza (868) have described a Tb-labeling system consisting of a DTPA adduct formed with p-aminosalicylic acid (DTPA-PAS), chelated with Tb, and coupled to DNA via one of the DTPA carboxylic acids. The use of a Eu-cryptate formed with Eu^{3+} and tris-bipyridine cryptand has been tested in dot-blot hybridization using biotinylated DNA-probes and cryptate-labeled streptavidin (1890).

The use of Ru-chelates has the advantage of inherited kinetic stability that Ru-chelates generally have, but on the other hand, the decay time of Ru is considerably shorter and causes a more profound background problem than is encountered with lanthanide chelates. Bannwarth et al. (895, 896) have developed labeling techniques for coupling Ru-bathophenanthroline to the 5′ terminus of DNA. By choosing suitable conditions (removing oxygen and modifying the buffer) for the measurement of Ru-chelate fluorescence, they were able to prolong the decay times from 1 μs to 7.5 μs, which makes the background rejection with time resolution easier (897).

Various homogeneous hybridization methods have also been developed (or patented) based on, for instance, an energy transfer from the intercalating fluor to the attached lanthanide chelates (81), from an FITC-labeled oligonucleotide to a Texas Red-labeled probe (within a distance of less than 5 nucleotides) (1891), or from 5′-end-coupled fluorescein on a complementary chain 3′-end-coupled pyrene or Texas Red (638). These solution-phase detections of DNA hybridizations are made possible by the development of PCR technology, the use of which enables the application of even less sensitive detection systems.

CHAPTER

11

MULTIPARAMETRIC IMMUNOASSAYS

During the 1970s the main emphasis in research on immunoassays was to develop alternative labels and techniques to replace radioimmunoassays with non-isotopic assays. Fluorescent compounds, among the others, were regarded as interesting and potentially suitable alternatives. The major objective was to employ fluorescent probes to develop simple homogeneous assays. The research resulted in a number of homogeneous FIA techniques, from which especially the fluorescence polarization assay, commercialized by Abbott, proved to be very successful. During the 1980s the main emphasis was directed toward development of more sensitive non-radioisotopic technologies in order to find real alternatives for RIA and IRMA assays. As a result, EIAs have found extensive applications, and after the use of fluorogenic and luminogenic substrates, enzyme-based technologies have reached very high assay sensitivities. Another highly sensitive technology developed during the '80s was the time-resolved fluorometric immunoassay with lanthanide chelate labels—a technology which also achieved sensitivities exceeding those of radioisotopic techniques. Toward the end of the 1980s and in the early 1990s, the main development trend seems to have been directed toward totally automated immunoassay systems, random-access automates where the analytes are measured with automatic systems in the order received by the laboratory.

The future direction of immunoassay development could be the development of remote immunosensors—devices able to monitor analytes continuously in biological fluids without taking samples. Another idea for a future system could be a multiparametric analyzing system able to measure whole panels of analytes from a single sample, a future prospect presented by Professor Ekins (524, 1892–1894). In the system he named "microspot multi-analyte ratiometric immunoassay" or "dual-signal pulsed light time-resolved ambient analyte fluoroimmunoassay," the catching antibodies are labeled with one fluorescent compound and are immobilized on tiny spots or spot arrows. The saturation level of catching antibodies is measured by measuring the fluorescence of fluorescent second antibody bound to the spot in ratio to the fluorescence of immobilized antibody, and that ratio is a function of the analyte concentration in the sample. By rapidly scanning the spots with scanning-laser fluorometry, a whole panel of analytes could in principle be measured from a droplet of sample.

Fluorescence is particularly well suited for multiparametric determinations, because fluorometric determination can combine several parameters simultaneously, such as excitation, emission, fluorescence lifetime, and spatial resolution.

11.1. DUAL-LABEL IMMUNOASSAYS

A number of analytes are customarily always measured together from the same samples, and therefore there is a need to develop dual-label assays to simplify their simultaneous determination. Typical analyte pairs frequently measured together include thyroid hormones, T_3 and T_4 (1895), T_4 and TSH (1896) or free T_4 and TSH, vitamins B_{12} and folate, FSH and LH (1897), estrogen glucuronide and pregnanediol-glucuronide in urine (prognosis of ovulation) (1898, 1899), AFP and hCG for diagnosis of Down's syndrome, and the screening of HBsAg and HIV-Abs from blood collected for transfusion.

Requirements for labels in double-label assays relate to spillover of their signals, which should be negligible (or it should be possible for the spillovers to be mathematically processed in order to avoid interferences). Label pairs routinely used in RIAs are iodine isotopes 125 and 131 (1900) and ^{57}Co and ^{125}I, used, for example, in commercial dual-label assays of T_4 and TSH (1901). Enzymes also can be used for double-label assays, provided that the two chromogenic substrates have different absorption maxima, as, for instance, o-nitrophenyl-β-D-galactoside (for βDG) and phenolphthalein-phosphate (for ALP) (1902). Also, colloidal particles, silver and gold, are used as labels in double-label assays (304), as are combinations of two totally unrelated assay technologies, such as RIA and LIA (1903).

Fluorescent compounds are traditionally used for double- and triple-label staining in IF and flow-cytometric applications (Chapters 6.5 and 8.2.3). The first pair of fluorochromes used for simultaneous determination of two parameters was FITC and TRITC, used for example, in detecting IgD and IgM on lymphocyte surfaces (534) and for identification of bacteria with a fluorescence microscope (1904). FITC and dansyl-chloride were used for detecting IgG and IgM on spleen cells (1905), and FITC and Texas Red were used in two-laser flow-cytometric identification of lymphoid cell populations (529). Mossberg and Ericsson (1906) tested the use of Lucifer Yellow, Texas Red, FITC, and TRITC for double-label staining in confocal scanning microscopic studies. The orange fluorescence of B-phycoerythrin (B-PE) provides a good contrast to the green emission of fluorescein, and B-PE has become a very popular fluorescent probe also in double- and triple-label stainings. B-PE and FITC were used for measuring Epstein-Barr virus receptors on different B-cell subpopulations with a flow cytometer (1907), and the pair also was used for quantitative flow-cytometric detection of IgG and IgM using on-line polymerized beads (533) and the staining of lymphoid node sections (1908). The problem encountered with B-PE is its high absorptivity, which in certain conditions can cause quenching of FITC, if the respective labeled antibodies are bound to the same cell, and can thus lead to misinterpretations of the results (1909).

Triple labeling is sometimes used in immunological stainings. Staines et al. (665) performed three-color immunofluorescence histochemistry with FITC-labeled antibodies, TRITC- or Texas Red-labeled antibodies, and DACM (diethylaminocoumarine)-labeled avidin. Another coumarine derivative, 7-amino-4-methyl-coumarine-3-acetic acid (AMCA), is used as the third, blue emitting label after coupling to streptavidin—used, for instance, in a three-color immunofluorescence staining (1910). Rothbarth et al. suggested the use of SITC as a third fluorochrome for triple-label IF in addition to FITC and TRITC (691). Festin et al. have made a triple-label flow-cytometric analysis using colloidal gold particles in addition to B-PE and FITC (306), and three-color flow-cytometric measurement of lymphocytes with a single-laser excitation of FITC, B-PE, and DuoCHROME™ (the trade name of Becton Dickinson, a tandem probe of Texas Red-conjugated B-PE) (1911). Allophycocyanin (A-PC) is used as the third probe together with B-PE and FITC in the triple-label flow-cytometric assay of B-cell maturation (1912), for the determination of IgM, IgD, and BLA-1 and BLA-2 antigens on lymphocytes (1913), and as a fourth label in four-color flow-cytometric studies of B-cell differentiation (732) in addition to FITC, B-PE, and Texas Red. The probes were excited with two lasers, at 488 nm with an argon-ion laser and at 605 nm with a dye laser. A-PC is also used as a fourth label in the flow-cytometric assay of NK cell subpopulations together with Texas Red, B-PE, and FITC (1914). The use of five different labels, FITC, B-PE (excited with an argon-ion laser at 488 nm), Texas Red, A-PC (excited with a rhodamine G dye laser tuned to 600 nm) and monochlorobimate (excited with an argon-ion laser tuned to UV) has been tested in a flow-cytometric application (530).

Cascade Blue and BOPIDY are new fluorescent probes developed and commercialized by Molecular Probes, Inc. They are reportedly suited especially well for triple-label stainings with Texas Red as the third probe.

So far there are only a few examples of actual quantitative double-label FIAs using conventional fluorescent probes. Sidki et al. (1074) made a double-label simultaneous Sep-FIA for primidone and phenobarbital, using FITC-labeled phenobarbital and XRITC-labeled primidone. Dean et al. (1326)

have developed a double-label SL-FIA using 4MUP-conjugated phenytoin (snake venom phosphodiesterase as the releasing enzyme) and 3-carboxy-coumarine-7-galactoside–conjugated phenobarbital (βDG as the releasing enzyme). The reason for the limited use of organic fluorescent probes in double-label assays might be the relatively high signal spillover between the signals.

By combining spectral resolution with temporal resolution, a feature made possible with time-resolved fluorometry, it is possible to increase the specificity of signal detection considerably (826). The sharp emission peaks of lanthanide chelates, in addition to the typical fluorescence decay times each ion has in the particular chelate solution, offers a way to make double- or triple-label TR-FIAs (Fig. 11.1). Eu^{3+} and Tb^{3+} are used as labels in double-label TR-IFMAs of LH and FSH (827) and adeno- and rotaviruses (828). Sm^{3+} is also used as a probe in TR-fluorometric immunoassays (823, 825). A labeling reagent has recently been introduced for Sm-labeling (841), and it can be measured in the dissociative fluorescence-enhancement solution already optimized for Eu^{3+}, even though with somewhat decreased sensitivity (822). Sm^{3+} has been used, together with Eu^{3+}, in double-label TR-IFMA of potato viruses (825, 1915).

In addition to the long decay times, the fluorescence of lanthanide chelates also has relatively long fluorescence rise times due to various energy transfer processes taking place prior to the actual emission (1916). Combining organic fluorescent probes that emit within 10 ns from the excitation with lanthanide chelates which emit within 1 μs to a few milliseconds from excitation means that their fluorescences can be totally distinguished from each other by temporal resolution, which gives an excellent opportunity for multiparametric analysis (1917).

11.2. MULTIPLE-SPACE IMMUNOASSAYS

Another way to make multi-analyte assays is to use different spaces for different immunoreactions and detection by high spatial resolution. A sort of multiple-space immunoassay has been developed for an RIA (1918) and for an EIA of cortisol and dehydroepiandrosterone sulfate by using transferable solid-phases (1919). Fluorometry is especially suitable for high resolution detection even from microscopic objectives, when utilizing lasers for excitation with microfluorometers, for instance, or with confocal fluorescence microscopes. Laser scanning devices allow for real multiparametric determinations, as in systems described by Ekins et al. (524).

Current multiparametric assays based on spatial resolution are primarily performed with microbeads as solid-phases. The assays introduced are based

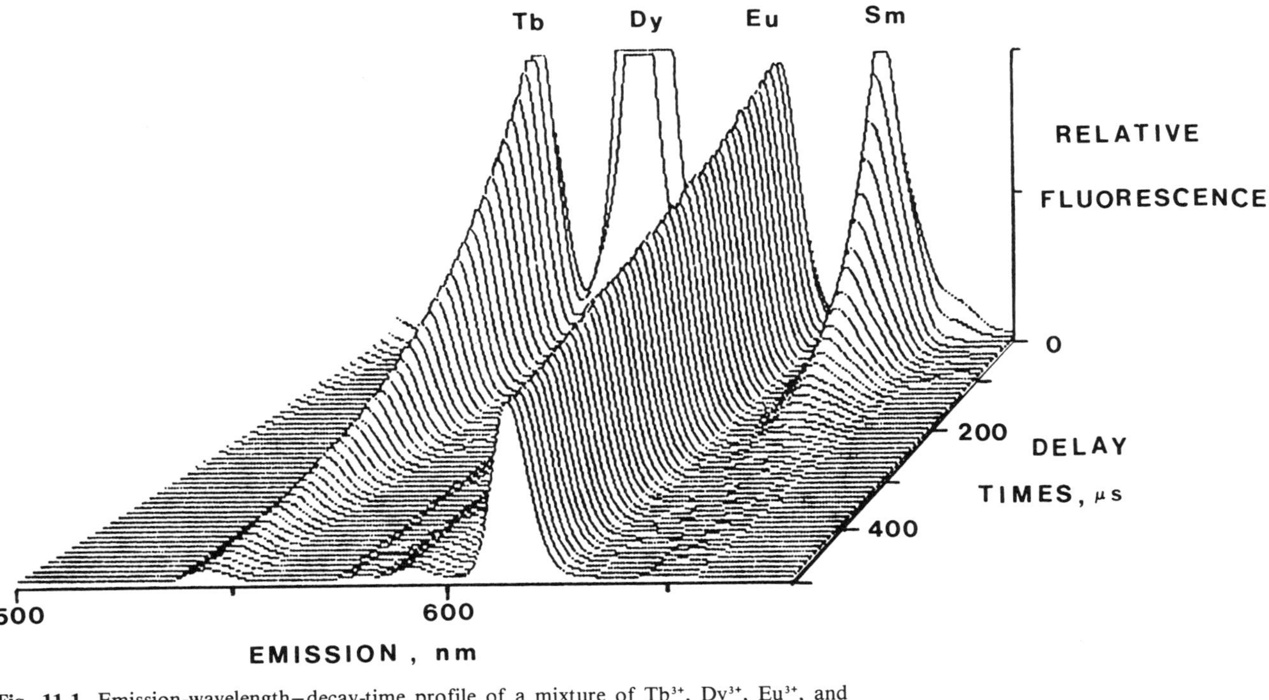

Fig. 11.1. Emission-wavelength–decay-time profile of a mixture of Tb^{3+}, Dy^{3+}, Eu^{3+}, and Sm^{3+} chelates with PTA.

on two or three sets of uniformly sized latex beads analyzed with flow cytometers able to measure bead-associated fluorescences separately from each size of beads (1019). Antibodies against cytomegalovirus and herpes simplex virus have been determined simultaneously using beads of 5 and 7 μm sizes (65) and three different antibodies against microbes using three different sets of beads of 5, 7, and 9.3 μm sizes (95).

REFERENCES

1. D. M. Weir, Ed., *Handbook of Experimental Immunology,* Blackwell Scientific Publication, Oxford, 1979.
2. I. Roit, J. Brostoff, and D. Male, *Immunology,* Churchill Livingstone, London, 1987.
3. L. Reiner, *Science,* **72,** 483 (1930).
4. M. Heidelberger and F. E. Kendall, *J. Exp. Med.,* **55,** 555 (1932).
5. A. H. Coons, H. J. Creech, and R. N. Jones, *Proc. Soc. Exptl. Biol. Med.,* **47,** 200 (1941).
6. A. H. Coons, H. J. Creech, R. N. Jones, and E. Berliner, *J. Immunol.,* **45,** 159 (1942).
7. S. A. Berson, R. S. Yalow, A. Bauman, M. A. Rothschild, and K. Newerly, *J. Clin. Invest.,* **35,** 170 (1956).
8. S. A. Berson and R. S. Yalow, *Adv. Biol. Med. Phys.,* **6,** 349 (1958).
9. K. Landsteiner, *The Specificity of Serological Reactions,* Harvard University Press, Cambridge, MA, 1946.
10. B. F. Erlanger, F. Borek, S. M. Beisen, and S. Lieberman, *J. Biol. Chem.,* **228,** 713 (1957).
11. W. H. Churchill and D. F. Tapley, *Nature,* **202,** 29 (1964).
12. R. P. Ekins, *Clin. Chim. Acta,* **5,** 453 (1960).
13. R. M. Barakat and R. P. Ekins, *Lancet,* **2,** 25 (1961).
14. A. J. Hodgkinson, A. M. Sidki, J. Landon, F. J. Rowell, and S. M. Mahmod, *Ann. Clin. Biochem.,* **22,** 519 (1985).
15. M. Sela, *Adv. Immunol.,* **5,** 29 (1966).
16. B. K. Van Weemen and A. H. W. M. Schuurs, *Immunochem.,* **12,** 667 (1975).
17. B. M. Jaffe and H. R. Behrman, *Methods of Hormone Radioimmunoassay,* 2nd ed., Academic Press, New York, 1979.
18. A. Tsuji, M. Maeda, H. Arakawa, S. Shimizu, T. Ike Gami, Y. Sudo, H. Hosoda, and T. Nambara, *J. Steroid Biochem.,* **27,** 33 (1987).
19. P. Aucouturier, J.-L. Preud'homme, and B. Lubochinsky, *Diagn. Immunol.,* **1,** 310 (1983).
20. H. Arakawa, M. Maeda, and A. Tsuji, *Anal. Biochem.,* **97,** 248 (1979).
21. Y. Kobayashi, T. Ogihara, K. Amitani, F. Watanabe, T. Kiguchi, I. Ninomiya, and Y. Kumahara, *Steroids,* **32,** 137 (1978).

22. H. Mikola and P. Miettinen, *Steroids,* **56,** 17 (1991).
23. L. X. Tiefenauer and R. Y. Andres, *J. Steroid. Biochem.,* **35,** 633 (1990).
24. G. Köhler and C. Milstein, *Nature,* **256,** 495 (1975).
25. E. D. Sevier, G. S. David, J. Martinis, W. J. Desmond, R. M. Bartholomew, and R. Wang, *Clin. Chem.,* **27,** 1797 (1981).
26. K. Siddle, "Properties and Applications of Monoclonal Antibodies," in W. P. Collins, Ed., *Alternative Immunoassays,* Wiley, Chichester, UK, 1985.
27. R. Ekins, *Nature,* **340,** 256 (1989).
28. C. A. Caulott, R. Boraston, C. Hill, P. W. Thompson, and J. R. Birch, "Production and Purification of Monoclonal Antibodies," in W. P. Collins, Ed., *Complementary Immunoassays,* Wiley, Chichester, UK, 1988.
29. J. P. A. M. Klerx, C. Jansen Verplanke, C. G. Blonk, and L. C. Twaalfhoven, *J. Immunol. Methods,* **111,** 179 (1988).
30. C. L. Reading, *J. Immunol. Methods,* **53,** 261 (1982).
31. R. A. Goldwasser and C. C. Shepard, *J. Immunol.,* **80,** 122 (1958).
32. H. L. Spiegelberg, *Adv. Immunol.,* **19,** 259 (1974).
33. W. J. Yount, M. M. Dorner, H. G. Kunkel, and E. A. Kabat, *J. Exp. Med.,* **127,** 633 (1968).
34. J. M. Teale and N. R. Klinman, "Control of the Production of Different Classes of Antibody," in W. E. Paul, Ed., *Fundamental Immunology,* Raven Press, New York, 1984.
35. H. L. Spiegelberg, *Methods Enzymol.,* **116,** 95 (1985).
36. G. Scatchard, *Ann. N.Y. Acad. Sci.,* **51,** 660 (1949).
37. T. M. Jackson and R. P. Ekins, *J. Immunol. Methods,* **87,** 13 (1986).
38. P. D. Gorevic, F. C. Prelli, and B. Frangione, *Methods Enzymol.,* **116,** 3 (1981).
39. W. A. L. Duijndam, J. Wiegant, P. Van Duijn, and J. J. Haaijman, *J. Immunol. Methods,* **109,** 289 (1988).
40. J. J. Langone, *J. Immunol. Methods,* **24,** 269 (1978).
41. P. Parnham, "Preparation and Purification of Active Fragments from Mouse Monoclonal Antibodies," in D. M. Weir, D. R. Parks, L. L. Lanier, and L. A. Herzenberg, Eds., *Handbook of Experimental Immunology,* Blackwell Scientific Publication, Oxford, 1986.
42. W. M. Hunter, J. G. Bennie, P. S. Budd, V. Van Heyningen, K. James, R. L. Micklem, and A. Scott, "Immunoradiometric Assays using Monoclonal Antibodies," in W. M. Hunter and J. E. T. Corrie, Eds., *Immunoassays for Clinical Chemistry,* 2nd ed., Churchill-Livingstone, Edinburgh, 1983.
43. J. A. Nisbet and S. Bird, *Clin. Chem.,* **32,** 201 (1986).
44. O. C. Boerman, M. F. G. Segers, L. G. Poels, P. Kenemans, and C. M. G. Thomas, *Clin. Chem.,* **36,** 888 (1990).
45. L. J. Kricka, D. Schmerfeld-Pruss, M. Senior, D. B. P. Goodman, and P. Kaladas, *Clin. Chem.,* **36,** 892 (1990).

46. A. Gardas and A. Lewartowska, *J. Immunol. Methods,* **106,** 251 (1988).
47. W. A. Ratcliffe and E. T. Corrie, *Clin. Chem.,* **28,** 1314 (1982).
48. P. Y. Wong, A. V. Mee, and F. F. K. Ho, *Clin. Chem.,* **25,** 914 (1979).
49. M. Hüfner and R.-D. Hesch, *Clin. Chim. Acta,* **44,** 101 (1973).
50. J. W. Kane, *Ann. Clin. Biochem.,* **16,** 209 (1979).
51. M. G. McConway, *Clin. Chim. Acta,* **158,** 59 (1986).
52. J. Seth and L. M. Brown, *Clin. Chim. Acta,* **86,** 109 (1978).
53. J. U. Eskola, V. Näntö, L. Meurling, and T. N.-E. Lövgren, *Clin. Chem.,* **31,** 1731 (1985).
54. E. Ezan, K. Drieu, and F. Dray, *J. Immunol. Methods,* **122,** 291 (1989).
55. M. S. Kumar, A. M. Safa, and S. D. Deodhar, *Clin. Chem.,* **22,** 1845 (1976).
56. L. B. Foster and R. T. Dunn, *Clin. Chem.,* **20,** 365 (1974).
57. M. J. Hasler, R. T. Painter, and G. D. Niswender, *Clin. Chem.,* **22,** 1850 (1976).
58. M. Wilchek and E. A. Bayer, *Anal. Biochem.,* **171,** 1 (1988).
59. F. Kohen, Y. Amir-Zaltsman, C. S. Strassburger, E. A. Bayer, and M. Wilchek, "The Avidin Biotin Reaction in Immunoassays," in W. P. Collins, Ed., *Complementary Immunoassays,* Wiley, Chichester, UK, 1988.
60. J.-L. Guesdon, T. Ternynck, and S. Avrameas, *J. Histochem. Cytochem.,* **27,** 1131 (1979).
61. S.-M. Hsu, L. Raine, and H. Fanger, *J. Histochem. Cytochem.,* **29,** 577 (1981).
62. J. W. Berman and R. S. Basch, *J. Immunol. Methods,* **36,** 335 (1980).
63. J. H. M. Cohen, J. P. Aubry, M. H. Jouvin, J. Wijdenes, J. Bancheran, M. Kazatchkine, and J. P. Revillard, *J. Immunol. Methods,* **99,** 53 (1987).
64. R. R. Hardy, K. Hayakawa, D. R. Parks, and B. A. Herzenberg, *Nature,* **306,** 270 (1983).
65. T. M. McHugh, R. C. Miner, L. H. Logan, and D. P. Stites, *J. Clin. Microbiol.,* **26,** 1957 (1988).
66. H. C. Loughrey, L. S. Choi, P. R. Cullis, and M. B. Bally, *J. Immunol. Methods,* **132,** 25 (1990).
67. R. H. Yolken, F. J. Leister, L. S. Whitcomb, and M. Santosham, *J. Immunol. Methods,* **56,** 319 (1983).
68. A. E. Ohworiole and T. J. Wilkin, *J. Immunol. Methods,* **115,** 99 (1988).
69. G. De Schrijver, R. J. Wieme, F. D'Haese, and D. Dean, *Anal. Chim. Acta,* **205,** 239 (1988).
70. M. Honda, S. Nagao, N. Yamamoto, Y. Tanaka, H. Tozawa, and T. Tokunaga, *J. Immunol. Methods,* **110,** 129 (1988).
71. F. P. Anderson and W. G. Miller, *Clin. Chem.,* **34,** 1417 (1988).
72. R. Bador, H. Dechaud, and F. Claustrat, *Clin. Chem.,* **34,** 596 (1988).
73. I. Hemmilä, J. Heikkilä, and P. Leivo, *Clin. Chem.,* **35,** 1206 (abs. 671) (1989).
74. E. P. Diamandis, *Clin. Biochem.,* **21,** 139 (1988).

75. L. Lärkfors and T. Ebendal, *J. Immunol. Methods,* **97,** 41 (1987).
76. J. J. Langone, *J. Immunol. Methods,* **18,** 281 (1977).
77. P. U. Baxi, A. Milon, J. Franz, and J.-J. Metzger, *J. Immunol. Methods,* **35,** 249 (1980).
78. H. Nakajima, Y. Nakata, and S. Saitoh, *J. Immunol. Methods,* **46,** 277 (1981).
79. I. Faiferman and D. Koffer, *Arthritis Rheumatism,* **25,** 799 (1982).
80. A. Ius, L. Ferrara, G. Meroni, and M. Bacigalupo, *Fres. Z. Anal. Chem.,* **322,** 509 (1985).
81. J. Stavrianopoulos, E. Rabbani, S. B. Abrams, and J. G. Wetmur, Eur. Patent Appl. No. 242,527 (1987).
82. S. Mansouri and J. S. Schultz, *Bio-technol.,* **2,** 885 (1984).
83. M. Slifkin and R. Cumbie, *J. Clin. Microbiol.,* **27,** 1036 (1989).
84. P. D. Patel and S. D. Haines, *Abstract of Papers Presented at the Sixth International Congress on Rapid Methods and Automation in Microbiology and Immunology,* No. 120, Espoo, Finland, July 1990.
85. A. Nagata and T. Komoda, *Clin. Chem.,* **36,** 1056 (abs. 490) (1990).
86. S. K. Skurkovich, A. J. Olshansky, R. S. Samoilova, and E. I. Eremkina, *J. Immunol. Methods,* **19,** 119 (1978).
87. J. Parkkinen and U. Oksanen, *Anal. Biochem.,* **177,** 383 (1989).
88. J. Parkkinen, *Clin. Chem.,* **35,** 1638 (1989).
89. Y. Suzuki, Y. Aoyagi, M. Muramatsu, K. Igarashi, A. Saito, M. Oguro, M. Isemura, and H. Asakura, *Ann. Clin. Biochem.,* **27,** 121 (1990).
90. M. Suter and J. E. Butler, *Immunol. Lett.,* **13,** 313 (1986).
91. W. D. Odell, J. Griffin, and R. Zahradnik, *Clin. Chem.,* **32,** 1873 (1986).
92. W. Schramm, T. Yang, and A. R. Midgley, *Clin. Chem.,* **33,** 1338 (1987).
93. B. Akerstrom, T. Brodin, K. Reis, and L. Bjorck, *J. Immunol.,* **135,** 2589 (1985).
94. M. M. Collins, C. H. Casavant, and D. P. Stites, *J. Clin. Microbiol.,* **15,** 456 (1982).
95. T. M. McHugh, D. P. Stites, C. H. Casavant, and M. J. Fulwyler, *J. Immunol. Methods,* **95,** 57 (1986).
96. A. P. Belozyorov, *Lab. Delo,* **3,** 24 (1989).
97. J. Oudin and M. J. Michel, *Exp. Med.,* **130,** 595 (1969).
98. I. M. Roitt, Y. M. Thanavala, D. K. Male, and F. C. Hay, *Immunology Today,* **6,** 265 (1985).
99. J. J. Langone and R. J. Bjercke, *Anal. Biochem.,* **182,** 187 (1989).
100. G. Barnard and F. Kohen, *Clin. Chem.,* **36,** 1945 (1990).
101. M. Brennan, P. F. Davison, and H. Paulus, *Science,* **229,** 81 (1985).
102. R. Hong and A. Nisonoff, *J. Biol. Chem.,* **240,** 388 (1965).
103. U. Hammerling, T. Auki, E. De-Harven, E. A. Boyse, and L. J. Old, *J. Exp. Med.,* **128,** 1461 (1968).

104. C. Milstein and A. C. Cuello, *Nature,* **305,** 537 (1983).
105. M. R. Suresh, A. C. Cuello, and C. Milstein, *Proc. Natl. Acad. Sci. USA,* **83,** 7989 (1986).
106. L. Karawajew, O. Behrsing, G. Kaiser, and B. Micheel, *J. Immunol. Methods,* **111,** 95 (1988).
107. H. Tada, Y. Toyoda, and S. Iwasa, *Hybridoma,* **8,** 73 (1989).
108. S. Roberts, J. C. Cheetham, and A. R. Rees, *Nature,* **328,** 731 (1987).
109. G. P. Moore, *Clin. Chem.,* **35,** 1849 (1989).
110. S. L. Morrison, S. Canfield, S. Porter, L. K. Tan, M.-H. Tao, and L. A. Wims, *Clin. Chem.,* **34,** 1668 (1988).
111. G. L. Boulianne, N. Hozumi, and M. J. Shulman, *Nature,* **312,** 643 (1984).
112. H. Dick, *Brit. Med. J.,* **291,** 762 (1985).
113. M. S. Neuberger, G. T. Williams, and R. O. Fox, *Nature,* **312,** 604 (1984).
114. K.-Z. Kameyama, K. Imai, T. Itoh, M. Taniguchi, K. Miura, and Y. Kurosawa, *FEBS Lett.,* **244,** 301 (1989).
115. J. E. Blalock and K. L. Bost, *Biochem. J.,* **234,** 679 (1986).
116. R. S. Yalow and S. A. Berson, *Nature,* **184,** 1648 (1959).
117. S. A. Berson and R. S. Yalow, *J. Clin. Invest.,* **38,** 1996 (1959).
118. R. S. Yalow and S. A. Berson, *J. Clin. Invest.,* **39,** 1157 (1960).
119. K. Landsteiner, *Klin. Woch.,* **6,** 103 (1927).
120. M. Heidelberger, F. E. Kendall, and C. M. Soo Hoo, *J. Exp. Med.,* **58,** 137 (1933).
121. L. Wide, H. Bennick, and S. G. O. Johansson, *Lancet,* **2,** 1105 (1967).
122. A. B. Stavitsky and E. R. Arquilla, *Fed. Proc.,* **12,** 461 (1953).
123. E. R. Arquilla and A. B. Stavitsky, *J. Clin. Invest.,* **35,** 458 (1956).
124. A. B. Stavitsky, *J. Immunol.,* **72,** 368 (1954).
125. R. S. Farr, *Fed. Proc.,* **16,** 412 (1957).
126. R. S. Farr, *J. Infect. Dis.,* **103,** 239 (1958).
127. R. T. Wold, F. E. Young, E. M. Tan, and R. S. Farr, *Science,* **161,** 806 (1968).
128. G. M. Grodsky, C. T. Peng, and P. H. Forsham, *Arch. Biochem.,* **81,** 264 (1959).
129. G. M. Grodsky and P. H. Hofstra, *J. Clin. Invest.,* **39,** 1070 (1960).
130. R. J. Weiler, D. Hofstra, A. Szentivanyi, R. Bleisdell, and D. W. Talmage, *J. Immunol.,* **85,** 130 (1960).
131. S. Lieberman, B. F. Erlanger, S. M. Beiser, and F. J. Agate, *Rec. Prog. Horm. Res.,* **15,** 165 (1959).
132. G. E. Abraham, *J. Clin. Endocrin. Metab.,* **29,** 866 (1969).
133. W. M. Hunter and F. C. Greenwood, *Nature,* **194,** 495 (1966).
134. S. I. Karonen, P. Morsley, M. Screin, and V. Senderling, *Ann. Biochem.,* **67,** 1 (1975).

135. J. I. Thorell and B. G. Johansson, *Biochim. Biophys. Acta,* **251,** 363 (1971).
136. V. Rosa, F. Pennisi, R. Bianchi, G. Federighi, and L. Donato, *Biochim. Biophys. Acta,* **133,** 486 (1967).
137. A. S. McFarlane, *Nature,* **182,** 53 (1958).
138. A. E. Bolton and W. M. Hunter, *Biochem. J.,* **133,** 529 (1973).
139. S. Udenfriend, L. Gerber, and N. Nelson, *Anal. Biochem.,* **161,** 494 (1987).
140. N. Bosworth and P. Towers, *Nature,* **341,** 167 (1989).
141. J. G. Ratcliffe, *Brit. Med. Bull.,* **30,** 32 (1974).
142. P. Cheret and P. Brossier, *Ann. Pharm. Fr.,* **44,** 203 (1986).
143. F. Mariet and P. Brossier, *Res. Comm. Chem. Pathol. Pharmacol.,* **68,** 251 (1990).
144. D. Schalch and M. Parker, *Nature,* **203,** 1141 (1964).
145. V. Herbert, K. S. Lou, and L. H. Gottlieb, *J. Clin. Endocrinol. Metab.,* **25,** 1375 (1965).
146. L. Lazarus and J. D. Young, *J. Clin. Endocrinol. Metab.,* **26,** 213 (1966).
147. E. Haber, E. B. Page, and F. F. Richards, *Anal. Biochem.,* **12,** 163 (1966).
148. K. Catt and G. W. Tregear, *Science,* **58,** 1570 (1967).
149. L. A. Cantarero, J. E. Butler, and J. W. Osborne, *Anal. Biochem.,* **105,** 375 (1980).
150. J. P. Rotmans and B. A. A. Scheven, *J. Immunol. Methods,* **70,** 53 (1984).
151. J. D. Conradie, M. Govender, and L. Visser, *J. Immunol. Methods,* **59,** 289 (1983).
152. K. Ruan, S. Hashida, S. Yoshitake, E. Ishikawa, O. Wakisaka, Y. Yamamoto, T. Ichioka, and K. Nakajima, *Ann. Clin. Biochem.,* **23,** 54 (1986).
153. E. Ishikawa, Y. Hamaguchi, M. Imagawa, M. Inada, H. Imura, N. Nakazawa, and H. Ogawa, *J. Immunoassay,* **1,** 385 (1980).
154. W. Hubl, G. Daxenbichler, and D. Meissner, *Clin. Chem.,* **34,** 2521 (1988).
155. R. K. Kobos, J. W. Eveleigh, and R. Arentzen, *Bio/Technol.,* **7,** 101 (1989).
156. P. Helsingius, I. Hemmilä, and T. Lövgren, *Clin. Chem.,* **32,** 1767 (1986).
157. E. P. Diamandis, V. Bhayana, K. Conway, E. Reichstein, and A. Papanastasiou-Diamandi, *Clin. Biochem.,* **21,** 291 (1988).
158. H. H. Sedlacek, K.-F. Mück, R. Rehkopf, S. Baudner, and F. R. Seiler, *J. Immunol. Methods,* **26,** 11 (1979).
159. W. K. Wang, L. T. Ho, Y. Chiang, and T. C. Chen, *J. Immunol. Methods,* **112,** 173 (1988).
160. J. C. Standefer and G. C. Saunders, *Clin. Chem.,* **24,** 1903 (1978).
161. B. S. Chessum and J. R. Denmark, *Lancet,* **1,** 161 (1978).
162. S. M. Burt, T. J. N. Carter, and L. J. Kricka, *J. Immunol. Methods,* **31,** 231 (1979).

163. D. F. Tallon, J. P. Gosling, P. M. Buckley, M. M. Dooley, W. F. Cleere, E. M. O'Dwyer, and P. F. Foitrell, *Clin. Chem.*, **30**, 1507 (1984).
164. R. M. Hendry and J. E. Herrmann, *J. Immunol. Methods,* **35**, 285 (1980).
165. A. Ali and R. Ali, *Clin. Biochem.*, **19**, 205 (1986).
166. J. A. Verschoor, N. M. J. Vermeuten, and L. Visser, *J. Immunol. Methods,* **127**, 43 (1990).
167. A. R. Neurath and N. Strick, *J. Virol. Methods,* **3**, 155 (1981).
168. A. R. Neurath, N. Strick, and S. Goodman, *J. Virol. Methods,* **4**, 297 (1982).
169. V. P. Chu and P. J. Tarcha, *J. Appl. Polym. Sci.*, **34**, 1917 (1987).
170. J. H. Peterman, P. J. Tarcha, V. P. Chu, and J. E. Butler, *J. Immunol. Methods,* **111**, 271 (1988).
171. M. Lynn, "Inorganic Support Intermediates: Covalent Coupling of Enzymes on Inorganic Supports," in H. H. Weetall, Ed., *Immobilized Enzymes, Antigens, Antibodies and Peptides: Preparation and Characterization,* Dekker, New York, 1975.
172. A. L. Plant, L. Locascio-Brown, M. W. Brizgys, and A. Durst, *Bio/Technol.*, **6**, 266 (1988).
173. J. P. Alarie, M. J. Sepaniak, and T. Vo-Dinh, *Anal. Chim. Acta,* **229**, 169 (1990).
174. K. Catt, H. D. Niall, and G. W. Tregear, *Biochem. J.*, **100**, 31 (1966).
175. P. H. Larsson, S. G. O. Johansson, A. Hult, and S. Göthe, *J. Immunol. Methods,* **98**, 129 (1987).
176. J. D. Place and H. R. Schroeder, *J. Immunol. Methods,* **48**, 251 (1982).
177. S. H. Lin, F. J. Regina, and J. M. Bolts, *Clin. Chem.*, **34**, 1156 (abs. 020) (1988).
178. W. G. Wood and A. Gadow, *J. Clin. Chem. Clin. Biochem.*, **21**, 789 (1983).
179. R. N. Hobbs, D. J. Lea, and D. J. Ward, *J. Immunol. Methods,* **65**, 235 (1983).
180. R. Axen, J. Porath, and S. Ernback, *Nature,* **214**, 1302 (1967).
181. L. Wide and J. Porath, *Biochim. Biophys. Acta,* **130**, 257 (1966).
182. E. Engvall and P. Perlmann, *Immunochemistry,* **8**, 871 (1971).
183. F. Paronetto, *Biol. Med.*, **113**, 394 (1963).
184. A. J. Toussaint, E. H. Fife, R. C. Parlett, L. F. Affronti, G. L. Wright, M. Reich, and W. C. Morse, *Am. J. Clin. Path.*, **52**, 708 (1969).
185. R. C. Aalberse, *Clin. Chim. Acta,* **48**, 109 (1973).
186. P. J. A. Capel and R. C. Aalberse, *J. Immunol. Methods,* **7**, 77 (1975).
187. J. J. Haaijman, F. J. Bloemmen, and C. M. Ham, *Ann. N.Y. Acad. Sci.*, **254**, 137 (1975).
188. J. P. R. van Dalen, W. Knapp, and J. S. Ploem, *J. Immunol. Methods,* **2**, 383 (1973).
189. A. M. Deelder and J. S. Ploem, *J. Immunol. Methods,* **4**, 239 (1975).

190. H.-O. Dauner, *GIT. Labor. Medizin,* **2,** 100 (1981).

191. R. S. Molday, W. J. Dreyer, A. Rembaum, and S. P. J. Yen, *J. Cell. Biol.,* **64,** 75 (1975).

192. D. J. Phillips, A. P. Kendal, R. G. Webster, P. M. Feorino, and C. B. Reimer, *J. Virol. Methods,* **1,** 275 (1980).

193. P. J. Robinson and P. Dunnill, *Biotechn. Bioeng.,* **15,** 603 (1973).

194. R. S. Kamel and J. Landon, *Clin. Chem.,* **25,** 1997 (1979).

195. M. Pourfarzaneh and R. D. Nargessi, *Clin. Chim. Acta,* **111,** 61 (1981).

196. R. D. Nargessi, J. Landon, M. Pourfarzaneh, and D. S. Smith, *Clin. Chim. Acta,* **89,** 455 (1978).

197. R. C. Birkmeyer, R. Diaco, D. K. Hutson, H. P. Lau, W. K. Miller, N. V. Neelkantan, T. J. Pankratz, S. Y. Tseng, D. K. Vickery, and E. K. Yang, *Clin. Chem.,* **33,** 1543 (1987).

198. B. Avner, B. P. Avner, B. Gaydos, S.-K. Liao, G. B. Thurman, and R. K. Oldham, *J. Immunol. Methods,* **113,** 123 (1988).

199. N. K. Kaufman, R. A. Harte, and A. B. Chen, US Patent No. 4,596,273 (1986).

200. R. A. Harte and M. Bart, US Patent No. 4,340,564 (1982).

201. H. Alfthan and U.-H. Stenman, *J. Chromatography,* **470,** 385 (1989).

202. B. H. Berne, *Clin. Chem.,* **29,** 1690 (1983).

203. K. Kato, Y. Umeda, F. Suzuki, D. Hayashi, and A. Kosaka, *Clin. Chem.,* **25,** 1306 (1979).

204. J. H. Livesey and R. A. Donald, *Clin. Chim. Acta,* **123,** 193 (1982).

205. S. M. Spinola and J. G. Cannon, *J. Immunol. Methods,* **81,** 161 (1985).

206. R. F. Vogt, D. L. Phillips, L. O. Henderson, W. Whitfield, and F. W. Spierto, *J. Immunol. Methods,* **101,** 43 (1987).

207. H. Hauri and K. Bucher, *Anal. Biochem.,* **159,** 386 (1986).

208. W. L. Hoffman and A. A. Jump, *Anal. Biochem.,* **181,** 318 (1989).

209. S. Hashida, K. Nakagawa, M. Imagawa, S. Inohe, S. Yoshitake, E. Ishikawa, Y. Endo, S. Ohtaki, Y. Ichioka, and K. Nakajima, *Clin. Chim. Acta,* **135,** 263 (1983).

210. A. Papanastasiou-Diamandi, T. K. Christopoulos, and E. P. Diamandis, *Clin. Chem. Enzym. Comms.,* **2,** 177 (1990).

211. H. C. B. Graves, *J. Immunol. Methods,* **111,** 157 (1988).

212. H. Graves, US Patent No. 4,829,009 (1989).

213. T. Kohno and E. Ishikawa, *Biochem. Biophys. Res. Commun.,* **147,** 644 (1987).

214. T. Kohno, T. Mitsukawa, S. Matsukura, and E. Ishikawa, *J. Clin. Lab. Anal.,* **2,** 209 (1988).

215. T. Kohno, T. Mitsukawa, S. Matsukura, Y. Tsunetoshi, and E. Ishikawa, *J. Clin. Lab. Anal.,* **3,** 163 (1989).

216. L. E. M. Miles and C. N. Hales, *Nature,* **219,** 186 (1968).

217. L. E. M. Miles and C. N. Hales, *Biochem. J.,* **108,** 611 (1968).
218. G. M. Addison and C. N. Hales, *Horm. Metab. Res.,* **3,** 59 (1971).
219. C. Readhead, G. M. Addison, C. N. Hales, and H. Lehnmann, *J. Endocr.,* **39,** 313 (1973).
220. B. K. Van Weeman and A. H. W. H. Schuurs, *FEBS Lett.,* **15,** 232 (1971).
221. E. Engvall and P. Perlmann, *J. Immunol.,* **109,** 129 (1972).
222. S. A. Berson and R. S. Yalow, *Clin. Chim. Acta,* **22,** 51 (1968).
223. J. L. Rudy, *Clin. Chem.,* **35,** 509 (1989).
224. C. J. Halfman and A. S. Schneider, *Anal. Chem.,* **53,** 654 (1981).
225. D. Rodbard, *Anal. Biochem.,* **90,** 1 (1978).
226. R. P. Ekins, G. B. Newman, P. Banks, and J. D. H. Slater, *J. Steroid. Biochem.,* **3,** 289 (1972).
227. R. P. Ekins, "The Precision Profile: Its Use in Assay Design, Assessment and Quality Control," in W. M. Hunter and J. E. T. Corrie, Eds., *Immunoassays for Clinical Chemistry,* Churchill-Livingstone, Edinburgh, 1983.
228. R. P. Ekins, "Current Concepts and Future Developments," in W. P. Collins, Ed., *Alternative Immunoassays,* Wiley, Chichester, UK, 1985.
229. M. Yanagishita and D. Rodbard, *Anal. Biochem.,* **88,** 1 (1978).
230. M. G. McConway, R. S. Chapman, G. H. Beastall, E. Brown, J. Tillman, J. A. Bonar, A. Hutchison, T. Allison, J. Finlayson, R. Weston, G. J. Beckett, G. D. Carter, E. Carlyle, R. Herbertson, G. Blundell, W. Edwards, A. C. A. Glen, and A. Reid, *Clin. Chem.,* **35,** 289 (1989).
231. H. A. Kemp, R. John, M. R. C. Path, and J. S. Woodhead, *Ligand Quarterly,* **5,** 27 (1982).
232. R. P. Ekins, "The Future Development of Immunoassay," in *Radioimmunoassay and Related Procedures in Medicine,* Proc. IAEA Symp., Vienna, 1978.
233. W. M. Hunter, "Recent Advances in Radioimmunoassays and Related Techniques," in *Radioimmunoassay and Related Procedures in Medicine,* Proc. IAEA Symp., Vienna, 1979.
234. D. Rodbard and G. H. Weiss, *Anal. Biochem.,* **52,** 10 (1973).
235. R. P. Ekins, *Brit. Med. Bull.,* **30,** 3 (1974).
236. J. S. Woodhead, G. M. Addison, and C. N. Hales, *Brit. Med. Bull.,* **30,** 44 (1974).
237. H. A. Kemp, R. John, and J. S. Woodhead, "Labelled Antibody Immunoassays," in W. R. Butt, Ed., *Practical Immunoassay,* Dekker, New York, 1984.
238. J. S. Woodhead, R. C. Brown, J. P. Aston, and I. Weeks, "Immunochemiluminometric Assays," in W. P. Collins, Ed., *Complementary Immunoassays,* Wiley, Chichester, UK, 1988.
239. S. Avrameas and J. Uriel, *C. R. Acad. Sci., Paris,* **262,** 2543 (1966).
240. S. Avrameas and B. Guilbert, *Eur. J. Immunol.,* **1,** 394 (1971).
241. E. Engvall and P. Perlmann, *J. Immunol. Methods,* **10,** 161 (1971).

242. K. E. Rubenstein, R. S. Schneider, and E. F. Ullman, *Biochem. Biophys. Res. Commun.,* **47**, 846 (1972).

243. C. C. Harris, R. H. Yolken, H. Krokan, and I. C. Hsu, *Proc. Natl. Acad. Sci. USA,* **76**, 5336 (1979).

244. E. Ishikawa and K. Kato, *Scand. J. Immunol.,* **8**, Suppl. 7, 43 (1978).

245. R. H. Yolken and P. J. Stopa, *J. Clin. Microbiol.,* **10**, 317 (1979).

246. E. Ishikawa, M. Imagawa, and S. Hashida, *Develop. Immunol.,* **18**, 219 (1983).

247. E. Ishikawa, *Clin. Biochem.,* **20**, 375 (1987).

248. G. G. Guilbault, P. J. Brignal, Jr., and M. Juneau, *Anal. Chem.,* **40**, 1256 (1968).

249. K. Puget, A. M. Michelson, and S. Avrameas, *Anal. Biochem.,* **79**, 447 (1977).

250. B. Rotman, *Proc. Natl. Acad. Sci. USA,* **47**, 1981 (1961).

251. K. Tanaka and E. Ishikawa, *Anal. Lett.,* **19**, 433 (1986).

252. H. R. Schroeder, P. O. Vogelhut, R. J. Carrico, R. C. Boguslaski, and R. T. Buckler, *Anal. Chem.,* **48**, 1933 (1976).

253. E. Soini, ''Instrumentation: Photometric and Photon Emission Immunoassays,'' in W. P. Collins, Ed., *Alternative Immunoassays,* Wiley, Chichester, UK, 1985.

254. A. K. Campbell, *Chemiluminescence, Principles and Applications in Biology and Medicine,* Ellis Horwood Ltd., Chichester, UK, 1986.

255. G. J. R. Barnard and W. P. Collins, *Med. Lab. Sci.,* **44**, 249 (1987).

256. H. R. Schroeder, R. J. Carrico, R. C. Boguslaski, and J. E. Christner, *Anal. Biochem.,* **72**, 283 (1976).

257. L. J. Kricka, *Anal. Biochem.,* **175**, 14 (1988).

258. G. H. G. Thorpe, L. J. Kricka, S. B. Moseley, and T. P. Whitehead, *Clin. Chem.,* **31**, 1335 (1985).

259. L. J. Kricka, R. A. W. Stott, and G. H. G. Thorpe, ''Enhanced Chemiluminescence Enzyme Immunoassay,'' in W. P. Collins, Ed., *Complementary Immunoassay,* Wiley, Chichester, UK, 1988.

260. J. C. Hummelen, T. M. Luider, and H. Wynberg, *Methods Enzymol.,* **133**, 531 (1987).

261. T. P. Whitehead, G. H. G. Thorpe, T. J. N. Carter, C. Groucutt, and L. J. Kricka, *Nature,* **305**, 158 (1983).

262. F. Kohen, M. Pazzagli, M. Serio, J. Boever, and D. Vandekerckhove, ''Chemiluminescence and Bioluminescence Immunoassay,'' in W. P. Collins, Ed., *Alternative Immunoassays,* Wiley, Chichester, UK, 1985.

263. I. Weeks, M. L. Sturgess, and J. S. Woodhead, *Clin. Sci.,* **70**, 403 (1980).

264. M. DeLuca, "Bioluminescence Assays," in B. D. Albertson and F. P. Haseltine, Eds., *Non-Radiometric Assays: Technology and Application in Polypeptide and Steroid Hormone Detection,* Alan R. Liss Inc., New York, 1988.

265. W. G. Wood, *J. Clin. Chem. Clin. Biochem.,* **22**, 905 (1984).

266. J. L. Riggs, R. J. Seiwald, J. H. Burckhalter, C. M. Downs, and T. G. Metcalf, *Am. J. Pathol.,* **34**, 1081 (1958).

267. R. Hiramoto, K. Engel, and D. Pressman, *Proc. Soc. Exp. Biol. Med.,* **97,** 611 (1958).

268. R. C. Mellors and R. Silver, *Science,* **114,** 356 (1951).

269. R. C. Mellors, A. Glassman, and G. N. Papanicolau, *Cancer,* **5,** 458 (1952).

270. M. Goldman, *Exp. Parasitol.,* **9,** 25 (1960).

271. J. S. Ploem, H. J. Tanke, I. Al, and A. M. Deelder, "Recent Developments in Immunofluorescence Microscopy," in W. Knapp, K. Holubar, and G. Wick, Eds., *Immunofluorescence and Related Staining Techniques,* Elsevier/North Holland Biomedical Press, Amsterdam, 1978.

272. A. J. Toussaint, C. J. Tarrant, and R. I. Anderson, *Proc. Soc. Exptl. Biol. Med.,* **120,** 783 (1965).

273. A. J. Toussaint and R. I. Anderson, *Appl. Microbiol.,* **13,** 552 (1965).

274. H. M. Shapiro, *Practical Flow Cytometry,* Alan R. Liss Inc., New York, 1985.

275. R. P. Tengerdy, *Anal. Chem.,* **35,** 1084 (1963).

276. R. P. Tengerdy, *J. Lab. Clin. Med.,* **65,** 859 (1965).

277. W. P. Dandliker and G. A. Feigen, *Biochem. Biophys. Res. Commun.,* **5,** 299 (1961).

278. A. R. Neurath, *Z. Naturforsch.,* **20b,** 974 (1965).

279. W. B. Dandliker, R. Alonso, and C. Y. Meyers, *Immunochemistry,* **4,** 295 (1967).

280. W. B. Dandliker, H. C. Shapiro, J. W. Meduski, R. Alonso, G. A. Feigen, and J. R. Hamrick, *Immunochemistry,* **1,** 165 (1964).

281. R. P. Tengerdy, *J. Lab. Clin. Med.,* **20,** 707 (1967).

282. W. B. Dandliker, R. J. Kelly, J. Dandliker, J. Farquhar, and J. Levin, *Immunochemistry,* **10,** 219 (1973).

283. R. D. Spencer, F. B. Toledo, B. T. Williams, and N. L. Yoss, *Clin. Chem.,* **19,** 838 (1973).

284. S. V. Boyden, *J. Exp. Med.,* **93,** 107 (1951).

285. D. Pressman, D. H. Campbell, and J. H. Pauling, *J. Immunol.,* **44,** 101 (1942).

286. N. R. Ling, *Immunology,* **4,** 49 (1961).

287. L. Gyenes and A. H. Schon, *Immunochemistry,* **1,** 43 (1964).

288. H. M. Johnson, K. Brenner, and H. E. Hall, *J. Immunol.,* **97,** 791 (1966).

289. L. Wide and C. A. Gemzell, *Acta Endocr. Copenh.,* **35,** 261 (1960).

290. O. Mäkelä, *Immunology,* **10,** 81 (1966).

291. J. Haimovich, E. Hurwitz, N. Novik, and M. Sela, *Biochim. Biophys. Acta,* **207,** 125 (1970).

292. S. Jormalainen, J. Aird, and O. Mäkelä, *Immunochemistry,* **8,** 450 (1971).

293. J. M. Andrieu, S. Mamas, and F. Dray, *Eur. J. Immunol.,* **4,** 417 (1974).

294. F. Dray, E. Maron, S. A. Tillson, and M. Sela, *Anal. Biochem.,* **50,** 399 (1972).

295. E. Maron and B. Bonavida, *Biochim. Biophys. Acta,* **229,** 273 (1971).

296. J. M. Singer and C. M. Plotz, *Am. J. Med.,* **21,** 888 (1956).

297. M. Sawai, T. Sudo, H. Okumura, S. Morita, S. Sato, S. Matsumoto, and S. Migita, *Prog. Symp. Chem. Physiol. Pathol. Annu. Meet. Jpn. Soc. Clin. Chem.,* **18,** 22 (1978).

298. C. L. Christian, R. M. Bryan, and D. L. Larson, *Proc. Soc. Exp. Med.,* **98,** 820 (1958).

299. C. L. Cambiaso, A. E. Leek, F. De Steenwinkel, J. Billen, and P. L. Masson, *J. Immunol. Methods,* **18,** 33 (1977).

300. D. Collet-Cassart, C. G. M. Magnusson, J. G. Ratcliffe, C. L. Cambiaso, and P. L. Masson, *Clin. Chem.,* **27,** 64 (1981).

301. C. G. M. Magnusson, D. Collet-Cassart, T. G. Merret, and P. L. Masson, *Clin. Allergy,* **11,** 453 (1981).

302. D. Collet-Cassart, C. G. M. Magnusson, C. L. Cambiaso, M. Lesna, and P. L. Masson, *Clin. Chem.,* **27,** 1205 (1981).

303. P. L. Masson, *J. Pharmaceut. Biomed. Anal.,* **5,** 113 (1987).

304. J. H. W. Leuvering, P. J. H. M. Thal, M. van der Waart, and A. H. W. M. Schuurs, *J. Immunoassay,* **1,** 77 (1980).

305. W. D. Geoghegan, *J. Clin. Immunoassay,* **11,** 11 (1988).

306. R. Festin, B. Björklund, and T. H. Tötterman, *J. Immunol. Methods,* **101,** 23 (1987).

307. R. K. Leute, E. F. Ullman, A. Goldstein, and L. A. Herzenberg, *Nature,* **236,** 93 (1972).

308. M. R. Montgomery, *Clin. Chem.,* **21,** 1323 (1975).

309. A. F. Esser, *Lab. Res. Methods Biol. Med.,* **4,** 213 (1980).

310. M. Cais, S. Dani, Y. Eden, O. Gandolfi, M. Horn, E. E. Isaacs, Y. Josephy, Y. Saar, E. Slovin, and L. Snarsky, *Nature,* **270,** 534 (1977).

311. A. A. Ismail, G. Jaouen, P. Cheret, and P. Brossier, *Clin. Biochem.,* **22,** 297 (1989).

312. I. Lavastre, J. Besancon, P. Brossier, and C. Moise, *Appl. Organomet. Chem.,* **4,** 9 (1990).

313. S. G. Weber and W. C. Purdy, *Anal. Lett.,* **12,** 1 (1979).

314. I. A. Alam and G. D. Christian, *Anal. Lett.,* **15,** 1449 (1982).

315. I. A. Alam and G. D. Christian, *Fresenius Z. Anal. Chem.,* **318,** 33 (1984).

316. I. A. Alam and G. D. Christian, *Fresenius Z. Anal. Chem.,* **320,** 281 (1985).

317. D. M. Hercules, Ed., *Fluorescence and Phosphorescence Analysis,* Wiley-Interscience, New York, 1965.

318. S. Udenfriend, *Fluorescence Assay in Biology and Medicine,* Academic Press, New York, 1969.

319. J. D. Winefordner, S. G. Schulman, and T. L. O'Haver, *Luminescence Spectrometry in Analytical Chemistry,* Wiley-Interscience, New York, 1972.

320. G. G. Guilbault, *Practical Fluorescence: Theory, Methods and Techniques,* Dekker, New York, 1973.

321. E. L. Wehry, Ed., *Modern Fluorescence Spectroscopy,* Plenum, New York, Vol. 1 and 2 (1976), Vol. 3 and 4 (1981).

322. S. G. Schulman, *Fluorescence and Phosphorescence Spectroscopy: Physicochemical Principles and Practice,* Pergamon, London, 1977.

323. S. G. Schulman, Ed., *Molecular Luminescence Spectroscopy: Methods and Applications,* Wiley-Interscience, New York, 1985.

324. A. Jablonski, *Z. Physik,* **94,** 38 (1935).

325. G. N. Lewis and M. J. Kasha, *J. Am. Chem. Soc.,* **66,** 2100 (1944).

326. C. A. Parker, C. G. Hatchard, and T. A. Joyce, *Nature,* **205,** 1282 (1965).

327. K. Kikuchi, H. Kokubun, and M. Koizumi, *Photochem. Photobiol.,* **7,** 499 (1968).

328. C. A. Parker, C. G. Hatchard, and T. A. Joyce, *Analyst,* **90,** 1 (1965).

329. A. N. Terenin and V. L. Ermolaev, *Dokl. Acad. Nauk. USSR,* **85,** 547 (1952).

330. A. Fernandez-Gutierrez and A. Muñoz De La Peña, "Determination of Inorganic Substances by Luminescence Methods," in S. G. Schulman, Ed., *Molecular Luminescence Spectroscopy,* Wiley-Interscience, New York, 1985.

331. M. Bajema, M. Gouterman, and C. B. Rose, *J. Mol. Spectrosc.,* **39,** 421 (1971).

332. L. A. Martarano, C.-P. Wong, W. DeW. Horrocks Jr., and A. M. Ponte Goncalves, *J. Phys. Chem.,* **80,** 2389 (1976).

333. T. Förster, *Ann. Physik,* **6,** 55 (1948).

334. L. Stryer and R. P. Haugland, *Proc. Natl. Acad. Sci. USA,* **58,** 719 (1967).

335. N. Ishibashi, T. Ogawa, T. Imasaka, and M. Kunitake, *Anal. Chem.,* **51,** 2096 (1979).

336. N. J. Dovichi, J. C. Martin, J. H. Jett, M. Trkula, and R. A. Keller, *Anal. Chem.,* **56,** 348 (1984).

337. T. Hirschfeld, *Applied Optics,* **15,** 2965 (1976).

338. R. A. Mathies and L. Stryer, "Single-Molecule Fluorescence Detection: A Feasibility Study Using Phycoerythrin," in D. L. Taylor, A. S. Waggoner, R. F. Murphy, F. Lanni, and R. R. Birge, Eds., *Applications of Fluorescence in the Biomedical Sciences,* Alan R. Liss Inc., New York, 1986.

339. D. C. Nguyen, R. A. Keller, J. H. Jett, and J. C. Martin, *Anal. Chem.,* **59,** 2158 (1987).

340. K. Peck, L. Stryer, A. N. Glazer, and R. A. Mathies, *Proc. Natl. Acad. Sci. USA,* **86,** 4087 (1989).

341. R. A. Mathies and K. Peck, *Anal. Chem.,* **62,** 1786 (1990).

342. E. Soini and I. Hemmilä, *Clin. Chem.,* **25,** 353 (1979).

343. M. Shaykh, N. Bazilinski, D. S. McCaul, S. Ahmed, A. Dubin, T. Musiala, and G. Dunea, *Clin. Chem.,* **31,** 1988 (1985).

344. S. A. Eremin, G. Gallacher, H. Lotey, D. S. Smith, and J. Landon, *Clin. Chem.,* **33,** 1903 (1987).

345. D. L. Colbert, G. Gallacher, A. M. Sidki, and R. W. Mainwaring-Burton, *J. Immunoassay,* **9,** 367 (1988).

346. I. Hemmilä, *Anal. Chem.,* **57,** 1676 (1985).

347. I. Hemmilä, *Scand. J. Clin. Lab. Invest.,* **48,** 389 (1988).

348. N. J. Turro, *Molecular Photochemistry,* WA Benjamin, New York, 1965.

349. R. F. Chen and J. R. Knutson, *Anal. Biochem.,* **172,** 61 (1988).

350. E. F. Ullman, N. N. Bellet, J. M. Brinkley, and R.F. Zuk, "Homogeneous Fluorescence Immunoassays," in R. M. Nakamura, W. R. Dito, and E. S. Tucker, Eds., *Immunoassays: Clinical Laboratory Techniques for the 1980s,* Alan R. Liss, Inc., New York, 1980.

351. E. J. Soini, "Theoretical Comparison of Alternative Labelling Techniques," in A. Ballows, R. C. Tilton, and A. Turano, Eds., *Rapid Methods and Automation in Microbiology and Immunology,* Brixia Academic Press, Brescia, Italy, 1989.

352. N. S. Allen and J. F. Kellar, *Photochemistry of Dyed and Pigmented Polymers,* Applied Science Publisher Ltd., London, 1980.

353. G. Böck, M. Hilchenbach, K. Schauenstein, and G. Wick, *J. Histochem. Cytochem.,* **33,** 699 (1985).

354. R. S. Davidson and J. E. Pratt, *J. Photochem. Photobiol.,* **1,** 361 (1988).

355. J. S. Ploem, *Ann. NY Acad. Sci.,* **177,** 414 (1971).

356. N. R. Bergquist and P. Nilsson, *Ann. NY Acad. Sci.,* **254,** 157 (1975).

357. D. Gill, *Experientia,* **35,** 400 (1979).

358. H. Giloh and J. W. Sedat, *Science,* **217,** 1252 (1987).

359. D. S. Kaplan and G. L. Picciolo, *J. Clin. Microbiol.,* **27,** 2008 (1989).

360. D. G. Johnson and G. M. De C. Nogueira Araujo, *J. Immunol. Methods,* **43,** 349 (1981).

361. K. D. Krenick, G. M. Kephart, K. P. Offord, S. L. Dunnette, and G. J. Gleich, *J. Immunol. Methods,* **117,** 91 (1989).

362. S. Fujita and M. Fukuda, *Histochem.,* **40,** 59 (1974).

363. A. H. Parola and E. E. Uzgiris, *Anal. Biochem.,* **138,** 386 (1984).

364. T. Hirschfeld, *J. Histochem. Cytochem.,* **27,** 96 (1979).

365. M. Lu-Steffes, G. W. Pittluck, M. E. Jolley, H. N. Panas, D. L. Olive, C.-H. J. Wang, D. D. Nyström, C. L. Keegan, T. P. Davis, and S. D. Stroupe, *Clin. Chem.,* **28,** 2278 (1982).

366. E. J. Shaw, R. A. A. Watson, and D. S. Smith, *Clin. Chem.,* **25,** 322 (1979).

367. R. S. Kamel, A. R. McGregor, J. Landon, and D. S. Smith, *Clin. Chim. Acta,* **89,** 93 (1978).

368. H. M. Friedman, N. B. Tustin, M. M. Hitchings, and S. A. Plotkin, *Am. J. Clin. Pathol.,* **76,** 305 (1981).

369. Y. Kobayashi, N. Tsubota, K. Miyai, and F. Watanabe, *Steroids,* **36,** 177 (1980).

370. Y. Kobayashi, K. Amitani, F. Watanabe, and K. Miyai, *Clin. Chim. Acta,* **92,** 241 (1979).

371. A. J. Munro, D. S. Smith, and E. J. Shaw, *J. Antimicrob. Chemother.,* **9,** 47 (1982).

372. A. R. McGregor, J. O. Crookall-Greening, J. Landon, and D. S. Smith, *Clin. Chim. Acta,* **83,** 161 (1978).

373. Y. Kobayashi, K. Miyai, N. Tsubota, and F. Watanabe, *Steroids,* **34,** 829 (1979).

374. J. Kam, R. A. Yoshida, US Patent No. 4,252,783 (1981).

375. E. F. Ullman, "Recent Advantages in Fluorescence Immunoassay Techniques," in J. Langan and J. J. Clapp, Eds., *Ligand Assay, Analysis of International Developments of Isotopic and Non-isotopic Immunoassay,* Masson Publishing, USA Inc., New York, 1981.

376. L. Winfrey and B. S. Wagman, *Am. Clin. Products,* **4,** 10 (1984).

377. C. J. Munro and B. L. Lasley, "Non-Radiometric Methods for Immunoassay of Steroid Hormones," in B. D. Alberson and F. P. Haseltine, Eds., *Non-Radiometric Assays, Technology and Application in Polypeptide and Steroid Hormone Detection,* Alan R. Liss, Inc., New York, 1988.

378. G. Osikowicz, I. Strarup-Brynes, B. Kucera, and A. S. Vanderbilt, *Clin. Chem.,* **33,** 885 (1987).

379. L. J. Blecka, AACC Therapeutic Drug Monitoring Continuing Education and Quality Control Program, 1 (1983).

380. C. H. Zeitvogel, G. J. Jackson, L. A. Cantrell, R. J. Brashear, J. B. Roberts, R. L. Schmidt, M. Adamczyk, D. A. Betebenner, and K. Vaughan, *Clin. Chem.,* **32,** 1171 (abs. 603) (1986).

381. G. J. Diebold and R. N. Zare, *Science,* **196,** 1439 (1977).

382. M. Fukuda, K. Nakanishi, I. Sawamura, and S. Fujita, *Histochem.,* **52,** 119 (1977).

383. I. Wieder, US Patent No. 4,150,295 (1979).

384. M. P. Bailey, B. F. Rocks, and C. Riley, "Chelated Terbium as a Label in Fluorescence Immunoassay," in T. T. Ngo, Ed., *Non-isotopic Immunoassay,* Plenum Press, New York, 1988.

385. T. C. O'Haver and J. D. Winefordner, *Anal. Chem.,* **38,** 1258 (1966).

386. J. D. Winefordner, *Acc. Chem. Res.,* **2,** 361 (1969).

387. W. Mueller and T. Hirschfeld, *Histochem. J.,* **9,** 121 (1977).

388. I. Wieder, "Background Rejection in Fluorescence Immunoassay," in W. Knapp, K. Holubar, and G. Wick, Eds., *Immunofluorescence and Related Staining Techniques,* Proc. Sixth Int. Conf., Vienna, Elsevier/North-Holland Biomedical Press, Amsterdam, 1978.

389. L. B. McGown, "Phase-Resolved Fluoroimmunoassay," in T. T. Ngo, Ed., *Non-isotopic Immunoassay,* Plenum Press, New York, 1988.

390. J. S. O'Neal and S. G. Schulman, *Anal. Chem.,* **56,** 2888 (1984).

391. L. Stryer, US Patent No. 4,542,104 (1985).

392. A. N. Glazer and L. Stryer, *Biophys. J.,* **43,** 383 (1983).
393. W. L. Hinze and H. Sing, *Anal. Chem.,* **3,** 193 (1984).
394. A. Sanz-Medel and J. Alonso, *Anal. Chim. Acta,* **165,** 159 (1984).
395. M. P. Bailey, B. F. Rocks, and C. Riley, *Ann. Clin. Biochem.,* **20,** 213 (1983).
396. C. J. Halfman, US Patent No. 4,640,898 (1987).
397. C. J. Halfman, F. C. L. Wong, and D. W. Jay, *Anal. Chem.,* **57,** 1928 (1985).
398. T. L. Keimig and L. B. McGown, *Talanta,* **33,** 653 (1986).
399. C. M. O'Donnell and J. D. Winefordner, *Clin. Chem.,* **21,** 285 (1975).
400. J. D. Winefordner, W. J. McCarthy, and P. A. John, *Methods Biochem. Anal.,* **15,** 363 (1967).
401. T. Vo-Dinh, *Room Temperature Phosphorimetry for Chemical Analysis,* Wiley-Interscience, New York, 1984.
402. E. M. Schulman and C. Walling, *Science,* **178,** 53 (1972).
403. R. A. Paynter, S. L. Wellons, and J. D. Winefordner, *Anal. Chem.,* **46,** 736 (1974).
404. G. J. Niday and P. G. Seybold, *Anal. Chem.,* **50,** 1577 (1978).
405. L. J. Clin Love, M. Scrilec, and J. G. Habarta, *Anal. Chem.,* **52,** 754 (1980).
406. S. Scypinski and L. J. Clin Love, *Anal. Chem.,* **56,** 322 (1984).
407. J. J. Aaron, J. J. Mousa, and J. D. Winefordner, *Talanta,* **20,** 279 (1973).
408. T. Vo-Dinh, E. L. Yen, and J. D. Winefordner, *Anal. Chem.,* **48,** 1186 (1976).
409. T. Vo-Dinh and M. Uziel, *Anal. Chem.,* **59,** 1093 (1987).
410. M. Fiore, J. Mitchell, T. Doan, R. Nelson, G. Winter, C. Grandone, K. Zeng, R. Haraden, J. Smith, K. Harris, J. Leszczynski, D. Berry, S. Safford, G. Barnes, A. Scholnick, and K. Ludington, *Clin. Chem.,* **34,** 1726 (1988).
411. J. H. Richardson, "Application of Lasers in Analytical Molecular Fluorescence Spectroscopy," in E. L. Wehry, Ed., *Modern Fluorescence Spectroscopy,* Vol. 4, Plenum Press, New York, 1981.
412. B. Kirsch, E. Voigtman, and J. D. Winefordner, *Anal. Chem.,* **57,** 2007 (1985).
413. F. E. Lytle, *J. Chem. Education,* **59,** 915 (1982).
414. M. J. Sepaniak, *Clin. Chem.,* **31,** 671 (1985).
415. S. Wohlstein, *Spectrosc. Int.,* **2,** 10 (1990).
416. J. H. Richardson and M. E. Ando, *Anal. Chem.,* **49,** 955 (1977).
417. A. B. Bradley and R. N. Zare, *J. Am. Chem. Soc.,* **98,** 620 (1976).
418. J. H. Richardson and S. M. George, *Anal. Chem.,* **50,** 616 (1978).
419. S. Yamada, K. Kano, and T. Ogawa, *Anal. Chim. Acta,* **134,** 21 (1982).
420. S. Yamada, F. Miyoshi, K. Kano, and T. Ogawa, *Anal. Chim. Acta,* **127,** 195 (1981).
421. T. Imakawa, H. Kadone, T. Okawa, and N. Ishibashi, *Anal. Chem.,* **49,** 667 (1977).
422. T. Imasaka and N. Ishibashi, *Anal. Chem.,* **62,** 363A (1990).

423. P. A. Johnson, T. E. Barber, B. W. Smith, and J. D. Winefordner, *Anal. Chem.*, **61**, 861 (1989).
424. T. Imasaka, A. Tsukamoto, and N. Ishibashi, *Anal. Chem.*, **61**, 2285 (1989).
425. T. Imasaka, H. Nakagawa, T. Okazaki, and N. Ishibashi, *Anal. Chem.*, **62**, 2405 (1990).
426. T. Kobayashi, Jpn. Patent No. 57-149965 (1982).
427. H. M. Shapiro, *Practical Flow Cytometry*, Alan R. Liss, Inc., New York, 1988.
428. G. I. Kaufman, J. F. Nester, and D. E. Wasserman, *J. Histochem. Cytochem.*, **19**, 469 (1971).
429. D. F. Nicoli, J. Briggs, and V. B. Elings, *Proc. Natl. Acad. Sci. USA*, **77**, 4904 (1980).
430. J. El Jabri, S. De Lauzon, N. Cittanova, P. Gervais, J. Mugnier, and B. Valeur, *Anal. Chim. Acta*, **227**, 129 (1989).
431. F. E. Lytle and M. S. Kelsey, *Anal. Chem.*, **46**, 855 (1974).
432. W. R. Seitz, *CRC Crit. Rev. Anal. Chem.*, **19**, 135 (1988).
433. T. Vo-Dinh, G. D. Griffin, and K. R. Ambrose, *Appl. Spectrosc.*, **40**, 696 (1986).
434. F. V. Bright, *Appl. Spectrosc.*, **42**, 1531 (1988).
435. D. Axelrod, T. P. Burghardt, and N. L. Thompson, *Ann. Rev. Biophys. Bioeng.*, **13**, 247 (1984).
436. T. Hirschfeld and M. J. Block, *Opt. Eng.*, **16**, 406 (1977).
437. T. Hirschfeld, M. J. Block, and W. Mueller, *J. Histochem. Cytochem.*, **25**, 719 (1977).
438. E. J. Ambrose, *Exp. Cell. Res.*, **8**, 54 (1961).
439. M. N. Kronick and W. A. Little, *J. Immunol. Methods*, **8**, 235 (1975).
440. M. N. Kronick and W. A. Little, US Patent No. 3,939,350 (1976).
441. N. L. Thompson and D. Axelrod, *Biophys. J.*, **43**, 103 (1983).
442. V. Hlady, D. R. Reinecke, and J. D. Andrade, *J. Colloid. Interface Sci.*, **111**, 555 (1986).
443. J. D. Andrade, R. A. Vanwagen, D. E. Gregonis, K. Newby, and J.-L. Lin, "Remote Fiber-Optic Biosensor Based on Evanescent-Excited Fluoroimmunoassay: Concept and Progress," IEEE Transact. Electr. Devic., ED-32, 1985.
444. D. J. Arndt-Jovin, M. Robert-Nicoud, S. J. Kaufman, and T. M. Jovin, *Science*, **230**, 247 (1985).
445. R. D. Allen, J. L. Travis, N. S. Allen, and H. Yilmaz, *Cell Motility*, **1**, 275 (1981).
446. T. M. Jovin and D. J. Arndt-Jovin, *Ann. Rev. Biophys. Chem.*, **18**, 271 (1989).
447. R. Rigler, *Acta Physiol. Scand.*, **67**, Suppl, 267 (1966).
448. J. J. Haaijman and J. P. R. Van Dalen, *J. Immunol. Methods*, **5**, 359 (1974).
449. R. H. Jensen, J. S. Greenspan, D. Moore II, N. Talar, and J. R. Roubinian, *J. Immunol. Methods*, **42**, 343 (1981).

450. D. S. Kaplan and G. L. Piccolo, *J. Clin. Microbiol.,* **27,** 442 (1989).

451. R. A. Velapoldi, J. C. Travis, W. A. Cassatt, and W. T. Yap, *J. Microscopy,* **103,** 293 (1975).

452. R. F. Vogt, Jr., G. D. Gross, L. O. Henderson, and D. L. Phillips, *Cytometry,* **10,** 294 (1989).

453. R. J. Kelly, W. B. Dandliker, and D. E. Williamson, *Anal. Chem.,* **48,** 846 (1976).

454. H. Maeda, *Clin. Chem.,* **24,** 2139 (1978).

455. S. R. Popelka, D. M. Miller, J. T. Holen, and D. M. Kelso, *Clin. Chem.,* **27,** 1198 (1981).

456. M. E. Jolley, S. D. Stroupe, K. S. Schwenzer, C. J. Wang, M. Lu-Steffes, H. D. Hill, S. R. Popelka, J. T. Holen, and D. M. Kelso, *Clin. Chem.,* **27,** 1575 (1981).

457. A. T. R. Williams, "Fluorescence Polarization Immunoassay," in W. P. Collins, Ed., *Complementary Immunoassays,* Wiley, Chichester, UK, 1988.

458. T. C. O'Haver and J. D. Winefordner, *Anal. Chem.,* **38,** 602 (1966).

459. S. I. Weissman, *J. Chem. Phys.,* **10,** 214 (1942).

460. G. D. R. Boutilier and J. D. Winefordner, *Anal. Chem.,* **51,** 1384 (1979).

461. R. P. Fisher and J. D. Winefordner, *Anal. Chem.,* **44,** 948 (1972).

462. C. G. Barnes and J. D. Winefordner, *Appl. Spectroscopy,* **38,** 214 (1984).

463. G. M. Klauminzer, *Laser Focus,* **11,** 35 (1975).

464. E. Soini and T. Lövgren, *CRC Critical Reviews in Analytical Chemistry,* **18,** 105 (1987).

465. S. M. Fernandez, "Time-Resolved Fluorescence Spectroscopy," in R. I. Sha'afi and S. M. Fernandez, Eds., *Fast Methods in Physical Biochemistry and Cell Biology,* Elsevier Science Publication, Amsterdam, 1983.

466. J. Yguerabide, H. F. Epstein, and L. Stryer, *J. Mol. Biol.,* **51,** 573 (1970).

467. C. A. Sacchi, O. Svelto, and G. Prenna, *Histochem. J.,* **6,** 251 (1974).

468. H. Schneckenburger, "Time-Resolved Microfluorescence in Biomedical Diagnosis," in *Proc. 16th Int. Congr. High Speed Photography,* The Society of Photo-optical Instrumentation Engineers, Bellingham, WA (USA), 1985.

469. H. Schneckenburger and E. Unsöld, "Time-Resolved Ultra-Sensitive Fluorescence Detection for Enzyme Analysis," in P. Brätter and P. Schramer, Eds., *Trace Element Analytical Chemistry in Medicine and Biology,* Vol. 2, Walter De Gruyter & Co., Berlin, 1983.

470. H. Schneckenburger, *Opt. Engin.,* **24,** 1042 (1985).

471. G. R. Haugen and F. E. Lytle, *Anal. Chem.,* **53,** 1554 (1981).

472. J. K. Weltman, R. P. Szaro, A. R. Frackelton, Jr., R. M. Dowben, J. R. Bunting, and R. E. Cathou, *J. Biol. Chem.,* **248,** 3173 (1973).

473. J. A. Knopp and G. Weber, *J. Biol. Chem.,* **244,** 6309 (1969).

474. C. Lovejoy, D. A. Holowka, and R. E. Cathou, *Biochemistry,* **16,** 3668 (1977).

475. E. Soini and H. Kojola, *Clin. Chem.,* **29,** 65 (1983).

476. H. J. Tanke, *J. Microscopy,* **155,** 405 (1989).

477. H. B. Beverloo, A. van Schadewijk, S. van Gelderen-Boele, and H. J. Tanke, *Cytometry,* **11,** 784 (1990).

478. J. R. Lakowicz, "A Review of Photon-Counting and Phase-Modulation Measurements of Fluorescence Decay Kinetics," in D. L. Taylor, A. S. Waggoner, R. F. Murphy, F. Lanni, and R. R. Birge, Eds., *Applications of Fluorescence in the Biomedical Sciences,* Alan R. Liss, Inc., New York, 1986.

479. L. B. McGown, *Anal. Chem.,* **61,** 839A (1989).

480. J. R. Lakowicz, R. Jayaweera, N. Joshi, and I. Gryczynski, *Anal. Biochem.,* **160,** 471 (1987).

481. F. V. Bright, *Anal. Chem.,* **60,** 1622 (1988).

482. J. R. Lakowicz, E. Gratton, H. Cherek, B. P. Maliwal, and G. Laczko, *J. Biol. Chem.,* **259,** 10967 (1984).

483. F. V. Bright and K. S. Litwiler, *Anal. Chem.,* **61,** 1510 (1989).

484. M. S. Artenstein and O. W. Dandridge, *J. Immunol.,* **100,** 831 (1968).

485. T. M. Li, J. E. Miller, F. E. Ward, and J. F. Burd, *Epilepsia,* **23,** 391 (1982).

486. D. L. Colbert, G. Gallacher, and R. W. Mainwaring-Burton, *Clin. Chem.,* **31,** 1193 (1985).

487. R. E. Coxon, G. Gallacher, J. Landon, and C. Rae, *Ann. Clin. Biochem.,* **25,** 49 (1988).

488. S. A. Eremin, D. E. Schiavetta, H. Lotey, D. S. Smith, and J. Landon, *Ther. Drug Monit.,* **10,** 327 (1988).

489. A. J. Hodgkinson, J. Landon, D. S. Smith, and A. M. Sidki, *Ther. Drug Monit.,* **8,** 236 (1986).

490. D. L. Colbert, D. S. Smith, J. Landon, and A. M. Sidki, *Ann. Clin. Biochem.,* **23,** 37 (1986).

491. A. M. Sidki, F. J. Rowell, and J. Landon, *Ann. Clin. Biochem.,* **20,** 227 (1983).

492. B. F. Rocks, V. M. R. Bertram, M. P. Bailey, C. Riley, and B. T. Thom, *Ann. Clin. Biochem.,* **25,** 522 (1988).

493. K. Izutsu, E. Truelove, S. Felton, I. Siegel, P. Madden, and M. Schubert, *J. Dent. Res.,* **59,** 1192 (1980).

494. C. M. O'Donnell, J. McBride, S. Suffin, and A. Broughton, *J. Immunoassay,* **1,** 375 (1980).

495. D. J. Phillips, G. G. Galland, C. B. Reimer, and A. P. Kendal, *J. Clin. Microbiol.,* **15,** 931 (1982).

496. J. T. Sundeen and R. S. Krakauer, *J. Immunol. Methods,* **26,** 229 (1979).

497. S. Hashida, K. Nakagawa, S. Yoshitake, M. Imagawa, E. Ishikawa, Y. Endo, S. Ohtaki, Y. Ichioka, and M. Nakajima, *Anal. Lett.,* **16,** 31 (1983).

498. F. Watanabe, N. Tsubota, Y. Kobayashi, O. Miyata, I. Ninomiya, and K. Miyai, *Steroids,* **40,** 393 (1982).

499. T. P. Gillis and J. J. Thompson, *J. Clin. Microbiol.,* **7**, 202 (1978).
500. J. W. Smith, T. P. Gillis, and J. J. Thompson, *J. Gen. Virol.,* **44,** 17 (1979).
501. Y. Yamaguchi, C. Hayashi, and K. Miyai, *Anal. Lett.,* **15/B8,** 731 (1982).
502. M. Muratsugu and M. Makino, *J. Clin. Chem. Clin. Biochem.,* **20,** 567 (1982).
503. P. Allain, A. Turcant, and A. Prémel-Cabil, *Clin. Chem.,* **35,** 469 (1989).
504. B. A. Warden, K. Allam, A. Sentissi, D. J. Cecchini, and R. W. Giese, *Anal. Biochem.,* **162,** 363 (1987).
505. F. Legros, M. Castillo, M. Praet, M. Vandenbranden, O. Lemoine, V. Cabiaux, J. P. Van Vooren, J. Nyabenda, P. Dierckx, M. Turneer, and J.-M. Ruysschaert, *J. Immunol. Methods,* **108,** 223 (1988).
506. M. A. Bacigalupo, A. Ius, G. Meroni, R. Saita, and C. Parini, *J. Steroid. Biochem.,* **19,** 1661 (1983).
507. H. Labrousse and S. Avrameas, *J. Immunol. Methods,* **103,** 9 (1987).
508. J. S. Ploem, "New Instrumentation for Sensitive Image Analysis of Fluorescence in Cells and Tissues," in D. L. Taylor, A. S. Waggoner, R. F. Murphy, F. Lanni, and R. R. Birge, Eds., *Applications of Fluorescence in the Biomedical Sciences,* Alan R. Liss, Inc., New York, 1986.
509. J. J. Haaijman and J. Slingerland-Teunissen, "Equipment and Preparative Procedures in Immunofluorescence Microscopy: Quantitative Study," in D. L. Taylor, A. S. Waggoner, R. F. Murphy, F. Lanni, and R. R. Birge, Eds., *Applications of Fluorescence in the Biomedical Sciences,* Alan R. Liss, Inc., New York, 1986.
510. M. Goldman, *Exp. Parasit.,* **9,** 25 (1960).
511. M. Goldman, *J. Histochem. Cytochem.,* **15,** 38 (1967).
512. C. E. O. Taylor and C. V. Heimer, *J. Biol. Standard.,* **2,** 11 (1974).
513. A. M. Deelder, H. J. Tanke, and J. S. Ploem, "Automated Quantitative Immunofluorescence Using the Aperture Defined Microvolume (ADM) Method," in W. Knapp, G. Holubar, and G. Wick, Eds., *Immunofluorescence and Related Staining Techniques,* Elsevier/North Holland Biomedical Press, Amsterdam, 1978.
514. H. J. Tanke, A. M. Deelder, M. H. Dresden, J. F. Jongkind, and J. S. Ploem, *Histochem. J.,* **17,** 797 (1985).
515. J. J. Haaijman and F. A. C. Wijnants, *J. Immunol. Methods,* **7,** 255 (1975).
516. J. E. DeJosselin De Jong, J. F. Jongkind, and H. R. Ywema, *Anal. Biochem.,* **102,** 120 (1980).
517. W. Knapp and J. S. Ploem, *J. Immunol. Methods,* **5,** 259 (1974).
518. H. Fiebach, W. Uckert, and B. Micheel, *Acta Biol. Med. Germ. Band.,* **41,** 689 (1982).
519. L. Hart, R. M. Donovan, E. Goldstein, and F. P. Brady, *Analyt. Quant. Cytol. Histol.,* **12,** 127 (1990).
520. H. Ueki, I. Yoskii, A. Ikeda, and N. Nohara, *Arch. Dermatol. Res.,* **265,** 189 (1979).

521. P. Vincent, M. Luciani, G. Farber, and H. Leclerc, "Recent Developments in Microscopic Automated Image Analysis," in A. Balows, R. C. Tilton, and A. Turano, Eds., *Rapid Methods and Automation in Microbiology and Immunology,* Brixia Academic Press, Brescia, 1989.

522. J. E. Sisken, G. H. Barrows, and S. D. Grasch, *J. Histochem. Cytochem.,* **34,** 61 (1986).

523. J. M. Basgen, T. E. Nevin, and A. F. Michael, *J. Immunol. Methods,* **124,** 77 (1989).

524. R. Ekins, F. Chu, and J. Micallef, *J. Biolum. Chemilum.,* **4,** 59 (1989).

525. H. M. Shapiro, E. R. Schildkraut, R. Curbelo, B. R. Turner, R. H. Webb, D. L. Brown, and M. J. Block, *J. Histochem. Cytochem.,* **25,** 836 (1977).

526. J. A. Steinkamp, *Rev. Sci. Instrum.,* **55,** 1375 (1984).

527. D. R. Parks and L. A. Herzenberg, *Methods Enzymol.,* **108,** 197 (1986).

528. D. R. Parks and L. L. Lanier, "Flow Cytometry and FACS," in D. M. Weir, D. R. Parks, L. L. Lanier, and L. A. Herzenberg, Eds., *Handbook of Experimental Immunology,* Blackwell Science Publisher, Oxford, 1986.

529. D. R. Parks, R. R. Hardy, and L. A. Herzenberg, *Immunology Today,* **4,** 145 (1983).

530. J. D. Woronicz and G. C. Rice, *J. Immunol. Methods,* **120,** 291 (1989).

531. L. Cook and D. Irving, *Clin. Immunoassay,* **12,** 36 (1989).

532. T. M. McHugh, Y. J. Wang, H. O. Chong, L. L. Blackwood, and D. P. Stites, *J. Immunol. Methods,* **116,** 213 (1989).

533. R. L. Houghton, N. Monji, J. Plastine, and J. Priest, *Clin. Chem.,* **32,** 1067 (1986).

534. M. R. Loken, D. R. Parks, and L. A. Herzenberg, *J. Histochem. Cytochem.,* **25,** 899 (1977).

535. P. Brandtzaeg, *Immunology,* **22,** 177 (1972).

536. G. Presani, S. Perticarari, and M. A. Mangiarotti, *J. Immunol. Methods,* **119,** 197 (1989).

537. J. M. Sligh, S. T. Roodman, and C. C. Tsai, *Am. J. Clin. Pathol.,* **91,** 210 (1989).

538. N. J. Dovichi, J. C. Martin, J. H. Jett, and R. A. Keller, *Science,* **219,** 845 (1983).

539. P. J. Lisi, C. W. Huang, R. A. Hoffman, and J. W. Teipel, *Clin. Chim. Acta,* **120,** 171 (1982).

540. C. Shellum and G. Gübitz, *Abstract of Papers Presented at the IIIrd International Symposium on Quantitative Luminescence Spectrometry in Biomedical Sciences,* Ghent, Belgium, May 1989.

541. R. A. Durst, L. Locascio-Brown, A. L. Plant, and M. V. Brizgys, *Clin. Chem.,* **34,** 1700 (1988).

542. C. S. Lim, J. N. Miller, and J. W. Bridges, *Anal. Chim. Acta,* **114,** 183 (1980).

543. S. D. Lidofsky, W. D. Hinsberg III, and R. N. Zare, *Proc. Natl. Acad. Sci. USA,* **78,** 1901 (1981).
544. S. D. Lidofsky, T. Imasaka, and R. N. Zare, *Anal. Chem.,* **51,** 1602 (1979).
545. H. Hosotsubo, K. Arai, and J.-I. Iwamura, *J. Immunol. Methods,* **85,** 115 (1985).
546. H. Hosotsubo, K. Arai, and J.-I. Iwamura, *J. Immunol. Methods,* **98,** 1 (1987).
547. M. F. Bryant, K. O'Keefe, and M. V. Malmstadt, *Anal. Chem.,* **47,** 2324 (1975).
548. M. E. Jolley, C.-H. J. Wang, S. J. Ekenberg, M. S. Zuelke, and D. M. Kelso, *J. Immunol. Methods,* **67,** 21 (1984).
549. R. E. Curry, H. Heitzman, D. H. Riege, R. V. Sweet, and M. G. Simonsen, *Clin. Chem.,* **25,** 1591 (1979).
550. M. G. Simonsen, *Clin. Biochem. Anal.,* **10,** 97 (1981).
551. S. M. Hall and A. W. Confer, *J. Clin. Microbiol.,* **25,** 350 (1987).
552. E. F. Ullman, M. Schwarzberg, and K. E. Rubenstein, *J. Biol. Chem.,* **251,** 4172 (1976).
553. T. M. Li, S. P. Robertson, T. H. Crouch, E. E. Pahuski, G. A. Bush, and S. J. Hydo, *Clin. Chem.,* **29,** 1628 (1983).
554. O. S. Khalil, W. S. Routh, K. Lingenfelter, D. B. Carr, and P. Labouceur, *Clin. Chem.,* **27,** 1586 (1981).
555. R. Polsky-Cynkin, *J. Clin. Immunoassay,* **11,** 69 (1988).
556. A. A. A. Ismael, P. M. West, and D. J. Goldie, *Clin. Chem.,* **24,** 571 (1978).
557. M. G. Pappas, "Dot Enzyme-Linked Immunosorbent Assays," in W. P. Collins, Ed., *Complementary Immunoassays,* Wiley, Chichester, UK, 1988.
558. V. Gordon, S. Ching, J. Hoijer, C. Jou, M. McMahow, D. Pacenti, D. Stimpson, and D. Zakula, *Abstract of Papers Presented in Sixth International Congress on Rapid Methods and Automation in Microbiology and Immunology,* Espoo, Finland, June 1990, abs. 145.
559. G. E. Valkirs and R. Barton, *Clin. Chem.,* **31,** 1427 (1985).
560. R. F. Zuk, V. K. Ginsberg, and T. Houts, *Clin. Chem.,* **31,** 1144 (1985).
561. W. E. Brown, *Clin. Chem.,* **33,** 1567 (1987).
562. G. Mould and V. Marks, *Clin. Pharmacokin.,* **14,** 65 (1988).
563. V. Ehrhardt, D. Neumeier, and H. D. Meyer, *J. Immunoassay,* **11,** 74 (1988).
564. L. Wu, G. Mylott, and B. Farrenkopf, *Clin. Chem.,* **36,** 1029 (abs. 0364) (1990).
565. G. Mylott, H. Jerome, B. Farrenkopf, K. Schwenzer, and R. A. Kaufman, *Clin. Chem.,* **36,** 1030 (abs. 0365) (1990).
566. N. B. Person, R. Caldwell, and C. McIntyre, *Clin. Chem.,* **36,** 1044 (abs. 0434) (1990).
567. H. Jerome, B. Farrenkopf, S. Vitone, T. Awdzeij, and R. A. Kaufman, *Clin. Chem.,* **36,** 1045 (abs. 0437) (1990).
568. G. Azzetti, M. Russolo, P. Fossati, and C. Musitelli, *Isr. J. Clin. Biochem. Lab. Sci.,* **4,** 31 (1985).

569. B. Fingerhut, R. Costanzo, Z. Chaudri, and S. Rizvi, *Clin. Chem.,* **27,** 1085 (abs. 309) (1981).

570. M. A. Pesce, *J. Clin. Lab. Autom.,* **3,** 327 (1983).

571. D. Plaut and C. Johnson, *J. Clin. Immunoassay,* **11,** 81 (1988).

572. N. Kameda and W. Y. Chen, *Clin. Chem.,* **34,** 1211 (abs. 286) (1988).

573. M. Sasaki and K. Ogura, *Clin. Chem.,* **36,** 1567 (1990).

574. W. E. Howard III, A. Greenquist, B. Walter, and F. Wogoman, *Anal. Chem.,* **55,** 878 (1983).

575. R. C. Boguslaski and A. C. Greenquist, *Diagn. Medicine,* **Oct.,** 73 (1983).

576. B. Walter, A. C. Greenquist, and W. E. Howard, *Anal. Chem.,* **55,** 873 (1983).

577. D. Fitzgerald, D. Richter, and J. Richards, *Clin. Chem.,* **35,** 1140 (abs. 351) (1989).

578. M. Knedel, G. Assmann, A. Courbe, L. van Impe, R. Kattermann, H. Keller, and M. Oellerich, *J. Clin. Chem. Clin. Biochem.,* **26,** 149 (1988).

579. M. S. Lifshitz and R. P. DeCresce, *Lab. Med.,* **18,** 472 (1987).

580. J. Boland, G. Carey, E. Krodel, and M. Kwiatkowski, *Clin. Chem.,* **36,** 1598 (1990).

581. I. Sakurabayashi, K. Sasak, Y. Yamagishi, and T. Kawai, *Clin. Chem.,* **36,** 1093 (abs. 661) (1990).

582. P. F. Laska, M. Adamich, C. C. Leflar, J. L. Seago, W. K. Miller, H. Umetsu, K. Imai, and H. Hashimoto, *Biochimica Clinica,* **13 Suppl. 1,** (abs. A34) (1989).

583. H. Ackermann, M. Staedter, J. Blackwood, S. Inbar, and G. Grenner, *Clin. Chem.,* **35,** 1180 (abs. 540) (1989).

584. S. Inbar, G. Grenner, J. Blackwood, E. Long, M. Bowen, and F. Meneghini, *Ann. Biol. Clin.,* **48,** 385 (1990).

585. G. Grenner, S. Inbar, F. A. Meneghini, E. W. Long, E. J. Yamartino, Jr., M. S. Bowen, J. J. Blackwood, A. J. Padilla, D. Maretsky, and M. Staedter, *Clin. Chem.,* **35,** 1865 (1989).

586. I. Badar, U. Vaupel, A. Case, K. Farrell, S. Inbar, and E. Metzmann, *Clin. Chem.,* **36,** 1028 (abs. 0359) (1990).

587. S. Dakubu, M. Tovey, M. Annunziato, G. Whiteley, and G. Grenner, *Clin. Chem.,* **35,** 1195 (abs. 611) (1989).

588. W. Hoover, D. Holmes, J. Pritchard, J. Richards, T. Sheehy, D. Waskiewicz, R. Wiitala, A. Bsalos, C. Grenz, L. Lenart, J. Nering, R. Tagliareni, and P. Webber, *Clin. Chem.,* **36,** 1209 (abs. 1202) (1990).

589. P. Wegfahrt, R. Cracauer, D. Duchon, D. Fitzgerald, R. Hart, W. Hoover, T. Larsen, W. Mahoney, L. Michels, J. Pumphrey, L. Raymond, and P. Werness, *Clin. Chem.,* **36,** 1094 (abs. 0667) (1990).

590. B. M. Krasovitskii and B. M. Bolotin, *Organic Luminescent Materials,* VCH Verlagsgeselschaft, Weinheim, GDR, 1989.

591. Y. Kanaoka, *Angew. Chem. Int. Ed. Engl.,* **16,** 137 (1977).

592. A. S. Waggoner, "Fluorescent Probes for Analysis of Cell Structure, Function, and Health by Flow and Imaging Cytometry," in D. L. Taylor, A. S. Waggoner, R. F. Murphy, F. Lanni, and R. R. Birge, Eds., *Applications of Fluorescence in the Biomedical Sciences,* Alan R. Liss, Inc., New York, 1986.

593. B. Rotman and B. W. Papermaster, *Proc. Natl. Acad. Sci. USA,* **55,** 134 (1966).

594. B. Micheel, P. Jantscheff, V. Böttger, G. Scharte, G. Kaiser, P. Stolley, and L. Karawajew, *J. Immunol. Methods,* **111,** 89 (1988).

595. J. Kang, C. Chang, R. Dondero, H. Graham, and D. Mochnal, *Clin. Chem.,* **32,** 1067 (abs. 089) (1986).

596. D. Ireland and D. Samuel, *J. Chemilum. Biolum.,* **2,** 215 (1988).

597. C. W. Parker, T. J. Yoo, M. C. Johnson, and S. M. Godt, *Biochemistry,* **6,** 3408 (1967).

598. A. P. Schaap, H. Akhavan, and L. J. Romano, *Clin. Chem.,* **35,** 1863 (1989).

599. H. Arakawa, M. Maeda, and A. Tsuji, *Chem. Pharm. Bull.,* **30,** 3036 (1982).

600. M. S. Abdel-Latif and S. G. Guilbault, *Anal. Chem.,* **60,** 2671 (1988).

601. A. Patel and A. K. Campbell, *Clin. Chem.,* **29,** 1604 (1983).

602. I. Hemmilä, *Appl. Fluor. Technol.,* **1,** 1 (1989).

603. R. F. Chen and C. H. Scott, *Anal. Lett.,* **18,** 393 (1985).

604. I. Hemmilä, *Clin. Chem.,* **31,** 359 (1985).

605. P. V. Tsyplenkov, V. I. Morozov, and V. A. Rogozkin, *Bioorg. Khimii,* **13,** 1605 (1987).

606. A. H. Coons and M. H. Kaplan, *J. Exptl. Med.,* **91,** 1 (1950).

607. T. H. Weller and A. H. Coons, *Proc. Soc. Exptl. Biol. Med.,* **86,** 789 (1954).

608. V. E. Barskii, V. B. Ivanov, Y. U. E. Sklyar, and G. I. Mikhailov, *Izv. Akad. Nauk. SSSR, Ser. Biol.,* **5,** 74 (1968).

609. D. Blakeslee and M. G. Baines, *J. Immunol. Methods,* **13,** 305 (1976).

610. A. N. De Belder and K. Granath, *Carbohydr. Res.,* **30,** 375 (1973).

611. R. F. Chen, *Arch. Biochem. Biophys.,* **133,** 263 (1969).

612. R. M. Watt and E. W. Voss, *Immunochemistry,* **14,** 533 (1977).

613. T. H. The and T. E. W. Feltkamp, *Immunology,* **18,** 865 (1970).

614. G. L. Rowley, T. Henriksson, A. Louie, P. H. Nguyen, M. Kramer, G. Der-Balian, and N. Kameda, *Clin. Chem.,* **33,** 1563 (1987).

615. S. Yaverbaum and J. Kusnetz, Canadian Patent No. 1,124,643 (1982).

616. J. P. Der-Balian, N. Kameda, and G. L. Rowley, *Anal. Biochem.,* **173,** 59 (1988).

617. S. H. Grossman, *J. Clin. Immunoassay,* **7,** 96 (1984).

618. R. Rodgers, M. Schwarzberg, P. Khanna, C.-H. Chang, and E. P. Ullman, *Clin. Chem.,* **24,** 1033 (abs. 225) (1978).

619. P. Van-Der Werf and C.-H. Chang, *J. Immunol. Methods,* **36,** 339 (1980).

620. M. T. Shipchandler, J. R. Fino, L. D. Klein, and C. L. Kirkemo, *Anal. Biochem.,* **162,** 89 (1987).

621. P. L. Khanna and E. F. Ullman, *Anal. Biochem.*, **108**, 156 (1980).
622. E. F. Ullman and P. L. Khanna, *Methods Enzymol.*, **74**, 28 (1981).
623. M. W. Elves, *J. Immunol. Methods*, **2**, 129 (1972).
624. G. R. Pullen, P. J. Chalmers, A. P. P. Nind, and R. C. Nairn, *J. Immunol. Methods*, **43**, 87 (1981).
625. J. W. Bruning, M. J. Kardol, and R. Arentzen, *J. Immunol. Methods*, **33**, 33 (1980).
626. J. S. Thompson, V. Overlin, C. D. Severson, T. J. Parsons, J. Herbick, R. G. Strauss, C. P. Burns, and F. H. J. Claas, *Transplant Proc.*, **12**, 26 (1980).
627. M. A. Kolber, R. R. Quinones, R. E. Gress, and P. A. Henkart, *J. Immunol. Methods*, **108**, 255 (1988).
628. U. Glagasigij, Y. Sato, and Y. Suzuki, *Chem. Pharm. Bull.*, **36**, 1086 (1988).
629. P. B. Garland and C. H. Moore, *Biochem. J.*, **183**, 561 (1979).
630. C. S. Chadwick, M. G. McEntergart, and R. C. Nairn, *Lancet*, **1**, 412 (1958).
631. P. Brandtzaeg, *Scand. J. Immunol.*, **2**, 273 (1973).
632. P. Brandtzaeg, *Scand. J. Immunol.*, **2**, 333 (1973).
633. M. J. Arnost, F. A. Meneghini, and P. S. Palumbo, Eur. Patent Appl. 0.285.179 (1988).
634. J. G. J. Bauman, J. Wiegant, P. Borst, and P. Van Duijn, *Exp. Cell. Res.*, **128**, 485 (1980).
635. D. Kramer, H. Klapper, and F. Miller, *Spectrosc. Lett.*, **3**, 23 (1968).
636. L. Mansbach, M. Becker, M. Gallagher, and S. Pearlman, *Clin. Chem.*, **31**, 930 (1985).
637. J. A. Titus, R. Haugland, S. O. Sharrow, and D. M. Segal, *J. Immunol. Methods*, **50**, 193 (1982).
638. L. E. Morrison, T. C. Halder, and L. M. Stols, *Anal. Biochem.*, **183**, 231 (1989).
639. Y. R. Tahboud and L. B. McGown, *Anal. Chim. Acta*, **182**, 185 (1986).
640. J. I. Braithwaite and J. N. Miller, *Anal. Chim. Acta*, **106**, 395 (1979).
641. R. Rezaei-Poor Kardost and E. W. Voss, *Mol. Immunol.*, **19**, 159 (1982).
642. R. Rezaei-Poor Kardost, P. A. Billing, and E. W. Voss, *Mol. Immunol.*, **19**, 963 (1982).
643. F. V. Bright, T. Betts, and K. S. Litwiler, *Anal. Chem.*, **62**, 1065 (1990).
644. J. S. O'Neal and S. G. Schulman, *Anal. Chim. Acta*, **170**, 143 (1985).
645. L. R. Yarbrough, J. G. Schlageck, and M. Baughman, *J. Biol. Chem.*, **254**, 12069 (1979).
646. M. Smolarsky, D. Teitelbaum, M. Sela, and C. Gitler, *J. Immunol. Methods*, **15**, 255 (1977).
647. R. E. Smith and R. MacQuarrie, *Anal. Biochem.*, **90**, 246 (1978).
648. J. C. Hummelen, T. M. Luider, and H. Wynberg, "Thermochemiluminescence Immunoassay," in W. P. Collins, Ed., *Complementary Immunoassay*, Wiley, Chichester, UK, 1988.

649. L. E. Morrison, US Patent No. 4,822,733 (1989).

650. L. E. Morrison, *Anal. Biochem.,* **174,** 101 (1988).

651. L. E. Morrison, T. C. Halder, and L. M. Stols, *Abstract of Papers Presented at the IIIrd International Symposium on Quantitative Luminescence Spectrometry in Biomedical Sciences,* Ghent, Belgium, May 1989.

652. R. P. Liburdy, US Patent No. 4,207,075 (1980).

653. R. P. Liburdy, *J. Immunol. Methods,* **28,** 233 (1979).

654. M. Aizawa, M. Tanaka, Y. Ikariyama, and H. Shinohara, *J. Biolumin. Chemilumin.,* **4,** 535 (1989).

655. Y. Ikariyama, H. Kunoh, and M. Aizawa, *Biochem. Biophys. Res. Commun.,* **128,** 987 (1985).

656. B. J. Tromberg, M. J. Sepaniak, J. P. Alarie, T. Vo-Dinh, and R. M. Santella, *Anal. Chem.,* **60,** 1901 (1988).

657. E. Koller, *Appl. Fluor. Technol.,* **1,** 13 (1989).

658. J. G. Molotkovsky and L. D. Bergelson, *Bioorg. Khimii,* **8,** 1256 (1982).

659. D. S. Wolfbeis, E. Koller, and P. Hoghmuth, *Bull. Chem. Soc. Japan,* **58,** 731 (1985).

660. G. S. Beddard, *J. Chem. Soc. Perkin Trans.,* **2,** 262 (1977).

661. R. H. Goodwin and F. Kavanagh, *Arch. Biochem.,* **36,** 442 (1951).

662. G. Fauler and E. Koller, *Abstract of Papers Presented at the IIIrd International Symposium on Quantitative Luminescence Spectrometry in Biomedical Sciences,* Ghent, Belgium, May 1989.

663. H. Khalfan, R. Abuknesha, M. Rand-Weaver, R. G. Price, and D. Robinson, *Histochem. J.,* **18,** 417 (1986).

664. J.-P. Aubry, I. Durand, P. De Paoli, and J. Banchereau, *J. Immunol. Methods,* **128,** 39 (1990).

665. W. A. Staines, B. Meister, T. Melander, J. I. Nagy, and T. Hökfelt, *J. Histochem. Cytochem.,* **36,** 145 (1988).

666. G. Fauler, *Appl. Fluor. Technol.,* **1,** 14 (1989).

667. D. Exley, *Pure Appl. Chem.,* **52,** 33 (1979).

668. G. I. Ekeke and D. Exley, "The Assay of Steroids by Fluoroimmunoassay," in S. B. Pal, Ed., *Enzyme Labelled Immunoassay of Hormones and Drugs,* Walter De Gruyter & Co., Berlin, 1978.

669. D. Exley and G. I. Ekeke, *J. Steroid. Biochem.,* **14,** 1297 (1981).

670. G. I. Ekeke, D. Exley, and R. Abuknesha, *J. Steroid. Biochem.,* **11,** 1597 (1979).

671. H. B. Chuang, *Diss. Abstract Int.,* **47,** 1963 (1986).

672. T. M. Li, J. L. Benovic, and J. F. Burd, *Anal. Biochem.,* **118,** 102 (1981).

673. J. F. Burd, R. J. Carrico, M. C. Fetter, R. T. Buckler, R. D. Johnson, R. C. Boguslaski, and J. E. Christner, *Anal. Biochem.,* **77,** 56 (1977).

674. J. F. Burd, R. C. Wong, J. E. Feeney, R. J. Carrico, and R. C. Boguslaski, *Clin. Chem.,* **23,** 1402 (1977).

675. M. Weigele, S. De Bernardo, W. Leimgruber, R. Cleeland, and E. Grunberg, *Biochem. Biophys. Res. Commun.*, **54**, 899 (1973).

676. R. F. Chen, *Anal. Lett.*, **7**, 65 (1974).

677. U. E. Handschin and W. J. Ritschard, *Anal. Biochem.*, **71**, 143 (1976).

678. I. N. Egwu and V. Kumar, *Med. Lab. Sci.*, **34**, 149 (1977).

679. P. Cukor, M. E. Woehler, C. Persiani, and A. Fermin, *J. Immunol. Methods*, **12**, 183 (1976).

680. S. Katsh, F. W. Leaver, J. S. Reynolds, and G. F. Katsh, *J. Immunol. Methods*, **5**, 179 (1974).

681. J. N. Miller, C. S. Lim, and J. W. Bridges, *Analyst*, **105**, 91 (1980).

682. G. Handley, J. N. Miller, and J. W. Bridges, *Proc. Analyt. Div. Chem. Soc.*, **16**, 26 (1979).

683. H. Thakrar and J. N. Miller, *Anal. Proc.*, **19**, 329 (1982).

684. P. B. Ghosh and M. W. Whitehouse, *Biochem. J.*, **108**, 155 (1968).

685. K. E. Carlson, M. Coppey, H. Magdalena, and J. A. Katzenellenbogen, *J. Steroid. Biochem.*, **32**, 345 (1989).

686. M. P. Bailey, B. F. Rocks, and C. Riley, *Ann. Clin. Biochem.*, **20**, 213 (1983).

687. D. N. Kirk and B. W. Miller, *J. Chem. Soc. Perkin Trans.*, **1**, 2979 (1988).

688. B. Desfosses, P. Urios, N. Christeff, K. M. Rajkowski, and N. Cittanova, *Anal. Biochem.*, **159**, 179 (1986).

689. M. P. Bailey, B. F. Rocks, and C. Riley, *Ann. Clin. Biochem.*, **21**, 59 (1984).

690. J. J. Haaijman, *Acta Histochem.*, **Suppl. 35**, 77 (1988).

691. P. H. Rothbarth, J. G. Olthof, and N. A. J. Mul, *Ann. N.Y. Acad. Sci.*, **254**, 65 (1975).

692. C. Parini, M. A. Bacigalupo, S. Colombi, L. Ferrara, F. Franceschetti, and R. Saita, *Steroids*, **46**, 903 (1985).

693. R. F. Chen, *Arch. Biochem. Biophys.*, **172**, 39 (1976).

694. V. A. Shibnev, M. P. Finogenova, A. I. Poletaev, and L. I. Marjash, *Bioorg. Khimii*, **10**, 921 (1984).

695. T. M. Li and J. F. Burd, *Biochem. Biophys. Res. Commun.*, **103**, 1157 (1981).

696. E. Berger, J. Pease, C. C. Chang, and L. Tarnowsky, *Abstracts of Papers Presented at the IIIrd International Symposium on Quantitative Luminescence Spectrometry in Biomedical Sciences*, Ghent, Belgium, May 1989.

697. P. L. Southwick, L. A. Ernst, E. W. Tauriello, S. R. Parker, R. B. Mujumdar, S. R. Mujumdar, H. A. Clever, and A. S. Waggoner, *Cytometry*, **11**, 418 (1990).

698. K. Sauda, T. Imasaka, and N. Ishibashi, *Anal. Chem.*, **58**, 2649 (1988).

699. J. E. Falk, *Porphyrins and Metalloporphyrins*, Elsevier Science Publishing Co., Amsterdam, 1964.

700. O. S. Wolfbeis, "Fluorescence of Organic Natural Products," in S. G. Schulman, Ed., *Molecular Luminescence Spectroscopy*, Wiley, New York, 1985.

701. D. Eastwood and M. Gouterman, *J. Mol. Spectrosc.*, **35**, 359 (1970).

702. T. J. Green, D. F. Wilson, J. M. Vanderkooi, and S. P. Defeo, *Anal. Biochem.*, **174**, 73 (1988).

703. D. D. Schmidt and H. Steffen, Eur. Patent No. 0 127,797, (1987).

704. P. J. Sims, A. S. Waggoner, C.-H. Wang, and J. F. Hoffman, *Biochemistry*, **13**, 3315 (1974).

705. J. L. Hendrix, Eur. Patent Appl. 0 071,991 (1983), and US Patent No. 4,707,454 (1987).

706. A. P. Savitsky, D. P. Papkovsky, I. V. Berezin, N. N. Ugarova, and G. V. Ponomarev, USSR Patent No. 1,313,172 (1988), *Chem. Abstract*, **109**, 34897G.

707. A. Waggoner, *Cytometry, Suppl. 4*, **4** (abs. 2) (1990).

708. D. Schindele, G. E. Renzoni, K. L. Fearon, M. W. Vandivor, R. J. Ekdahl, and B. V. Pepich, *Cytometry, Suppl. 4*, **4** (abs. 3) (1990).

709. P. S. Forgione and W. A. Henderson, UK Patent Appl. 2,063,469 (1981), US Patent No. 4,375,972 (1983).

710. D. J. Recktenwald, US Patent No. 4,876,190 (1989).

711. J. L. Hendrix, *Clin. Chem.*, **29**, 1003 (1983).

712. D. B. Papkovsky, A. P. Savitsky, N. N. Ugarova, I. V. Berezin, and G. V. Ponomarev, *Prikl. Biokihim. Mikrobiol.*, **25**, 548 (1989) (Russ.).

713. A. P. Savitsky, D. B. Papkovsky, and I. V. Berezin, *Dokl. Akad. Nauk. SSSR*, **293**, 744 (1987).

714. V. T. Ivanova, O. A. Stafayeva, A. P. Savitsky, and M. A. Yachno, *Voprosy Virologii*, **3**, 362 (1988).

715. D. P. Papkovsky, A. P. Savitsky, and V. Ya. Byhovsky, *Probl. Endokrinol.*, **34**, 58 (1988) (Russ.).

716. S. M. Krylova, O. A. Stafeva, A. P. Savitsky, M. M. Dikov, and G. A. Yermolin, *Vopr. Med. Khimii SSSR*, **36**, 47 (1990) (Russ.).

717. A. P. Savitsky, D. P. Papkovsky, and G. V. Ponomarev, *Dokl. Acad. Nauk. SSSR*, **304**, 1005 (1989).

718. D. Mew, C.-K. Wat, G. H. N. Towers, and J. G. Levy, *J. Immunol.*, **130**, 1473 (1983).

719. A. P. Savitsky, K. Lopatin, T. V. Cherednikova, E. A. Lukyanets, M. G. Galpern, and V. L. Solovyeva, *Abstracts of Papers Presented at the International Conference of Photodynamic Therapy*, (abs. 117) Sofia, Bulgaria, 1989.

720. A. N. Glazer and L. Stryer, *Trends Biochem. Sci.*, **9**, 423 (1984).

721. A. N. Glazer, *Ann. Rev. Biophys. Chem.*, **14**, 47 (1985).

722. V. T. Oi, A. N. Glazer, and L. Stryer, *J. Cell. Biol.*, **93**, 981 (1982).

723. M. N. Kronick, *J. Immunol. Methods*, **92**, 1 (1986).

724. M. N. Kronick, "Phycobiliproteins as Labels in Immunoassay," in T. T. Ngo, Ed., *Non-isotopic Immunoassay*, Plenum Press, New York, 1988.

725. L. Stryer, A. N. Glazer, and V. T. Oi, US Patent No. 4,520,110 (1985).

726. J. Grabowski and E. Gantt, *Photochem. Photobiol.*, **28**, 39 (1978).

727. A. N. Glazer and L. Stryer, *Biophys. J.,* **43,** 383 (1983).

728. J. C. White and L. Stryer, *Anal. Biochem.,* **161,** 442 (1987).

729. S. Walsh Yeh, L. J. Ong, J. H. Clark, and A. N. Glazer, *Cytochemistry,* **8,** 91 (1987).

730. M. N. Kronick and P. D. Grossman, *Clin. Chem.,* **29,** 1582 (1983).

731. H. M. Shapiro, A. N. Glazer, L. Christenson, J. M. Williams, and T. B. Strom, *Cytometry,* **4,** 276 (1983).

732. R. R. Hardy, K. Hayakawa, D. R. Parks, and L. A. Herzenberg, *J. Exp. Med.,* **159,** 1169 (1984).

733. P. Khanna, *Abstract of Papers Presented at the Conference of Phycobiliproteins in Biology and Medicine,* Seattle, WA, 1985.

734. B. Francis, D. W. Buck, L. L. Lanier, M. F. LaFoe, D. R. Bethell, and M. E. Jolley, *Abstract of Papers Presented at the Conference of Phycobiliproteins in Biology and Medicine,* Seattle, WA, 1985.

735. W. E. Woods, C.-J. Wang, P. K. Houtz, H.-H. Tai, T. Wood, T. J. Weckman, J.-M. Yang, S.-L. Chang, J. W. Blake, T. Tobin, J. McDonald, S. Kalita, V. D. Bass, P. Weege, B. DeLeon, C. Brockus, S. Wie, R. A. Chung, J. Brecht, J. Conner, P. Dahl, E. Lewis, C. A. Prange, F. J. Ozog, and M. T. Green, *Res. Commun. Chem. Pathol. & Pharmacology,* **61,** 111 (1988).

736. C. A. Prange, S. Wie, C. L. Brockus, P. A. Dahl, E. L. Lewis, J. M. Brecht, J. C. Connor, R. A. Chung, J. McDonald, V. D. Bass, S. Merchant, S. Kwiatkowski, W. E. Woods, D. S. Watt, H.-H. Tai, J. W. Blake, S.-L. Chang, and T. Tobin, *Res. Commun. Subst. Abuse,* **9,** 129 (1988).

737. T. Lindmo, O. Børmer, J. Ugelstad, and K. Nustad, *J. Immunol. Methods,* **126,** 183 (1990).

738. C. F. Meares and T. G. Wensel, *Accts. Chem. Res.,* **17,** 202 (1984).

739. C. J. Beinlich, J. A. Piper, J. C. O'Neal, and O. D. White, *Clin. Chem.,* **31,** 2014 (1985).

740. R. W. Kozak, R. A. Atcher, O. A. Gansow, A. M. Friedman, J. J. Hines, and T. A. Waldmann, *Proc. Natl. Acad. Sci. USA,* **83,** 474 (1986).

741. L. H. DeRiemer and C. F. Meares, *J. Med. Chem.,* **22,** 1019 (1979).

742. D. J. Hnatowich, W. W. Layne, R. L. Childs, D. Lanteigne, and M. A. Davis, *Science,* **220,** 613 (1983).

743. M. W. Brechbiel, O. A. Gansow, R. A. Atcher, J. Schlom, J. Esteban, D. E. Simpson, and D. Colcher, *Inorg. Chem.,* **25,** 2772 (1986).

744. M. W. Sundberg, C. F. Meares, D. A. Goodwin, and C. I. Diamanti, *J. Med. Chem.,* **17,** 1304 (1974).

745. R. B. Lauffer, T. J. Brady, R. D. Brown, C. Baglin, and S. H. Koenig, *Magn. Reson. Med.,* **3,** 541 (1986).

746. E. C. Unger, W. G. Totty, D. M. Neufeld, F. L. Otsuka, W. A. Murphy, M. S. Welsh, J. M. Connet, and G. W. Philpott, *Invest. Radiol.,* **20,** 693 (1985).

747. Y. Manabe, C. Longley, and P. Furmanski, *Biochim. Biophys. Acta,* **883,** 460 (1986).

748. A. D. Sherry, W. P. Cacheris, and K.-T. Kuan, *Magn. Reson. Med.,* **8,** 180 (1988).

749. M. J. Doyle, H. B. Halsall, and W. R. Heineman, *Anal. Chem.,* **54,** 2318 (1982).

750. P. Brossier, *Bull. Trav. Soc. Pharm. Lyon,* **28,** 33 (1984).

751. M. Cais, US Patent No. 4,205,952 (1980).

752. H. G. Brittain, "Bioinorganic Luminescence Spectroscopy," in S. G. Schulman, Ed., *Molecular Luminescence Spectroscopy,* Wiley, New York, 1985.

753. R. S. Davidson and S. D. Votier, PCT Patent No. WO 87/04,523 (1987).

754. M. K. Moi, C. F. Meares, M. J. McCall, W. C. Cole, and S. J. Denardo, *Anal. Biochem.,* **148,** 249 (1985).

755. G. A. Crosby, E. R. Whan, and M. R. Alire, *J. Chem. Phys.,* **34,** 743 (1961).

756. W. DeW. Horrocks, Jr., and M. Albin, *Prog. Inorg. Chem.,* **31,** 1 (1984).

757. R. E. Whan and G. A. Crosby, *J. Mol. Spectrosc.,* **8,** 315 (1962).

758. G. A. Crosby and A. R. Peacock, *Biopolymers,* **6,** 1225 (1968).

759. N. Filipescu, G. Mushrush, C. Hurt, and N. McAvoy, *Nature,* **211,** 960 (1966).

760. C. C. Bryden and C. N. Reilley, *Anal. Chem.,* **54,** 610 (1987).

761. W. DeW. Horrocks, Jr., and D. R. Sudnick, *J. Amer. Chem. Soc.,* **101,** 334 (1979).

762. J.-C. G. Bünzli and G. R. Choppin, *Lanthanide Probes in Life, Chemical and Earth Sciences, Theory and Practice,* Elsevier Science Publisher, Amsterdam, 1989.

763. C. H. Evans, *Trends Biochem. Sci.,* **8,** 445 (1983).

764. J. Reuben, "Bioinorganic Chemistry: Lanthanides as Probes in Systems of Biological Interest," in K. A. Gschneider, Jr., and L. Eyring, Eds., *Handbook on the Physics and Chemistry of Rare Earths,* North Holland Publishing Co., Amsterdam, 1979.

765. P. B. O'Hara, *Photochem. Photobiol.,* **46,** 1067 (1987).

766. F. S. Richardson, *Chem. Rev.,* **82,** 541 (1982).

767. J. M. Wolfson and D. R. Kearns, *Biochemistry,* **14,** 1436 (1975).

768. T. D. Barela, S. Burchett, and D. E. Kizer, *Biochemistry,* **14,** 4887 (1975).

769. G. Yonuschot and G. W. Mushrush, *Biochemistry,* **14,** 1677 (1975).

770. W. DeW. Horrocks, Jr., and D. R. Sudnick, *Science,* **206,** 1194 (1979).

771. C. K. Luk, *Biochemistry,* **10,** 2838 (1971).

772. W. DeW. Horrocks, Jr., and J. M. Tingey, *Biochemistry,* **27,** 413 (1988).

773. P. Gangola and A. E. Shamoo, *Eur. J. Biochem.,* **162,** 357 (1987).

774. D. Axelrod and M. P. Klein, *Biochem. Biophys. Res. Commun.,* **57,** 927 (1974).

775. R. B. Mikkelsen and D. F. H. Wallach, *Biochim. Biophys. Acta,* **363,** 211 (1974).

776. N.-E. L. Saris, *Chem. Phys. Lipids,* **34,** 1 (1983).

777. J. Wilschut, N. Düzgünes, R. Fraley, and D. Papahadjopoulos, *Biochemistry,* **19,** 6011 (1980).

778. J. N. Miller and C. Thirkettle, *Biochem. Medicine,* **13,** 98 (1975).

779. I. Romslo, *Clin. Chim. Acta,* **75,** 171 (1977).

780. L. M. Hirschy, E. V. Dose, and J. D. Winefordner, *Anal. Chim. Acta,* **147,** 311 (1983).

781. L. A. Files, L. Hirschy, and J. D. Winefordner, *J. Pharmaceut. Biomed. Analysis,* **3,** 95 (1985).

782. T. J. Wenzel, L. M. Collette, D. T. Dahlen, S. M. Hendrickson, and L. W. Yarmaloff, *J. Chromatogr. Biomed. Appl.,* **433,** 149 (1988).

783. P. R. Haddad, *Talanta,* **24,** 1 (1977).

784. C. C. Hinckley, *J. Amer. Chem. Soc.,* **91,** 5160 (1969).

785. A. P. B. Sinha, "Fluorescence and Laser Action in Rare Earth Chelates," in C. N. R. Rao and J. R. Ferrano, Eds., *Spectroscopy in Inorganic Chemistry,* Academic Press, London, 1971.

786. R. B. Green, *Amer. Lab.,* **3,** 47 (1971).

787. R. M. Dagnall, R. Smith, and T. S. West, *Analyst,* **92,** 358 (1967).

788. N. S. Poluektov, L. A. Alakaeva, and M. A. Tischenko, *Zh. Anal. Khimii,* **28,** 1621 (1973).

789. T. D. Barela and A. D. Sherry, *Anal. Biochem.,* **71,** 351 (1976).

790. S. J. Lyle and N. A. Za'tar, *Anal. Chim. Acta,* **162,** 305 (1984).

791. M. A. Tishchenko, G. I. Gerasimenko, and N.S. Poluektov, *Zavod. Lab.,* **40,** 935 (1974).

792. N. S. Poluektov, L. A. Alakaeva, and M. A. Tishchenko, *Zavod. Lab.,* **37,** 1077 (1971).

793. A. Lempicki and H. Samelson, *Phys. Lett.,* **4,** 133 (1963).

794. J. L. Reid and M. Calvin, *J. Amer. Chem. Soc.,* **72,** 2948 (1950).

795. R. Belcher, R. Perry, and W. I. Stephen, *Analyst,* **94,** 26 (1969).

796. T. Taketatsu and A. Sato, *Anal. Chim. Acta,* **108,** 429 (1979).

797. T. Shigematsu, M. Matsui, and R. Wake, *Anal. Chim. Acta,* **46,** 101 (1969).

798. W. L. Scaff, Jr., D. L. Dyer, and K. Mori, *J. Bacteriol.,* **98,** 246 (1969).

799. J. R. Anderson and D. Westmoreland, *Soil. Biol. Biochem.,* **3,** 85 (1971).

800. J. R. Anderson and J. M. Slinger, *Soil. Biol. Biochem.,* **7,** 205 (1975).

801. B. G. Johnen and E. A. Drew, *Soil. Biol. Biochem.,* **10,** 487 (1978).

802. B. G. Johnen, *Soil. Biol. Biochem.,* **10,** 495 (1978).

803. T. Taketatsu, *Talanta,* **29,** 397 (1982).

804. R. P. Fisher and J. D. Winefordner, *Anal. Chem.,* **43,** 454 (1971).

805. F. Halverson, J. S. Brinen, and J. R. Leto, *J. Chem. Phys.,* **41,** 157 (1964).

806. T. Kareseva and V. E. Karesev, *Koord. Khimii,* **1,** 926 (1975).

807. H. G. Brittain, *Inorg. Chem.,* **19,** 640 (1980).

808. I. Hemmilä, S. Dakubu, V.-M. Mukkala, H. Siitari, and T. Lövgren, *Anal. Biochem.,* **137,** 335 (1984).

809. R. C. Leif, S. P. Clay, H. G. Gratzner, H. G. Haines, L. M. Vallarino, and I. Wieder, "Markers for Instrumental Evaluation of Cells of the Female Reproductive Tract: Existing and New Markers," in G. L. Wied, G. F. Bahr, and P. H. Bartels, Eds., *Proc. Int. Conf. Automation of Uterine Cancer Cytology,* Tutorials of Cytology, Chicago, 1967.

810. R. C. Leif, R. A. Thomas, T. A. Yopp, B. D. Watson, V. R. Guarino, D. H. K. Hindman, N. Lefkovc, and M. Vallarino, *Clin. Chem.,* **23,** 1492 (1977).

811. L. M. Vallarino, B. D. Watson, D. H. K. Hindman, V. Jagodil, and R. C. Leif, "Quantum Dyes: A New Tool for Cytology Automation," in N. J. Pressman and G. L. Wied, Eds., *Proc. 2nd Int. Conf. Automation of Cancer Cytology and Cell Image Analysis,* Tutorials of Cytology, Chicago, 1979.

812. I. Wieder and K. O. Hidgson, Germ. Patent No. 2,628,158 (1977).

813. A.-T. Hansson and J. Carlsson, Swedish Patent Appl. 8602840-4 (1986).

814. A. G. Goryushko, N. K. Davidenko, L. S. Kudryavtseva, M. O. Lozinskii, L. N. Lugina, and Y. A. Fialkov, *Russ. J. Inorg. Chem.,* **25,** 1327 (1980).

815. A. G. Goryushko and N. K. Davidenko, *Russ. J. Inorg. Chem.,* **25,** 1470 (1980).

816. E. Soini and I. Hemmilä, US Patent No. 4,374,120 (1983).

817. E. Soini, I. Hemmilä, and T. Lövgren, Eur. Patent Appl. 103,558 (1984).

818. I. Wieder and R. H. Wollenberg, Germ. Patent No. 3,033,691 (1981), US Patent No. 4,352,751 (1982).

819. I. Wieder and R. L. Hale, PCT Patent Appl. WO 87/07,955 (1987).

820. I. E. Svetlova, N. A. Dobrynina, N. S. Smirnova, L. I. Martynenko, A. M. Yevseyef, and A. P. Savitsky, *Zh. Neorg. Khimii,* **34,** 52 (1989).

821. I. Hemmilä and S. Dakubu, US Patent No. 4,565,790 (1986).

822. I. Hemmilä and M. Latva, *Clin. Immunoassay,* **13,** 58 (abs. 31) (1990).

823. R. Bador, H. Déchaud, F. Claustrat, and C. Desuzinges, *Clin. Chem.,* **33,** 48 (1987).

824. I. Hemmilä and E. Markela, *Clin. Chem.,* **36,** 1094 (abs. 664) (1990).

825. M. Saarma, L. Järvekülg, I. Hemmilä, H. Siitari, and R. Sinijärv, *J. Virol. Methods,* **23,** 47 (1989).

826. I. A. Hemmilä, *ISI Atlas of Sci. Immunology,* **1,** 231 (1988).

827. I. Hemmilä, S. Holttinen, K. Pettersson, and T. Lövgren, *Clin. Chem.,* **33,** 2281 (1987).

828. H. Siitari, *J. Virol. Methods,* **28,** 179 (1990).

829. J. A. Keelan, J. T. France, and P. M. Barling, *Clin. Chem.,* **33,** 2292 (1987).

830. P. Degan, G. Montagnoli, and C. P. Wild, *Clin. Chem.,* **35,** 2308 (1989).

831. R. P. Ekins and S. Dakubu, PCT Int. Patent Appl. 88/02,489 (1988).

832. S. Dakubu, R. Hale, A. Lu, J. Quick, D. Solas, and J. Weinberg, *Clin. Chem.,* **34,** 2337 (1988).

833. Y. Xu, Y. Wang, and X. Liu, *CA,* **109,** 33434 (1988).

834. J.-H. Yang, G.-Y. Zhu, and H. Wang, *Analyst,* **114,** 1417 (1989).

835. Y.-X. Ci and Z.-H. Lan, *Anal. Chem.,* **61,** 1063 (1989).

836. G. E. Krejcarek and K. L. Tucker, *Biochem. Biophys. Res. Commun.,* **77,** 581 (1977).

837. C. H. Paik, M. A. Ebbert, P. R. Murphy, C. R. Lassman, R. C. Reba, W. C. Eckelman, K. Y. Pak, J. Powe, Z. Steplenski, and H. Koprowski, *J. Nucl. Med.,* **24,** 1158 (1983).

838. K. Pettersson, H. Siitari, I. Hemmilä, E. Soini, T. Lövgren, V. Hänninen, P. Tanner, and U.-H. Stenman, *Clin. Chem.,* **29,** 60 (1983).

839. V.-M. Mukkala, H. Mikola, and I. Hemmilä, *Anal. Biochem.,* **176,** 319 (1989).

840. H. Mikola, V.-M. Mukkala, and I. Hemmilä, Eur. Patent No. 139,675 (1987) and US Patent No. 4,808,541 (1989).

841. I. Hemmilä, E. Markela, H. Mikola, and T. Stahlberg, *Abstracts of Papers Presented at the Sixth International Congress on Rapid Methods and Automation in Microbiology and Immunology,* No. 146, Helsinki, Espoo, Finland, June 1990.

842. K. Blomberg, C. Granberg, I. Hemmilä, and T. Lövgren, *J. Immunol. Methods,* **86,** 225 (1986).

843. M. Kwiatkowski, C. Sund, J. Ylikoski, V.-M. Mukkala, and I. Hemmilä, Eur. Patent Appl. 298,939 (1989).

845. C. Sund, J. Ylikoski, P. Hurskainen, and M. Kwiatkowski, *Nucleosides & Nucleotides,* **7,** 655 (1988).

846. A. Oser, W. K. Roth, and G. Valet, *Nucl. Acids Res.,* **16,** 1181 (1988).

847. D. Engelhardt, E. Rabbani, S. Kline, J. G. Stavrianopoulos, and D. Kirtikar, Eur. Patent Appl. 285,057 (1988).

848. D. S. Frank and M. W. Sundberg, Eur. Patent Appl. 2,963 (1979).

849. D. S. Frank and M. W. Sundberg, US Patent No. 4,283,382 (1981).

850. B. A. Burdick and S. J. Danielson, Eur. Patent Appl. 195,624 (1986).

851. J. R. Schaeffer, B. J. Chen, and M. A. Schen, Eur. Patent Appl. 195,623 (1986).

852. M. Hayashi, K. Makiguchi, and Y. Nomura, Jpn. Patent No. 61,258,172 (CA 106; 172480e) (1986).

853. D. B. Wagner and R. A. Baffi, Eur. Patent App. 191,575 (1986).

854. D. B. Wagner and R. A. Baffi, US Patent No. 4,698,263 (1987).

855. D. B. Wagner and R. A. Baffi, US Patent No. 4,707,453 (1987).

856. T. J. Mercolino, G. P. Vonk, D. B. Wagner, "Fluorescent Immunoassay Using Liposomes that Incorporate a Water-Insoluble Europium Chelate," in *Proceedings of the 7th Int. Congress on Immunology,* Berlin, July 1989. Abs. 121–41, G. Fisher Verlag, Stuttgart, 1989.

857. N. J. Wilmott, J. N. Miller, and J. F. Tyson, *Analyst,* **109,** 343 (1984).

858. R. A. Evangelista and A. Pollak, Eur. Patent Appl. 171,978 (1986).

859. R. A. Evangelista and A. Pollak, US Patent No. 4,772,563 (1988).

860. R. A. Evangelista, A. Pollak, B. Allore, E. F. Templeton, R. C. Morton, and E. P. Diamandis, *Clin. Biochem.,* **21,** 173 (1988).

861. E. P. Diamandis and A. J. Lowden, Eur. Patent Appl. 290,269 (1988).

862. E. P. Diamandis and R. C. Morton, *J. Immunol. Methods,* **112,** 43 (1988).

863. A. D. Elster, S. C. Jackels, N. S. Allen, and R. C. Marrache, *Am. J. Neuroradiol.,* **10,** 1137 (1989).

864. K. H. Milby and R. N. Zare, *Int. Clin. Products,* **10,** 10 (1984).

865. J. E. Kuo, K. H. Milby, W. D. Hinsberg III, P. R. Poole, V. L. McGuffin, and R. N. Zare, *Clin. Chem.,* **31,** 50 (1985).

866. M. P. Bailey, B. F. Rocks, and C. Riley, *Analyst,* **109,** 1449 (1984).

867. M. P. Bailey, B. F. Rocks, and C. Riley, *Analyst,* **110,** 603 (1985).

868. S. S. Saavedra and E. G. Picozza, *Analyst,* **114,** 835 (1989).

869. J. Siepak, *Analyst,* **114,** 529 (1989).

870. A. Canfi, M. P. Bailey, and B. F. Rocks, *Analyst,* **114,** 1407 (1989)

871. A. Canfi, M. P. Bailey, and B. F. Rocks, *Analyst,* **114,** 1405 (1989).

872. E. G. Picozza and S. S. Saavedra, Eur. Patent Appl. 340,675 (1989).

873. J. C. Hinshaw, J. L. Toner, and G. A. Reynolds, Eur. Patent Appl. 68,875 (1983).

874. J. L. Toner, Eur. Patent Appl. 288,256 (1988).

875. J. L. Toner, US Patent No. 4,837,169 (1989).

876. R. L. Hale and D. W. Solas, Eur. Patent Appl. 195,413 (1986).

877. J. Kankare, H. Takalo, and P. Pasanen, Eur. Patent Appl. 203,047 (1986).

878. M. Kwiatkowski, V.-M. Mukkala, M. Helenius, J. Ylikoski, and P. Dahlén, *Abstract of Papers Presented at the Sixth International Congress on Rapid Methods and Automation in Microbiology and Immunology,* No. 293, Espoo, Finland, June 1990.

879. E. J. Soini, L. J. Pelliniemi, I. A. Hemmilä, V.-M. Mukkala, J. J. Kankare, and K. Fröjdman, *J. Histochem. Cytochem.,* **36,** 1449 (1988).

880. I. Hemmilä and A. Båtsman, *Clin. Chem.,* **34,** 1163 (abs. 054) (1988).

881. I. Hemmilä, O. Malminen, H. Mikola, and T. Lövgren, *Clin. Chem.,* **34,** 2320 (1988).

882. G. Barnard, F. Kohen, H. Mikola, and T. Lövgren, *J. Biolum. Chemilum.,* **4,** 177 (1989).

883. J.-M. Lehn, *Pure & Appl. Chem.,* **49,** 857 (1977).

884. N. Sabbatini, S. Dellonte, M. Ciano, A. Bonazzi, and V. Balzani, *Chem. Phys. Lett.,* **107,** 212 (1984).

885. B. Alpha, J.-M. Lehn, and G. Mathis, *Angew. Chem.,* **99,** 259 (1987).

886. B. Alpha, V. Balzani, J.-M. Lehn, S. Perathoner, and N. Sabbatini, *Angew. Chem. Int. Ed. Engl.,* **26,** 1266 (1987).

887. G. Blasse, G. J. Dirksen, D. Van Der Voort, N. Sabbatini, S. Perathoner, J.-M. Lehn, and B. Alpha, *Chem. Phys. Lett.,* **146,** 347 (1988).

888. G. Mathis and J.-M. Lehn, French Patent No. 2,570,703 (1986).

889. J.-M. Lehn, G. Mathis, B. Alpha, R. Deschenaux, and E. Jolu, Eur. Patent Appl. 321,353 (1988).

890. G. Mathis, M. Amoravain, A. Dedieu, F. Socquet-Clerc, E. J. P. Jolu, R. Deschenaux, and J.-M. Lehn, *Abstract of Papers Presented at the IIIrd International Symposium on Quantitative Luminescence Spectrometry in Biomedical Sciences,* Ghent, Belgium, May 1989.

891. G. Valet and A. Oser, *Cytometry,* **Suppl. 2,** 23 (abs. 116) (1990).

892. N. Sabbatini, M. Guardigli, V. Balzani, E. Ghidini, A. Pochini, and R. Ungaro, *Abstract of Papers Presented at the Interdisciplinary Meeting on Luminescence Fundamentals and Applications,* No. 41, Bologna, Italy, May 1989.

893. L. M. Vallarino, *J. Less-Common Metals,* **149,** 121 (1989).

894. F. Müller, and D. Schmidt, Eur. Patent No. 178,450 (1986).

895. W. Bannwarth, D. Schmidt, R. L. Stallard, C. Hornung, R. Knorr, and F. Müller, *Helv. Chim. Acta,* **71,** 2085 (1988).

896. W. Bannwarth and D. Schmidt, *Tetrahedr. Lett.,* **30,** 1513 (1989).

897. W. Bannwarth, D. Schmidt, R. L. Stallard, C. Hornung, R. Knorr, and F. Müller, *Abstracts of Papers Presented at the Sixth International Congress on Rapid Methods and Automation in Microbiology and Immunology,* No. 285, Espoo, Finland, July 1990.

898. R. B. Thompson and L. M. Vallarino, *Proc. SPIE-Int. Soc. Opt. Eng.,* **909,** 426 (1988).

899. L. DeCola, F. Barigelletti, V. Balzani, P. Belser, A. von Zelewsky, F. Vögte, F. Ebmeyer, and S. Grammenudi, *J. Amer. Chem. Soc.,* **110,** 7210 (1988).

900. S. G. Weber, US Patent No. 4,293,310 (1981).

901. A. J. Bard and G. M. Whitesides, PCT Int. Patent Appl. WO 86/02,734 (1986).

902. R. J. Massey, M. J. Powell, P. A. Mied, P. Feng, and L. Della Ciana, PCT Int. Patent Appl. WO 87/06,706 (1987).

903. P. Del Castillo, A. R. Llorente, A. Gómez, J. Gosálvez, V. J. Goyanes, and J. C. Stockert, *Anal. Quant. Cytol. Histol.,* **12,** 11 (1990).

904. T. Hirschfeld, *Appl. Optics,* **15,** 3135 (1976).

905. S. M. Krylova, I. Y. Sakharov, M. A. Slinkin, A. P. Savitsky, A. L. Klibanov, V. P. Torchilin, and I. V. Berezin, *Vopr. Med. Khimii,* **34,** 116 (1988).

906. K. Guy, D. N. Crichton, and J. A. Ross, *J. Immunol. Methods,* **112,** 261 (1988).

907. H. Schmitz and D. Kampa, *J. Immunol. Methods,* **26,** 173 (1979).

908. T. Lövgren, *J. Steroid. Biochem.,* **27,** 47 (1987).

909. R. R. Gonzales, O. Mäentausta, J. Solyom, and R. Vihko, *Clin. Chem.,* **36,** 1667 (1990).

910. F. J. Lücke and W. Schlegel, *Fresenius J. Anal. Chem.,* **337,** 97 (1990).

911. S. Rasi, E. Suvanto, L. M. Vilpo, and J. A. Vilpo, *J. Immunol. Methods,* **117,** 33 (1989).

912. A.-C. Höglund, K. Blomberg, H. Mikola, and T. Lövgren, "Direct Measurement of T4 in Blood Spots Using a Time-Resolved Fluoroimmunoassay: Comparison of Different Tracers," in B. J. Schmidt, A. J. Diament, and N. S. Loghin-Grosso, Eds., *Current Trends in Infant Screening: Proceedings of the 7th International Screening Symposium,* Elsevier Science Publisher BV, Amsterdam, 1989.

913. A. R. M. Azad, S. J. Kirchanski, and M. C. Brown, Eur. Patent Appl. 77,671 (1983).

914. D. F. Ranney, PCT. Int. Patent Appl. WO 87/02,893 (1987).

915. S. C. Wang, M. G. Wickström, D. L. White, J. Klaveness, E. Holtz, P. Rongved, M. E. Moseley, and R. Brasch, *Radiology,* **175,** 483 (1990).

916. K. Blomberg, H. Mikola, and T. Lövgren, "Optimization of a Time-Resolved Fluorometric Assay for 17-α-OH-progesterone in Blood Spots Using Multiple Labeled 17-OHP as Tracer," in B. J. Schmidt, A. J. Diament, and N. S. Loghin-Grosso, Eds., *Current Trends in Infant Screening: Proceedings of the 7th International Screening Symposium,* Elsevier Science Publisher BV, Amsterdam, 1989.

917. J. Ylikoski, P. Hurskainen, P. Dahlén, C. Sund, T. Lövgren, and M. Kwiatkowski, PCT. Int. Patent Appl. WO 88/02,784 (1988).

918. P. Mar, K. Pachmann, K. Reinecke, B. Emmerich, and E. Thiel, *Blood,* **74,** 638 (1989).

919. R. C. Morton and E. P. Diamandis, *Anal. Chem.,* **62,** 1841 (1990).

920. T. K. Christopoulos, E. S. Lianidou, and E. P. Diamandis, *Clin. Chem.,* **36,** 1094 (abs. 665) (1990).

921. J. U. Eskola, V. Näntö, and T. Lehto, *Biochimica Clinica,* **13,** Suppl. 1/8, 164 (abs. A51) (1989).

922. A. D. Baugham, M. M. Standish, and J. D. Watkins, *J. Mol. Biol.,* **13,** 238 (1965).

923. L. D. Mayer, M. J. Hope, P. R. Cullins, and A. S. Janoff, *Biochim. Biophys. Acta,* **817,** 193 (1985).

924. C. Kirby and G. Gregoriadis, *Bio/Technol.,* **2,** 979 (1984).

925. R. L. Shew and D. W. Deamer, *Biochim. Biophys. Acta,* **816,** 1 (1985).

926. T. D. Heatlh, B. A. Macher, and D. Papahadjopoulos, *Biochim. Biophys. Acta,* **640,** 66 (1981).

927. F. J. Martin and D. Papahadjopoulos, *J. Biol. Chem.,* **257,** 286 (1982).

928. K. Hashimoto, J. E. Loader, and S. C. Kinsky, *Biochim. Biophys. Acta,* **856,** 556 (1986).

929. A. L. Plant, L. Locascio-Brown, and R. A. Durst, *Abstracts of Papers Presented at the IIIrd International Symposium on Quantitative Luminescence Spectrometry in Biomedical Sciences,* No. 35, Ghent, Belgium, May 1989.

930. T. Kataoka, K. Inoue, S. Galanos, and S. C. Kinsky, *Eur. J. Biochem.,* **24,** 123 (1971).
931. S. C. Kinsky, *Biochim. Biophys. Acta,* **265,** 1 (1972).
932. S. C. Kinsky, *Methods Enzymol.,* **32,** 501 (1974).
933. A. Truneh, P. Machy, and P. K. Horan, *J. Immunol. Methods,* **100,** 59 (1987).
934. A. G. Gray, J. Morgan, D. C. Linch, and E. R. Huehns, *J. Immunol. Methods,* **121,** 1 (1989).
935. A. Truneh and P. Machy, *Cytometry,* **8,** 562 (1987).
936. J. N. Wenstein, P. Yoshikamis, R. Henkart, W. A. Blumenthal, and W. A. Hagins, *Science,* **195,** 489 (1977).
937. R. B. Thompson and B. P. Gaber, *Anal. Lett.,* **18,** 1847 (1985).
938. M. L. Elliot, M. Erali-Woodward, C. Hixson, and T. R. Witty, *Clin. Chem.,* **31,** 929 (1985).
939. B. Axelsson, H. Eriksson, C. Borrebäck, B. Mattiasson, and H. O. Sjögren, *J. Immunol. Methods,* **41,** 351 (1981).
940. A. Rembaum and W. J. Dreyer, *Science,* **208,** 364 (1980).
941. W. J. Dreyer, US Patent No. 4,108,972 (1978).
942. D. Bourel, A. Rolland, R. Le Verge, and B. Genetet, *J. Immunol. Methods,* **106,** 161 (1988).
943. T. J. Higgins, H. C. O'Neill, and C. R. Parish, *J. Immunol. Methods,* **47,** 275 (1981).
944. J. Mirro, Jr., J. F. Schwartz, and C. I. Civin, *J. Immunol. Methods,* **47,** 39 (1981).
945. J. Y. Bonnefoy, J. Banchereau, J. P. Aubry, and J. Wijdenes, *J. Immunol. Methods,* **88,** 25 (1986).
946. G. C. Saunders, J. H. Jett, and J. C. Martin, *Clin. Chem.,* **31,** 2020 (1985).
947. H. J. Tanke, J. C. Slats, and J. S. Ploem, PCT. Int. Patent Appl. WO 87/00,926 (1987).
948. H. J. Tanke, A. van Schadewijk, and S. van Gelderen, *Abstract of Papers Presented at the Meeting of New Frontiers in Cytometry,* No. 126, Sienna, Feb. 1989.
949. N. P. Verwoerd, J. Bonnet, H. B. Beverloo, and H. J. Tanke, *Cytometry,* **Suppl. 2,** 83 (abs. 501A) (1990).
950. H. J. Tanke, J. Bonnet, R. Runia, N. P. Verwoerd, and H. B. Beverloo, *Royal Micr. Soc.,* **24,** 348 (1989).
951. E. Ishikawa, S. Hashida, T. Kohno, and K. Tanaka, "Methods for Enzyme-Labeling of Antigens, Antibodies, and Their Fragments," in T. T. Ngo, Ed., *Non-isotopic Immunoassay,* Plenum Press, New York, 1988.
952. P. Hösli, *Clin. Chem.,* **23,** 1476 (1977).
953. P. Hösli, S. Avrameas, A. Ullmann, E. Vogt, and M. Rodrigot, *Clin. Chem.,* **24,** 1325 (1978).

954. F. C. Grenier, E. N. Granados, B. C. Schick, L. Kolaczkowski, and T. A. Pry, *Clin. Chem.,* **33,** 1570 (1987).

955. R. Armenta, T. Tarnowski, I. Gibbons, and E. F. Ullman, *Anal. Biochem.,* **146,** 211 (1985).

956. M. Numazawa, A. Haryu, K. Kurosaka, and T. Nambarat, *FEBS Lett.,* **79,** 396 (1977).

957. F. Von Hofmann, L. Hofmann, W. Hubl, and D. Meissner, *Z. Med. Labor. Diagn.,* **25,** 14 (1984).

958. M. Imagawa, S. Hashida, E. Ishikawa, H. Mori, C. Nakai, Y. Ichioka, and K. Nakajima, *Anal. Lett.,* **16,** B19, 1509 (1983).

959. A. Tsuji, M. Maeda, H. Arakawa, K. Matsuoka, N. Kato, H. Naruse, and M. Irie, "Enzyme Immunoassay of Hormones and Drugs by Using Fluorescence and Chemiluminescence Reaction," in S. B. Pal, Ed., *Enzyme Labelled Immunoassay of Hormones and Drugs,* Walter de Gruyter & Co., Berlin, 1978.

960. K. Matsuoka, M. Maeda, and A. Tsuji, *Chem. Pharm. Bull.,* **28,** 1864 (1980).

961. A. S. Ferrer, J. S. Santema, R. Hilhorst, and A. J. W. G. Visser, *Anal. Biochem.,* **187,** 129 (1990).

962. C.-L. Lee, M. C. Wang, G. P. Murphy, and T. M. Chu, *Cancer Res.,* **38,** 2871 (1978).

963. R. Moser and E. Koller, *Abstracts of Papers Presented at the IIIrd International Symposium on Quantitative Luminescence Spectrometry in Biomedical Sciences,* Ghent, Belgium, May 1989.

964. R. Klem and W. Marvin, *Clin. Chem.,* **36,** 1125 (abs. 806) (1990).

965. A. P. Schaap, *J. Biolum. Chemilum.,* **2,** 253 (1988).

966. F. Kohen, Z. Hollander, and R. C. Boguslaski, *J. Steroid. Biochem.,* **11,** 161 (1979).

967. F. Kohen, Z. Hollander, J. F. Burd, and R. C. Boguslaski, *Research on Steroids,* **8,** 147 (1979).

968. J. S. O'Neal, K. B. Sloan, and S. G. Schulman, *J. Pharmaceut. Biomed. Analysis,* **4,** 103 (1986).

969. E. Ishikawa, *J. Biochem.,* **73,** 1319 (1973).

970. M. T. Makler, A. C. Bakke, and R. C. Piper, *J. Immunol. Methods,* **108,** 137 (1988).

971. R. M. Nakamura, "Fluorescent Antibody Methods: Quality Assurance Procedures," in R. M. Nakamura, Ed., *Immunoassays in the Clinical Laboratory,* Alan R. Liss, Inc., New York, 1979.

972. S. S. Hipp, Y. Han, and D. Murphy, *J. Clin. Microbiol.,* **25,** 1938 (1987).

973. M. R. Hammerschlag, P. J. Rettig, and M. E. Shields, *Pediatr. Infect. Dis. J.,* **7,** 11 (1988).

974. S.-P. Wang and J. T. Grayston, *Am. J. Ophthalmol.,* **70,** 367 (1970).

975. L. R. Krylov, L. Marcoux, and H. D. Isenberg, *J. Clin. Microbiol.,* **26,** 377 (1988).
976. B. Hennes, W. Kruse, H. Hofmann, and D. Petzoldt, *Hautarzt.,* **37,** 662 (1986).
977. R. C. Moseley, L. Corey, D. Benjamin, C. Winter, and M. L. Remington, *J. Clin. Microbiol.,* **13,** 913 (1981).
978. N. J. Schmidt, J. Dennis, and E. H. Lennette, *J. Clin. Microbiol.,* **7,** 576 (1978).
979. S. Arista, L. Giovannelli, M. Balsano, and R. Stefano, *Quad. Sclavo Diagn.,* **20,** 258 (1984).
980. S. H. Guenthner and C. C. Linnemann, Jr., *Lab. Medicine,* **19,** 581 (1988).
981. J. Luka, R. C. Chase, and G. R. Pearson, *J. Immunol. Methods,* **67,** 145 (1984).
982. H. W. Wilkinson, *Yale J. Biol. Med.,* **57,** 567 (1984).
983. V. Borghi, M. De-Palma, M. Vecchi, F. Pellegrino, N. Mongiardo, I. Cocchi, B. De-Rienzo, and F. Squadrini, *Microbiologica,* **11,** 81 (1988).
984. S. F. Lyons, G. M. McGillivray, A. P. Coppin, and B. D. Schoub, *S. Afr. Med. J.,* **68,** 575 (1985).
985. B. L. Elder and T. F. Smith, *Am. J. Clin. Pathol.,* **87,** 230 (1987).
986. E. M. Peterson, R. Oda, P. Tse, C. Gastaldi, S. C. Stone, and L. M. De La Maza, *J. Clin. Microbiol.,* **27,** 350 (1989).
987. T. G. Wreghitt and M. Sillis, *Isr. J. Med. Sci.,* **23,** 704 (1987).
988. J. K. Robinson and R. Gottschalk, *Arch. Dermatol.,* **120,** 199 (1984).
989. D. Koffler, P. H. Schur, and H. G. Kunkel, *J. Exp. Med.,* **126,** 607 (1967).
990. F. Kozin, M. Fowler, and S. M. Koethe, *Am. J. Clin. Pathol.,* **74,** 785 (1980).
991. W. D. Mercer, M. E. Lippman, T. M. Wahl, C. A. Carlson, D. A. Wahl, D. Lezotte, and P. O. Teague, *Cancer,* **46,** 2859 (1980).
992. E. H. Fife, Jr., R. H. Kruse, A. J. Toussaint, and E. V. Staab, *Lab. Anim. Care,* **20,** 969 (1970).
993. T. C. Chawla, A. Sharma, U. Kiran, D. K. Shriniwas, and B. N. Tandon, *Tubercle,* **67,** 55 (1986).
994. A. J. Toussaint, *Exp. Parasit.,* **19,** 71 (1966).
995. W. A. Hook and E. H. Fife, Jr., *Appl. Microbiol.,* **15,** 350 (1967).
996. R. W. Gore and E. H. Sadun, *Experim. Parasitol.,* **23,** 287 (1968).
997. E. H. Clinard, *Am. J. Vet. Res.,* **36,** 615 (1975).
998. J. A. Garnham, B. N. Wilkie, K. Nielsen, and J. Thorsen, *J. Immunol. Methods,* **14,** 147 (1977).
999. R. E. Duxbury and E. H. Sadun, *Experim. Parasitol.,* **20,** 77 (1967).
1000. B. Micheel, U. Karsten, and H. Fiebach, *J. Immunol. Methods,* **46,** 41 (1981).
1001. B. Micheel, U. Karsten, and H. Fiebach, *Acta Histochem.,* **71,** 15 (1982).
1002. N. C. Fisher, N. Hinds-Aldrich, J. E. Haddow, and G. A. Hudson, *Thromb. Res.,* **31,** 145 (1983).

1003. L. D. Cles, K. Bruch, and W. E. Stamm, *J. Clin. Microbiol.,* **26,** 1735 (1988).

1004. W. Knapp, "Preparation and Use of Defined Antigenic Substrates for Standardized Immunofluorescence," in G. Wick, K. N. Traill, and K. Schauenstein, Eds., *Immunofluorescence Technology: Selected Theoretical and Clinical Aspects,* Elsevier Biomedical Press, Amsterdam, 1982.

1005. F. J. Bloemmen, J. Rádl, J. J. Haaijman, P. Van Der Berg, H. R. E. Schuit, and W. Hijmans, *J. Immunol. Methods,* **10,** 337 (1976).

1006. W. Knapp, J. Menzel, and C. Steffen, *Z. Immunitaetsforsch.,* **148,** 132 (1974).

1007. A. M. Deelder and J. S. Plocm, *Experim. Parasitol.,* **37,** 173 (1975).

1008. G. Koch, K. Nooter, B. Bentvelzen, and J. J. Haaijman, *Eur. J. Cancer,* **13,** 1397 (1977).

1009. W. Knapp and H. Ludwig, *Z. Immunitaetsforsch.,* **151,** 61 (1976).

1010. J. J. Haaijman and J. Brinkhof, *J. Immunol. Methods,* **14,** 213 (1977).

1011. T. Oonishi, K. Sakashita, and N. Uyesaka, *J. Immunol. Methods,* **115,** 159 (1988).

1012. M. Y. Hoven, L. De Leij, F. K. Keij, and T. H. The, *J. Immunol. Methods,* **117,** 275 (1989).

1013. A. Caruso, L. Terlenghi, A. Scalzini, R. Verardi, I. Foresti, P. Pollard, C. Bonfanti, G. Ravizzola, N. Manca, and A. Turano, *J. Immunol. Methods,* **113,** 27 (1988).

1014. C. F. Garcia, L. M. Weiss, J. Lowder, C. Komoroske, M. P. Link, R. Levy, and R. A. Warnke, *Am. J. Clin. Pathol.,* **87,** 470 (1987).

1015. K. B. Alonso and N. R. Brownlee, *Clin. Chem.,* **25,** 1077 (abs. 074) (1979).

1016. M. R. Wilson and J. S. Wotherspoon, *J. Immunol. Methods,* **107,** 225 (1988).

1017. M. R. Wilson, S. P. Mulligan, and R. L. Raison, *J. Immunol. Methods,* **107,** 231 (1988).

1018. L. Aurelian, *Diagn. Gynecol. Obstet.,* **4,** 375 (1982).

1019. M. J. Fulwyler, T.-M. McHugh, R. Schwadron, J. J. Scillian, D. Lau, M. P. Busch, S. Roy, and G. N. Vyas, *Cytometry,* **2,** Suppl. 19 (abs. 104) (1988).

1020. Y. Suzuki, T. Oite, T. Yamamoto, T. Morita, and I. Kimara, *Japan J. Exp. Med.,* **49,** 179 (1979).

1021. B. L. Allman, F. Short, and V. H. T. James, *Clin. Chem.,* **27,** 1167 (1981).

1022. R. J. Playford, A. Dawnay, W. R. Cattell, and J. Landon, *Ann. Clin. Biochem.,* **22,** 166 (1985).

1023. E. J. Shaw, R. A. A. Watson, and D. S. Smith, *Eur. J. Drug. Metab. Pharmacokin.,* **4,** 191 (1977).

1024. T. Chard and A. Sykes, *Clin. Chem.,* **25,** 973 (1979).

1025. M. Schwalbe, E. Dorn, and K. Beyermann, *J. Agric. Food. Chem.,* **32,** 734 (1984).

1026. A. Reyes, M. Morell, and J. J. Laserna, *Anal. Chim. Acta,* **170,** 133 (1985).

1027. J. H. Chen and N. Kameda, *Clin. Chem.,* **32,** 1160 (abs. 547) (1986).

1028. W. Lee, T. Wong, F. Kamal, G. Ayanoglu, and N. Kameda, *Clin. Chem.,* **32,** 1171 (abs. 602) (1986).

1029. H. T. Karnes, J. C. Gudat, C. M. O'Donnell, and J. D. Winefordner, *Clin. Chem.,* **26,** 970 (abs. 56) (1980).

1030. H. T. Karnes, J. C. Gudat, C. M. O'Donnell, and J. D. Winefordner, *Clin. Chem.,* **27,** 249 (1981).

1031. C. M. O'Donnell, J. H. McBride, A. Broughton, and S. C. Suffin, *Clin. Chem.,* **25,** 1077 (abs. 73) (1979).

1032. M. J. Kurtz, M. Billings, T. Koh, G. Olander, T. Tyner, B. Weaver, and L. Stone, *Clin. Chem.,* **29,** 1015 (1983).

1033. M. A. Pfaller, D. J. Krogstad, G. G. Granich, and P. Murray, *J. Clin. Microbiol.,* **20,** 311 (1984).

1034. W. L. T. Wong, J. H. Chen, and N. Kameda, *Clin. Chem.,* **32,** 1085 (abs. 178) (1986).

1035. R. E. Coxon, C. Rae, G. Gallacher, and J. Landon, *Clin. Chim. Acta,* **175,** 297 (1988).

1036. A. Louie, P. Nguyen, M. Kramer, T. Henriksson, and G. L. Rowley, *Clin. Chem.,* **32,** 1146 (abs. 478) (1986).

1037. T. Henriksson, M. Kramer, A. Louie, P. H. Nguyen, and G. L. Rowley, *Clin. Chem.,* **33,** 918 (abs. 187) (1987).

1038. A. Louie, P. H. Nguyen, W. Woo, T. Henriksson, and G. L. Rowley, *Clin. Chem.,* **33,** 919 (abs. 191) (1987).

1039. J. Chesham, S. W. Anderton, and C. F. M. Kingdon, *Clin. Chem.,* **32,** 669 (1986).

1040. J. M. Yoder, L. A. Schick, and R. P. Moore, *Thrombosis Res.,* **24,** 51 (1981).

1041. I. Spilberg, A. Gallacher, B. Mandell, B. Hahn, and J. Mehta, *Amer. J. Med. Sci.,* **272,** 83 (1976).

1042. H. Hosotsubo, K. Arai, and J.-I. Iwamura, *Chromatographia,* **25,** 129 (1988).

1043. A. Sykes and T. Chard, *Clin. Chem.,* **26,** 1224 (1980).

1044. L. A. Kaplan, I. W. Chen, N. Gau, J. Fearn, H. Maxon, C. Volle, and E. A. Stein, *Clin. Biochem.,* **14,** 182 (1981).

1045. D. H. Riege, R. V. Sweet, and R. E. Curry, *Clin. Chem.,* **25,** 1133 (abs. 353) (1979).

1046. Y. Kobayashi, M. Yamata, F. Watanabe, and K. Miyai, *J. Steroid. Biochem.,* **16,** 521 (1982).

1047. R. L. Chan, L. M. Krausz, and R. V. Sweet, *Clin. Chem.,* **27,** 1085 (abs. 308) (1981).

1048. G. C. Blanchard and R. Garder, *Clin. Chem.,* **24,** 808 (1978).

1049. E. A. H. Hische, H. J. Van Der Helm, and T. Out, *Clin. Chim. Acta,* **97,** 93 (1979).

1050. N. J. Verhoef, *Clin. Chem.,* **28,** 2185 (1982).

1051. T. Takeoka, Y. Shinohara, K. Mori, and K. Furumi, *J. Neurol. Sci.,* **96,** 229 (1990).

1052. T. Takeoka, Y. Shinohara, K. Mori, and K. Furumi, *J. Neurol. Sci.,* **96,** 229 (1990).

1053. M. W. Burgett, S. J. Fairfield, and J. F. Monthony, *Clin. Chim. Acta,* **78,** 277 (1977).

1054. M. W. Burgett, S. J. Fairfield, and J. F. Monthony, *J. Immunol. Methods,* **16,** 211 (1977).

1055. J. H. Liu, F. E. Klink, and J. D. Nichol, *J. Forensic Sci.,* **25,** 686 (1980).

1056. T. M. Saba, E. Cho, and F. A. Blumenstock, *Exp. Mol. Pathol.,* **41,** 81 (1984).

1057. S. De Lauzon, J. El Jabri, N. Cittanova, P. Gervais, J. Mugnier, J. Pouget, and B. Valeur, *Abstract of Papers Presented at the IIIrd International Symposium on Quantitative Luminescence Spectroscopy in Biomedical Sciences,* Ghent, Belgium, May 1989.

1058. F. P. Anderson and W. G. Miller, *Clin. Chem.,* **32,** 1063 (abs. 68) (1986).

1059. C. B. Reimer, D. J. Phillips, C. M. Black, and T. W. Wells, "Standardization of Ligand Binding Assay for Alpha Phetoprotein," in W. Knapp, K. Holubar, and G. Wick, Eds., *Immunofluorescence and Related Staining Techniques,* Elsevier/North Holland Biomedical Press, Amsterdam, 1978.

1060. J. C. Hierholzer, D. J. Phillips, D. D. Humphrey, R. A. Coombs, and C. B. Reimer, *Arch. Virol.,* **80,** 1 (1984).

1061. E. N. Fox, *Proc. Soc. Exptl. Biol. Med.,* **109,** 577 (1962).

1062. A. Van Aert, L. Uytterhaegen, P. Brioen, B. Rombaut, R. De Geyter, and A. Boeye, *Vet. Immunol. Immunopathol.,* **9,** 183 (1985).

1063. R. D. Nargessi, M. Pourfarzaneh, and J. Landon, *Clin. Chim. Acta,* **111,** 65 (1981).

1064. A. T. M. Al-Ani, M. H. H. Al-Hakiem, and T. Chard, *Clin. Chim. Acta,* **112,** 91 (1981).

1065. M. Pourfarzaneh, G. W. White, J. Landon, and D. S. Smith, *Clin. Chem.,* **26,** 730 (1980).

1066. B. A. El-Gamal, S. A. Eremin, D. S. Smith, and J. Landon, *Ann. Clin. Biochem.,* **25,** 35 (1988).

1067. G. I. Ekeke, J. Landon, C. R. W. Edwards, G. W. White, and F. Shridi, *Clin. Chim. Acta,* **109,** 31 (1981).

1068. R. D. Nargessi, J. Ackland, M. Hassan, G. C. Forrest, D. S. Smith, and J. Landon, *Clin. Chem.,* **26,** 1701 (1980).

1069. R. S. Kamel, M. K. Abdul Majid, and F. J. Dhahir, *Clin. Chem.,* **32,** 1160 (abs. 548) (1986).

1070. F. A. Shridi, A. Chitranukroh, M. Pourfarzaneh, B. H. Billing, and G. Ekeke, *Ann. Clin. Biochem.,* **17,** 188 (1980).

1071. M. H. H. Al-Hakiem, R. D. Nargessi, M. Pourfarzaneh, G. N. White, D. S. Smith, and A. J. Hodgkinson, *J. Clin. Chem. Clin. Biochem.,* **20,** 151 (1982).

1072. R. S. Kamel, J. Landon, and D. S. Smith, *Clin. Chem.,* **26,** 1281 (1980).

1073. A. M. Sidki, J. Landon, and F. Rowell, *Clin. Chem.,* **30,** 1348 (1984).

1074. A. M. Sidki, D. S. Smith, and J. Landon, *Ther. Drug. Monit.,* **7,** 101 (1985).

1075. I. H. Al-Abdulla, A. M. Sidki, J. Landon, and F. J. Rowell, *Southeast Asian J. Trop. Med. Public Health,* **20,** 361 (1989).

1076. I. H. Al-Abdulla, G. W. Mellor, M. S. Childerstone, A. M. Sidki, and D. S. Smith, *J. Immunol. Methods,* **122,** 253 (1989).

1077. A. M. Sidki, I. H. Al-Abdulla, and F. J. Rowell, *Clin. Chem.,* **33,** 463 (1987).

1078. M. H. H. Al-Hakiem, G. W. White, D. S. Smith, and J. Landon, *Ther. Drug. Monit.,* **3,** 159 (1981).

1079. F. J. Rowell, S. M. Hui, and R. S. Kamel, *Clin. Chem.,* **27,** 1249 (1981).

1080. K. Staley, R. Coxon, G. Gallacher, and J. Landon, *Ther. Drug. Monit.,* **10,** 321 (1988).

1081. R. E. Coxon, A. J. Hodgkinson, A. M. Sidki, J. Landon, and G. Gallacher, *Ther. Drug. Monit.,* **9,** 478 (1987).

1082. D. L. Colbert, A. M. Sidki, G. Gallacher, and J. Landon, *Analyst,* **112,** 1483 (1987).

1083. D. L. Colbert, G. Gallacher, P. Ayling, and G. J. Turner, *Clin. Chim. Acta,* **171,** 37 (1988).

1084. R. D. Nargessi, B. Shine, and J. Landon, *J. Immunol. Methods,* **71,** 17 (1984).

1085. B. Shine and F. Begumbaig, *Clin. Chem.,* **32,** 2105 (1986).

1086. L. Viinikka, J. Landon, and M. Pourfarzaneh, *Clin. Chim. Acta,* **114,** 1(1981).

1087. C. M. Black, L. Pine, C. B. Reimer, R. F. Benson, and T. W. Wells, *J. Clin. Microbiol.,* **15,** 1077 (1982).

1088. N. Monji, C.-A. Cole, and S. M. Schreiner, *Clin. Chem.,* **32,** 1175 (abs. 621) (1986).

1089. J. McDonald, R. Gall, P. Wiedenbach, V. D. Bass, B. Deleon, C. Brockus, D. Stobert, S. Wie, C. A. Prange, J.-M. Yang, C. L. Tai, T. J. Weckman, W. E. Woods, H.-H. Tai, J. W. Blake, and T. Tobin, *Res. Commun. Chem. Pathol. Pharmac.,* **57,** 389 (1987).

1090. J.-M. Yang, C.-L. Tai, T. J. Weckman, H.-H. Tai, J. W. Blake, T. Tobin, J. McDonald, R. Gall, P. Wiedenbach, V. D. Bass, B. DeLeon, C. Brockus, D. Stobert, S. Wie, and C. A. Prange, *Res. Commun. Subst. Abuse,* **8,** 59 (1987).

1091. C. A. Prange, C. Brockus, S. Wie, R. A. Chung, J. M. Brecht, J. C. Conner, P. A. Dahl, E. L. Lewis, J. McDonald, S. Kalita, F. J. Ozog, M. T. Green, S. Kwiatkowski, J. P. Goodman, L. Sturma, S. D. Stanley, J.-M. Yang, T. Wood, P. Henry, T. J. Weckman, W. E. Woods, D. J. Watt, H.-H. Tai, S.-L. Chang, J. W. Blake, and T. Tobin, *Res. Commun. Subst. Abuse,* **10,** 1 (1989).

1092. M. C. Custer and M. T. Lotze, *J. Immunol. Methods,* **128,** 109 (1990).

1093. B. J. Del Tito, Jr., D. W. Zabriskie, and E. J. Arcuri, *J. Immunol. Methods,* **107,** 67 (1988).

1094. F. Islam, Y. Urade, Y. Watanabe, and O. Hayaishi, *Arch. Biochem. Biophys.,* **277,** 290 (1990).

1095. J. D. Peterson, J. Y. Kim, R. W. Melvold, S. D. Miller, and C. Waltenbaugh, *J. Immunol. Methods,* **119,** 83 (1989).

1096. T. J. Quade, T. W. Pitts, and W. G. Tarpley, *Biochem. Biophys. Res. Commun.,* **163,** 172 (1989).

1097. D. R. Bethel, M. Dawson, and M. J. Lafoe, *BioTechniques,* **3,** 465 (1985).

1098. B. Avner, B. Gaydos, S.-K. Liao, and B. P. Avner, *Fed. Proc.,* **46,** 1060 (abs. 4334) (1987).

1099. M. J. Lafoe, M. E. Jolley, and D. R. Bethell, *Hybridoma,* **4,** 67 (1985).

1100. M. Liebert, L. Laino, and R. L. Wahl, *J. Immunol. Methods,* **101,** 85 (1987).

1101. H. Inoue, S. Hirohashi, Y. Shimosato, M. Enjoji, and S.-I. Hakamori, *Eur. J. Immunol.,* **19,** 2197 (1989).

1102. G. Laszlo and H. B. Dickler, *Hybridoma,* **9,** 111 (1990).

1103. J. Mayus, K. Macke, P. Shackelford, J. Kim, and M. Nahm, *J. Immunol. Methods,* **88,** 65 (1986).

1104. M. H. Nahm, M. G. Scott, and P. G. Shackelford, *Ann. Clin. Lab. Sci.,* **17,** 183 (1987).

1105. J. D. Peterson, J. Y. Kim, R. W. Melvold, S. D. Miller, and C. Waltenbaugh, *J. Immunol. Methods,* **119,** 83 (1989).

1106. J. V. Madassery, O. H. Kwon, S. Y. Lee, and H. Nahm, *Clin. Chem.,* **34,** 1407 (1988).

1107. J. D. Peterson, S. D. Miller, and C. Waltenbaugh, *J. Virol. Methods,* **27,** 189 (1990).

1108. M. Dawson, M. E. Jolley, and D. R. Bethell, *Hybridoma,* **3,** 80 (1984).

1109. W. R. Schwan, C. Waltenbaugh, and J. L. Duncan, *J. Immunol. Methods,* **126,** 247 (1990).

1110. O. Berg and L. Hemmingsen, *Scand. J. Clin. Lab. Invest.,* **41,** 323 (1981).

1111. B. I. Bluestein, A. J. Famulare, and T. E. Worthy, US Patent No. 4,780,423 (1988).

1112. R. M. Hull, *Lab. World,* **29,** 79 (1978).

1113. R. Wang, B. Merrill, and E. T. Maggio, *Clin. Chim. Acta,* **102,** 169 (1980).

1114. T.-H. Nguyen and R. J. Dockhorn, *Ann. Allergy,* **46,** 8 (1981).

1115. N. Kameda, R. A. Harte, and F. H. Deindoerfer, *Clin. Chem.,* **22,** 1200 (abs. 212) (1976).

1116. G. S. Zaatari, S. R. Hamilton, J. Jacobs, and T. B. Datiles, *Clin. Chim. Acta,* **103,** 357 (1980).

1117. R. W. Stevens, D. Elmendorf, M. Gourlay, E. Stroebel, and H. A. Gaafar, *J. Clin. Microbiol.,* **10,** 346 (1979).

1118. H. S. Rock, M. W. Burgett, and J. D. Allen, *Clin. Chem.,* **25,** 1078 (abs. 75) (1979).

1119. G. C. Blanchard and R. E. Gardner, *J. Immunol. Methods,* **52,** 81 (1982).

1120. N. M. Burdash, A. D. Ponzio, and C. B. Loadholt, *J. Rheumatology,* **8,** 837 (1981).

1121. G. W. Cannon, M. J. Egger, J. R. Ward, L. J. Blonquist, and L. B. Collette, *Am. J. Clin. Pathol.,* **87,** 223 (1987).

1122. A. B. Carpenter and C. D. Bartkowiak, *Clin. Chem.,* **35,** 464 (1989).

1123. S. S. Levison and J. Goldman, *Clin. Chem.,* **32,** 1069 (abs. 95) (1986).

1124. M. Koelle and W. E. Bartholomew, *J. Clin. Microbiol.,* **16,** 271 (1982).

1125. M. K. Fleetwood, B. A. Maier, and S. H. Lewis, *Clin. Chem.,* **27,** 503 (1981).

1126. R. Harte, N. Kameda, and J. Chang, *Clin. Chem.,* **24,** 1033 (abs. 227) (1978).

1127. Z. Rudzki, L. J. Tunbridge, and J. V. Lloyd, *Thromb. Res.,* **16,** 577 (1979).

1128. K. H. Wiedmann, A. Melms, and P. A. Berg, *Liver,* **3,** 369 (1983).

1129. N. Kameda, J. Chang, and F. Deindoerfer, *Clin. Chem.,* **24,** 1033 (abs. 226) (1978).

1130. C. H. Casavant, A. C. Hart, and D. P. Stites, *J. Clin. Microbiol.,* **10,** 712 (1979).

1131. B. H. Berne, K. T. DeBlock, and O. J. Lawless, *Arthritis Rheum.,* **25,** 997 (1982).

1132. B. H. Berne, K. T. Galland, and R. C. Welton, *Clin. Chem.,* **30,** 757 (1984).

1133. R. Klein, J. Lindenborn-Fotinos, and P. A. Berg, *J. Immunol. Methods,* **11,** 227 (1983).

1134. A. S. Weissfeld, W. D. Gehle, and A. C. Sonnenwirth, *J. Clin. Microbiol.,* **16,** 82 (1982).

1135. N. E. Cremer, S. J. Hagens, and C. Cossen, *J. Clin. Microbiol.,* **11,** 746 (1980).

1136. S. L. Fayram, A. Nakasone, S. Aarnaes, M. Zartarian, E. M. Peterson, and L. De La Maza, *J. Clin. Microbiol.,* **17,** 685 (1983).

1137. J. P. Brody, J. H. Binkley, and S. A. Harding, *J. Clin. Microbiol.,* **10,** 708 (1979).

1138. G. A. Castellano, D. L. Madden, G. T. Hazzard, L. S. Cleghorn, D. V. Vails, A. C. Ley, N. R. Tzan, and J. L. Sever, *J. Infect. Dis.,* **143,** 578 (1981).

1139. S. L. Fayram, S. Akin, S. L. Aarnaes, E. M. Peterson, and L. M. De La Maza, *J. Clin. Microbiol.,* **25,** 178 (1987).

1140. J. M. Echevarria, F. De Ory, and R. Najera, *J. Clin. Microbiol.,* **22,** 428 (1985).

1141. K. W. Walls and E. R. Barnhart, *J. Clin. Microbiol.,* **7,** 234 (1978).

1142. B. Hyde, M. W. Burgett, and E. T. Maggio, *Clin. Chim. Acta,* **103,** 393 (1980).

1143. S. A. Violand, T. G. Mitchell, and K. T. Kleeman, *J. Clin. Microbiol.,* **16,** 341 (1982).

1144. L. G. Carlson and J. J. Plorde, *Diagn. Microbiol. Infect. Dis.,* **1,** 233 (1983).

1145. E. Falcioni, N. W. Brattig, and P. A. Berg, *Clin. Chem.,* **19,** 289 (1986).

1146. M. Wilson, D. A. Ware, and K. W. Walls, *J. Clin. Microbiol.,* **25,** 2262 (1987).

1147. W. B. Benjamin, S. C. Specter, T. W. Klein, M. Hitchings, and H. Friedman, *J. Clin. Microbiol.,* **12,** 558 (1980).

1148. T. G. Roesing, J. Meeker, B. Carfinkce, A. Gray, and M. Hitchings, *J. Biol. Standardiz.,* **9,** 401 (1981).

1149. S. C. Pflugfelder, J. Suelflow, M. E. Pflugfelder, and D. W. Parke, *Ann. Ophthalmol.,* **20,** 355 (1988).

1150. F. De Ory, J. M. Echevarria, and C. J. Domingo, *Diagn. Microbiol. Infect. Dis.,* **10,** 61 (1988).

1151. A. W. Confer, J. C. Wright, J. M. Cummins, R. J. Panciera, and R. E. Corstvet, *J. Clin. Microbiol.,* **18,** 866 (1983).

1152. A. W. Confer, J. C. Fox, P. R. Newman, G. W. Lawson, and R. E. Corstvet, *Can. J. Comp. Med.,* **47,** 37 (1983).

1153. H. J. Gittelman, R. B. Grieve, M. M. Hitchings, R. H. Jacobson, and R. H. Cypess, *J. Clin. Microbiol.,* **13,** 309 (1981).

1154. G. B. Estes, M. Munoz, N. M. Burdash, and G. Virella, *J. Immunol. Methods,* **35,** 105 (1980).

1155. G. Burges, H. P. Holley, Jr., and G. Virella, *Diagn. Immunol.,* **4,** 43 (1986).

1156. R. W. Stevens and R. F. Schell, *J. Clin. Microbiol.,* **15,** 191 (1982).

1157. M. F. Cole, S. D. Hsu, and W. H. Bowen, *J. Immunol. Methods,* **53,** 335 (1982).

1158. K. E. Hechemy, H. L. Harris, J. A. Wethers, R. W. Stevens, B. R. Stock, A. A. Reilly, and J. L. Benach, *J. Clin. Microbiol.,* **27,** 1854 (1989).

1159. D. R. Pennell, P. J. Wand, and R. F. Schnell, *J. Clin. Microbiol.,* **25,** 2218 (1987).

1160. T. A. Thompson and H. W. Wilkinson, *J. Clin. Microbiol.,* **16,** 202 (1983).

1161. K. W. Walls and M. Wilson, *Ann. N.Y. Acad. Sci.,* **420,** 422 (1983).

1162. S. M. Hall, A. W. Confer, L. B. Tabatabai, and B. L. Deyoe, *J. Clin. Microbiol.,* **20,** 1023 (1984).

1163. B. Gerson, L. Dean, and F. Bell, *Ther. Drug. Monit.,* **3,** 167 (1981).

1164. Y.-G. Tsay and R. J. Palmer, *Clin. Chim. Acta,* **109,** 151 (1981).

1165. D. A. Bruckner, J. A. Hindler, W. J. Martin, and R. Palmer, *Antimicr. Agents Chemother.,* **21,** 107 (1982).

1166. W. L. T. Wong and N. Kameda, *Clin. Chem.,* **34,** 1251 (abs. 481) (1988).

1167. G. L. Rowley, A. S. Louie, T. M. Henriksson, and P. H. Nguyen, *Clin. Chem.,* **34,** 1210 (abs. 282) (1988).

1168. R. N. Hobbs, *J. Immunol. Methods,* **117,** 257 (1989).

1169. H.-P. Wang, H.-T. Ho, F. Davouzadeh, and H. Wang, *Clin. Chem.,* **35,** 1189 (abs. 583) (1989).

1170. M. C. La-Regina, J. Lonigro, L. Woods, W. C. Hall, and R. E. Doyle, *J. Clin. Microbiol.,* **26,** 573 (1988).

1171. C. Lucas, S. Frie, R. Peters, and J. Parker, *Lab. Anim. Sci.,* **37,** 51 (1987).

1172. C. Glad, *Appl. Biochem. Biotechnol.,* **7,** 75 (1982).

1173. A. Padilla, D. Maretsky, J. Blackwood, S. Inbar, and G. Grenner, *Clin. Chem.,* **35,** 1196 (abs. 618) (1989).

1174. M. Staedter, D. Maretsky, J. Finneran, K. Penta, M. Shae, S. Inbar, J. Blackwood, and G. Grenner, *Clin. Chem.,* **35,** 1196 (abs. 616) (1989).

1175. J. Cox, M. Staedter, J. Blackwood, S. Inbar, and E. Metzmann, *Clin. Chem.,* **36,** 1036 (abs. 0397) (1990).

1176. H. Ackermann, E. Steva, J. Blackwood, S. Inbar, and E. Metzmann, *Clin. Chem.,* **36,** 1038 (abs. 0404) (1990).

1177. M. Shea, P. D'Eon, J. Blackwood, S. Inbar, and E. Metzmann, *Clin. Chem.,* **36,** 1045 (abs. 0439) (1990).

1178. W. K. Wang, L. T. Ho, and Y. Chiang, *Isr. J. Clin. Biochem. Lab. Sci.,* **4,** 53 (1985).

1179. R. A. Harte, A. B. Chen, and N. K. Kaufman, US Patent No. 4,540,660 (1985).

1180. W. K. Wang, L. T. Ho, and Y. Chiang, *Clin. Chem.,* **36,** 1092 (abs. 0658) (1990).

1181. S. M. Toler, W. H. Porter, and M. H. H. Chandler, *Ther. Drug Monit.,* **12,** 300 (1990).

1182. F. Perrin, *J. Phys. Radium.,* **7,** 390 (1926).

1183. F. V. Bright, *Anal. Chem.,* **61,** 309 (1989).

1184. W. B. Dandliker, M.-L. Hsu, J. Levin, and B. R. Rao, *Methods Enzymol.,* **74,** 3 (1981).

1185. G. Weber, *Biochem. J.,* **51,** 145 (1952).

1186. W. B. Dandliker, R. J. Brawn, H.-L. Hsu, P. N. Brawn, J. Levin, C. Y. Meyers, and V. M. Kolb, *Cancer Res.,* **38,** 4212 (1978).

1187. W. B. Dandliker, M.-L. Hsu, and W. P. Vanderlaan, "Fluorescence Polarization Immunoassays/Receptor Assays," in R. M. Nakamura, W. R. Dito, and E. S. Tucker, Eds., *Immunoassays: Clinical Laboratory Techniques for the 1980s,* Alan R. Liss, Inc., New York, 1980.

1188. P. Urios, N. Cittanova, and M.-F. Jayle, *FEBS Lett.,* **94,** 54 (1978).

1189. H. R. Lukens, C. B. Williams, J. A. Lewison, W. B. Dandliker, D. Marayama, and R. C. Baron, *Environ. Sci. Technol.,* **11,** 292 (1977).

1190. M. E. Jolley, *J. Anal. Toxicol.,* **5,** 236 (1981).

1191. D. Haidukewych, *Immunoassay Technology,* **2,** 71 (1986).

1192. M. E. Jolley, S. D. Stroupe, C.-H. Wang, H. N. Panas, C. L. Keegan, R. L. Schmidt, and K. S. Schwenzer, *Clin. Chem.,* **27,** 1190 (1981).

1193. J. M. Andrews and R. Wise, *J. Antimicrob. Chemother.,* **14,** 509 (1984).

1194. P. R. Oeltgen, W. A. Shank, Jr., R. A. Blouin, and T. Clark, *Ther. Drug. Monit.,* **6,** 360 (1984).

1195. T. Fujimoto, Y. Tsuda, R. Tawa, and S. Hirose, *Clin. Chem.,* **35,** 867 (1989).

1196. O. S. Tayed, A. T. El-Tahawy, and S. I. Islam, *Ther. Drug. Monit.,* **8,** 232 (1986).

1197. B. E. Bleske, T. A. Larson, and J. C. Rotschafer, *Ther. Drug. Monit.,* **9,** 48 (1987).

1198. K. S. Schwenzer and J. P. Anhalt, *Antimicr. Agents Chemother.,* **23,** 683 (1983).

1199. C. Van Remmerden, J. R. Brouwers, J. A. Berk, and R. J. Boskma, *Pharm. Weekbl. Sci.,* **6,** 68 (1984).

1200. T. Uematsu, A. Mizuno, Y. Suzuki, R. Sato, T. Yamazaki, and M. Nakashima, *Ther. Drug. Monit.,* **10,** 459 (1988).

1201. B. H. Filburn, V. H. Shull, Y. M. Tempera, and J. D. Dick, *Antimicrob. Agents Chemother.,* **24,** 216 (1983).

1202. T. Uematsu, R. Sato, A. Mizuno, M. Nishimoto, S. Nagashima, and M. Nakashima, *Clin. Chem.,* **34,** 1880 (1988).

1203. M. Lu-Steffes, G. W. Pittluck, M. E. Jolley, H. N. Panas, D. L. Olive, C. H. Wang, D. D. Nyström, C. L. Keegan, T. P. Davis, and S. D. Stroupe, *Clin. Chem.,* **28,** 2278 (1982).

1204. N. Ratnaraj, V. D. Goldberg, and P. T. Lascelles, *Analyst,* **111,** 517 (1986).

1205. D. E. Beck, J. A. Farringer, W. R. Ravis, and C. A. Robinson, *Clin. Pharm.,* **6,** 888 (1987).

1206. D. Haidukewych, *Clin. Chem.,* **30,** 1425 (1984).

1207. M. I. A. Peña and E. S. Lope, *J. Pharmaceut. Biomed. Anal.,* **6,** 1035 (1988).

1208. D. Haidukewych, *Clin. Chem.,* **31,** 156 (1985).

1209. B. H. Chen, E. H. Taylor, E. Kennedy, B. Ackerman, K. Olsen, and A. A. Pappas, *Clin. Chim. Acta,* **175,** 107 (1988).

1210. B. H. Ackerman, K. M. Olsen, E. E. Kennedy, E. H. Taylor, B. H. Chen, D. Jordan, and D. J. Ackerman, *Pharmacotherapy,* **9,** 220 (1989).

1211. M. Tod, G. Resplandy, R. Farinotti, Y. Provost, and A. Dauphin, *J. Pharmaceut. Biomed. Anal.,* **8,** 279 (1990).

1212. E. Bertol, F. Mari, and F. Torracca, *J. Anal. Toxicol.,* **11,** 122 (1987).

1213. T. Horiuchi, I. Johno, S. Kitazava, and M. Goto, *Drug Intellig. Clin. Pharmacy,* **22,** 507 (1988).

1214. M. Littlefield, L. Kolaczkowski, P. Wang, and T. Schroeder, *Clin. Chem.,* **34,** 1159 (abs. 031) (1988).

1215. H. D. Hill, M. E. Jolley, C. H. J. Wang, C. J. Quille, C. L. Keegan, D. D. Nyström, D. L. Olive, H. N. Panas, and S. D. Stroupe, *Clin. Chem.,* **27,** 1086 (abs. 310) (1981).

1216. S. H. Y. Wong and N. Marzouk, *Clin. Chem.,* **31,** 1576 (1985).

1217. R. L. Lalonde, M. B. Bottorff, and A. B. Straughn, *Ther. Drug. Monit.,* **7,** 442 (1985).

1218. T. Schulte, A. V. Berg, W. Buhr, and D. Berdel, *Atemweg Lungenkrauk,* **14,** 320 (1988).

1219. P. Bianchi, *Clin. Chem.,* **32,** 2099 (1986).

1220. L. F. Ferreri, V. A. Raisys, and K. E. Opheim, *J. Anal. Toxicol.,* **8,** 138 (1984).

1221. N. Rawal, F. Y. Leung, and A. R. Henderson, *Clin. Chem.,* **29,** 586 (1983).

1222. H. Nakashima, K. Tsutsumi, M. Hashiguchi, Y. Kumagai, and A. Ebihara, *J. Chromatogr.,* **489,** 425 (1989).

1223. C. Keegan, N. Wang, D. Heiman, J. Simpson, D. Backes, and M. Aden, *Clin. Chem.,* **32,** 1055 (abs. 026) (1986).

1224. H. Schutz and W. R. Schneider, *Z. Rechtsmed.,* **99,** 181 (1987).

1225. Y. H. Caplan and B. Levine, *Clin. Chem.,* **34,** 1271 (abs. 578) (1988).

1226. R. J. Straka, T. J. Hoon, R. L. Lalonde, J. A. Pieper, and M. B. Bottorff, *Clin. Chem.,* **33,** 1898 (1987).

1227. F. Koizumi, T. Kawamura, A. Ishimori, H. Ebina, and M. Satoh, *Tohoku J. Exp. Med.,* **155,** 159 (1988).

1228. N. Liappis, *Klin. Pediatr.,* **198,** 33 (1986).

1229. P. Wang, M. A. Morrison, and N. Wang, *Clin. Chem.,* **32,** 1061 (abs. 059) (1986).

1230. W. Vogt and I. Welsch, *Clin. Chem.,* **34,** 1459 (1988).

1231. P. Wang, V. Meucci, E. Simpson, M. Morrison, S. Lunetta, M. Zajac, and R. Boeckx, *Transplant. Proc.,* **22,** 1186 (1990).

1232. M. Plebani, L. Sciacovelli, C. D. Paleari, and A. Burlina, *Clin. Chem.,* **34,** 1183 (abs. 150) (1988).

1233. A. Sanghvi, W. Diven, H. Seltman, and T. Starzl, *Clin. Chem.,* **34,** 1904 (1988).

1234. T. J. Schroeder, A. J. Pesce, F. M. Hassan, J. R. Wermeling, A. Warner, K. T. Schlueter, and M. R. First, *Transplant. Proc.,* **20,** Suppl. 2, 345 (1988).

1235. B. G. Joyce and R. Bacchus, *Annals Saudi Medicine,* **9,** 52 (1989).

1236. R. Rondanelli, M. B. Regazzi, L. Gastaldi, P. Legnazzi, and P. Abelli, *Ther. Drug. Monit.,* **12,** 182 (1990).

1237. C. Montojo, M. V. Calvo, and A. Dominguez-Gil, *J. Clin. Pharm. Ther.,* **1,** 45 (1990).

1238. Y. Hayashi, N. Shibata, T. Minouchi, H. Shibata, T. Ono, and H. Shimakawa, *Ther. Drug. Monit.,* **11,** 205 (1989).

1239. W. Mraz, C. Müller, B. Molnar, and M. Knedel, *Transplant. Proc.,* **21,** 885 (1989).

1240. A. J. Pesce, T. J. Schroeder, and M. R. First, *Transplant. Proc.,* **22,** 1171 (1990).

1241. K. L. Napoli and B. D. Kahan, *Transplant. Proc.,* **22,** 1175 (1990).

1242. K. L. Napoli and B. D. Kahan, *Transplant. Proc.,* **22,** 1181 (1990).

1243. M. Plebani, C. D. Paleari, M. Masiero, D. Faggian, and A. Burlina, *Ther. Drug. Monit.,* **12,** 284 (1990).

1244. R. E. Dubler, D. Heiman, and D. Raden, *Clin. Chem.,* **32,** 1054 (abs. 013) (1986).

1245. T. Gates and M. Jenkins, *Clin. Chem.,* **34,** 1167 (abs. 070) (1988).

1246. P. Kinz, A. Tracqui, P. Mangin, A. Lugnier, and A. Chaumont, *Clin. Chem.,* **34,** 2374 (1988).

1247. J. Ramsey, T. Gates, K. Hranitzky, M. Jenkins, and J. Melerski, *Clin. Chem.,* **34,** 1167 (abs. 071) (1988).

1248. D. Nam, F. Ungemach, O. Meek, D. Backes, and J. Simpson, *Clin. Chem.,* **32,** 1057 (abs. 039) (1986).

1249. J. De Kanel, L. Dunlap, and T. D. Hall, *Clin. Chem.,* **35,** 2110 (1989).

1250. A. Poklis, *J. Anal. Toxicol.,* **11,** 228 (1987).

1251. C. E. McCord and J. R. McCutcheon, *J. Anal. Toxicol.,* **12,** 295 (1988).

1252. D. R. Sellers, M. Franklin, R. Behling, and P. Buchaklian, *Clin. Chem.,* **34,** 1206 (abs. 270) (1988).

1253. P. Painter, J. Evans, W. Law, Sr., and W. Law, Jr., *Clin. Chem.,* **34,** 1212 (abs. 290) (1988).

1254. L. K. Law, L. K. Cheung, and R. Swaminathan, *Clin. Chem.,* **34,** 1918 (1988).

1255. D. Armbruster, R. Harris, R. Scarbrough, and C. Tamez, *J. Clin. Lab. Anal.,* **2,** 3 (1988).

1256. D. R. Sellers, M. Kashik, and R. Behling, *Clin. Chem.,* **34,** 1209 (abs. 278) (1988).

1257. J. C. Ritchie, B. M. Belkin, K. R. Krishnan, C. B. Nemeroff, and B. J. Carroll, *Biol. Psychiatry,* **15,** 159 (1990).

1258. M. K. Gupta, C. E. Pippenger, K. Seifarth, and S. Hahn, *Clin. Chem.,* **34,** 1216 (abs. 310) (1988).

1259. I. Strarup-Brynes, G. Osikowicz, A. S. Vanderbilt, J. Fino, and M. T. Shipchandler, *Clin. Chem.,* **34,** 1170 (abs. 596) (1986).

1260. R. J. Brashear, C. H. Zeitvogel, G. J. Jackson, C. A. Flentge, L. L. Janulis, L. A. Cantrell, B. Schmidt, M. Adamczyk, D. A. Betebenner, and K. S. Vaughan, *Clin. Chem.,* **35,** 355 (1989).

1261. D. B. Gordon, *Clin. Exp. Hypertens., Part A,* **A10,** 485 (1988).

1262. L. G. Bennett and E. G. Chiapetta, Eur. Patent Appl. No. 210,410 (1987).

1263. M. G. Buitrago, F. Cava, A. G. Del-Campo, J. C. Moyano, and J. A. Navajo, *Clin. Chem.,* **34,** 595 (1988).

1264. C. Benattar, J. Francoual, J. F. Magny, and A. Lindenbaum, *Ann. Biol. Clin.,* **47,** 181 (1989).

1265. N. Gässler and W. G. Wood, *Ärztl. Lab.,* **35,** 165 (1989).

1266. R. A. A. Watson, J. Landon, E. J. Shaw, and D. J. Smith, *Clin. Chim. Acta,* **73,** 51 (1976).

1267. A. M. Sidki, K. Staley, H. Boyes, J. Landon, and A. H. Williams, *J. Clin. Chem. Clin. Biochem.,* **26,** 69 (1988).

1268. G. Gallacher, R. Coxon, J. Landon, C. J. Rae, and R. Abukinesha, *Ann. Clin. Biochem.,* **25,** 42 (1988).

1269. A. M. Sidki, I. H. Al-Abdulla, J. Landon, and F. J. Rowell, *J. Trop. Med. Public Health,* **18,** 149 (1987).

1270. A. P. Bennett, G. Gallacher, and J. Landon, *Ann. Clin. Biochem.,* **24,** 374 (1987).

1271. G. Gallacher, M. Hansell, and J. Landon, *Ther. Drug. Monit.,* **11,** 607 (1989).

1272. D. L. Colbert, D. S. Smith, J. Landon, and A. M. Sidki, *Clin. Chem.,* **30,** 1765 (1984).

1273. D. L. Colbert and M. Childerstone, *Clin. Chem.,* **33,** 1921 (1987).

1274. M. C. Hansell, F. J. Rowell, J. Landon, and A. M. Sidki, *Ann. Clin. Biochem.,* **23,** 596 (1986).

1275. G. W. Mellor and G. Gallacher, *Clin. Chem.,* **36,** 110 (1990).

1276. G. G. Granini, M. R. Eveland, and D. J. Krogstad, *Antimicr. Agents Chemother.,* **33,** 1275 (1989).

1277. A. A. Al-Ansari, D. S. Smith, and J. Landon, *J. Steroid. Biochem.,* **19,** 1475 (1983).

1278. M. Sawada, T. Yamaguchi, T. Sugimoto, S. Matsuura, and T. Nagatsu, *Clin. Chim. Acta,* **138,** 275 (1984).

1279. A. A. K. Al-Ansari, M. Massoud, L. A. Perry, and D. S. Smith, *Clin. Chem.,* **29,** 1803 (1983).

1280. D. A. Herold and M. H. Margrey, *Clin. Chem.,* **32,** 1112 (abs. 311) (1986).

1281. I. S. Kampa and J. I. Jarzabek, *Clin. Chem.,* **32,** 1054 (abs. 023) (1986).

1282. V. M. Haver, N. Audino, S. Burris, and M. Nelson, *Clin. Chem.,* **35,** 138 (1989).

1283. T. N. Awdziej, H. Y. Yee, B. Farrenkopf, R. A. Kaufman, P. S. Manchard, and P. S. Belica, *Clin. Chem.,* **32,** 1050 (abs. 002) (1986).

1284. G. F. Kapke and B. B. Bustamante, *Clin. Chem.,* **32,** 1054 (abs. 024) (1986).

1285. M. A. Chiarizia and S. C. Lewis, *Clin. Chem.,* **32,** 1079 (abs. 146) (1986).

1286. M. Y. Yee, R. A. Kaufman, C. B. Zanhoff, and A. Focella, *Clin. Chem.,* **32,** 1085 (abs. 179) (1986).

1287. B. Farrenkopf, R. A. Kaufman, and S. J. Salamone, *Clin. Chem.,* **32,** 1080 (abs. 151) (1986).

1288. K. Nithipatikom and L. B. McGown, *Talanta,* **36,** 305 (1989).

1289. P. Urios and N. Cittanova, *Anal. Biochem.,* **185,** 308 (1990).

1290. J. F. Burd, *Methods Enzymol.,* **74,** 79 (1981).

1291. R. C. Boguslaski, T. M. Li, J. L. Benovic, T. T. Ngo, J. F. Burd, and R. C. Carrico, "Substrate Labeled Homogeneous Fluorescent Immunoassay for Haptens and Proteins," in R. M. Nakamura, W. R. Dito, and E. S. Tucker III, Eds., *Immunoassays: Clinical Laboratory Techniques for the 1980s,* Alan R. Liss, Inc., New York, 1980.

1292. R. C. Wong, J. F. Burd, R. J. Carrico, R. T. Buckler, J. Thoma, and R. C. Boguslaski, *Clin. Chem.,* **25,** 686 (1979).

1293. J. F. Burd, *Clin. Chem.,* **25,** 1077 (abs. 071) (1979).

1294. J. F. Burd, R. J. Carrico, H. M. Kramer, and C. E. Denning, "Homogeneous Substrate-Labeled Fluorescent Immunoassay for Determining Tobramycin Concentrations in Human Serum," in S. B. Pal, Ed., *Enzyme Labelled Immunoassay of Hormones and Drugs,* Walter de Gruyter & Co., Berlin, 1978.

1295. A. G. Buchanan, E. Witwicki, and W. L. Albritton, *Am. J. Med. Technol.,* **49,** 437 (1983).

1296. G. R. Gotelli, M. F. Winter, and M. Mitchell, *Clin. Chem.,* **30,** 1110 (1984).

1297. J. F. Burd, R. C. Wong, J. E. Feeney, R. J. Carrico, and R. C. Boguslaski, *Clin. Chem.,* **23,** 1402 (1977).

1298. W. Hospes, R. J. Boskma, and J. R. B. J. Brouwers, *Pharm. Weekbl. Sci. Ed.,* **4,** 32 (1982).

1299. S. G. Thompson and J. F. Burd, *Antimicrob. Agents Chemother.,* **18,** 264 (1980).

1300. L. O. White, M. J. Bywater, and D. S. Reeves, *J. Antimicrob. Chemother.,* **12,** 403 (1983).

1301. U. Klotz, *Ther. Drug. Monit.,* **6,** 355 (1984).

1302. P. A. Toseland, J. F. Wicks, and R. G. Newall, *Ther. Drug. Monit.,* **5,** 501 (1983).

1303. G. Gonzales, A. Cid-Amador, B. Steele, and A. Castro, *Clin. Chem.,* **28,** 1494 (1982).

1304. S. J. Davis and V. Marks, *Ann. Clin. Biochem.,* **20,** 274 (1983).

1305. L. M. Krausz, J. B. Hitz, R. T. Buckler, and J. F. Burd, *Ther. Drug. Monit.,* **2,** 261 (1980).

1306. R. D. Johnson, L. J. Messenger, L. M. Krausz, R. T. Buckler, and J. F. Burd, *Clin. Chem.,* **27,** 1093 (abs. 348) (1981).

1307. D. B. Smith and G. F. Carl, *Arch. Neurol.,* **39,** 363 (1982).

1308. G. F. Carl, D. B. Smith, and L. P. Dunn, *Clin. Biochem.,* **15,** 298 (1982).

1309. T. M. Li, J. L. Benovic, R. T. Buckler, and J. F. Burd, *Clin. Chem.,* **27,** 22 (1981).

1310. B. Walter, *Clin. Chem.,* **27,** 1086 (abs. 311) (1981).

1311. K. Borner, *Fresenius Z. Anal. Chem.,* **301,** 112 (1980).

1312. A. Castro and B. Steele, *Clin. Biochem.,* **16,** 281 (1983).

1313. E. J. Coombes, T. R. Gamlen, G. F. Batstone, and S. T. Holgate, *Clin. Chim. Acta,* **136,** 187 (1984).

1314. J. J. MacKichan, J. D. Coyle, B. J. Shields, H. Boudoulas, and J. J. Lima, *Clin. Chem.,* **30,** 768 (1984).

1315. J. J. Lima, B. J. Shields, L. H. Howell, and J. J. MacKichan, *Ther. Drug. Monit.,* **6,** 203 (1984).

1316. H. Feinstein, H. Hovav, B. Fridlender, D. Inbar, and R. T. Buckler, *Clin. Chem.,* **28,** 1665 (1982).

1317. S. Tosoni, C. Signorini, and A. Albertini, *Ther. Drug. Monit.,* **7,** 236 (1985).
1318. J. D. Place and S. G. Thompson, *Antimicrob. Agents Chemother.,* **24,** 240 (1983).
1319. S. Pearson, J. M. Smith, and V. Marks, *Ann. Clin. Biochem.,* **21,** 208 (1984).
1320. S. M. Walker and R. E. Hill, *Clin. Chem.,* **29,** 1567 (1983).
1321. J. Patinkin, D. Inbar, C. Ben-Gigi, S. Derfler, Y. Klausner, and B. Fridlender, *J. Immunoassay,* **4,** 159 (1983).
1322. T. T. Ngo, R. J. Carrico, R. C. Boguslaski, and J. F. Burd, *J. Immunol. Methods,* **42,** 93 (1981).
1323. D. Worah, K. K. Yeung, F. E. Ward, and R. J. Carrico, *Clin. Chem.,* **27,** 673 (1981).
1324. A. C. Greenquist, B. Walter, and T. M. Li, *Clin. Chem.,* **27,** 1614 (1981).
1325. S. Tosoni, C. Signorini, and A. Albertini, *Clin. Chem.,* **29,** 991 (1983).
1326. K. J. Dean, S. G. Thompson, J. F. Burd, and R. T. Buckler, *Clin. Chem.,* **29,** 1051 (1983).
1327. F. Kohen, J. B. Kim, G. Barnard, and H. R. Lindner, *Biochim. Biophys. Acta,* **629,** 328 (1980).
1328. F. Kohen, J. B. Kim, H. R. Lindner, Z. Eshhar, and B. Green, *FEBS Lett.,* **111,** 427 (1980).
1329. R. A. Yoshida, Eur. Patent No. 15,695 (1980).
1330. E. F. Ullman, US Patent No. 3,998,943 (1976) and US Patent No. 4,161,515 (1979).
1331. R. F. Zuk, I. Gibbons, G. L. Rowley, and E. F. Ullman, US Patent No. 4,281,061 (1981).
1332. D. S. Smith, Eur. Patent No. 34,050 (1981).
1333. C. W. Parker, T. J. Yoo, M. C. Johnson, and S. M. Godt, *Biochemistry,* **11,** 3408 (1981).
1334. D. S. Smith, *FEBS Lett.,* **77,** 25 (1977).
1335. E. J. Shaw, R. A. A. Watson, J. Landon, and D. S. Smith, *J. Clin. Path.,* **30,** 526 (1977).
1336. D. S. Smith, Germ. Patent No. 2,716,276 (1977).
1337. L. O. White, L. M. Scammell, and D. S. Reeves, *J. Antimicrob. Chemother.,* **6,** 267 (1980).
1338. D. F. J. Brown, S. F. Birks, G. D. W. Curtis, and E. Perks, *J. Antimicrob. Chemother.,* **7,** 205 (1981).
1339. A. Broughton and M. Frazier, *Clin. Chem.,* **24,** 1033 (abs. 224) (1978).
1340. R. F. Müller, R. Palluk, K. Ehlenz, and M. A. Kempfle, *Studia Biophysica,* **123,** 19 (1988).
1341. A. J. Portman, S. A. Levison, and W. B. Dandliker, *Biochem. Biophys. Res. Commun.,* **43,** 207 (1971).
1342. D. E. Lopatin and E. W. Voss, Jr., *Biochemistry,* **10,** 208 (1971).

1343. D. S. Smith, M. H. H. Al-Hakiem, and J. Landon, *Ann. Clin. Biochem.,* **18,** 253 (1981).

1344. R. D. Nargessi and J. Landon, *Methods Enzymol.,* **74,** 60 (1981).

1345. R. F. Zuk, G. L. Rowley, and E. F. Ullman, *Clin. Chem.,* **25,** 1554 (1979).

1346. M. Hassan, J. Landon, and D. S. Smith, *J. Immunoassay,* **3,** 1 (1982).

1347. R. D. Nargessi, J. Landon, and D. S. Smith, *Clin. Chim. Acta,* **89,** 461 (1978).

1348. R. D. Nargessi, J. Landon, and D. S. Smith, *J. Immunol. Methods,* **26,** 307 (1979).

1349. J. M. Brinkley, G. L. Rowley, P. Singh, and E. F. Ullman, *Clin. Chem.,* **25,** 1077 (abs. 072) (1979).

1350. E. F. Ullman and M. Schwarzberg, US Patent No. 3,996,345 (1976).

1351. P. L. Khanna, "Fluorescence Energy Transfer Immunoassay," in T. T. Ngo, Ed., *Non-isotopic Immunoassays,* Plenum Press, New York, 1988.

1352. P. L. Khanna and E. F. Ullman, Eur. Patent No. 50,684 (1982) and US Patent No. 4,318,846 (1982).

1353. J. Calvin, K. Burling, C. Blow, I. Barnes, and C. P. Price, *J. Immunol. Methods,* **86,** 249 (1986).

1354. C. A. Fisher, P. C. Hsu, and G. M. Daffern, *Clin. Chem.,* **26,** 987 (1980).

1355. W. M. Eimstad, M. Schwarzberg, R. Rodgers, P. Khanna, C.-H. Chang, and E. F. Ullman, *Clin. Chem.,* **24,** 1015 (abs. 138) (1978).

1356. P. C. Hsu, S. D. King, T. J. Tarlow, and N. F. Bellet, *Clin. Chem.,* **26,** 1072 (1980).

1357. C. Tuttle, C.-J. Hsu, and L. Winfrey, *Clin. Chem.,* **26,** 1070 (1980).

1358. A. Lakshmi, W. Eimstad, N. Bellet, and C. Fisher, *Clin. Chem.,* **27,** 1075 (1981).

1359. K. Thorp, *Clin. Chem.,* **29,** 1189 (abs. 321) (1983).

1360. D. Quinn and P. McWhirter, *Clin. Chem.,* **29,** 1190 (abs. 323) (1983).

1361. C. S. Lim, J. N. Miller, and J. W. Bridges, *Anal. Biochem.,* **108,** 176 (1980).

1362. M. A. Phillips and I.-J. Ford, *Clin. Chem.,* **29,** 1190 (abs. 324) (1983).

1363. N. Bellet, L. Winfrey, A. Horton, A. Syed, P. Khanna, and W. Colvin, *Clin. Chem.,* **27,** 1071 (abs. 236) (1981).

1364. A. Duncan and W. Colvin, *Clin. Chem.,* **29,** 1190 (abs. 322) (1983).

1365. F. P. Anderson and W. G. Miller, *Clin. Chem.,* **34,** 1187 (abs. 169) (1988).

1366. D. J. Litman, Z. Harel, and E. F. Ullman, US Patent No. 4,318,707 (1982).

1367. G. Mathis and T. Davin, PCT Int. Patent Appl. WO 87/00927 (1987).

1368. R. Luedtke, C. S. Owen, and F. Karush, *Biochemistry,* **19,** 1182 (1980).

1369. C. J. Halfman, R. J. Dowe, and A. S. Schneider, *Clin. Chem.,* **34,** 1703 (1988).

1370. I. Wieder and R. L. Hale, PCT Int. Patent Appl. WO 87/07955 (1987).

1371. T. Kataoka, J. R. Williamson, and S. C. Kinsky, *Biochim. Biophys. Acta,* **298,** 158 (1973).

1372. W. J. Litchfield, J. W. Freytag, and M. Adamich, *Clin. Chem.,* **30,** 1441 (1984).

1373. H. R. Six, W. W. Young, Jr., K. Uemura, and S. C. Kinsky, *Biochemistry,* **13,** 4050 (1974).

1374. J. P. O'Connell, R. L. Campbell, B. M. Fleming, T. J. Mercolino, M. D. Johnson, and D. A. McLaurin, *Clin. Chem.,* **31,** 1424 (1985).

1375. J. Szebeni, E. E. Dilorio, H. Hauser, and K. H. Winterhalter, *Biochemistry,* **24,** 2827 (1985).

1376. G. K. Humphries and H. M. McConnell, *Proc. Natl. Acad. Sci. USA,* **71,** 1691 (1974).

1377. T. R. Hesketh, S. N. Payne, and J. H. Humphrey, *Immunology,* **23,** 705 (1972).

1378. B. Geiger and M. Smolarsky, *J. Immunol. Methods,* **17,** 7 (1977).

1379. J. W. Freytag and W. J. Litchfield, *J. Immunol. Methods,* **70,** 133 (1984).

1380. F. Szoka and D. Papahadjopoulos, *Proc. Natl. Acad. Sci. USA,* **75,** 4194 (1978).

1381. N. K. Childers, S. M. Michalek, J. H. Eldridge, F. R. Denys, A. K. Berry, and J. R. McGhee, *J. Immunol. Methods,* **119,** 135 (1989).

1382. K. Rokugawa, Y. Takiguchi, Y. Ishimori, T. Tsuneyoshi, M. Koyama, F. Watanabe, H. Matsuda, Y. Inui, and S. Sekine, *Clin. Chem.,* **34,** 1164 (abs. 056) (1988).

1383. J. N. Weinstein, S. Yoshikama, P. Henkart, R. Blumenthal, and W. A. Hagins, *Science,* **195,** 489 (1977).

1384. M. Fiechtner, M. Wong, C. Bieniarz, and M. T. Shipchandler, *Anal. Biochem.,* **180,** 140 (1989).

1385. D. A. Kendall and R. C. MacDonald, *Anal. Biochem.,* **134,** 26 (1983).

1386. F. S. Ligler, R. Bredehorst, A. Talebian, L. C. Shriver, C. F. Hammer, J. P. Sheridan, C.-W. Vogel, and B. P. Gaber, *Anal. Biochem.,* **163,** 369 (1987).

1387. M. Umeda, T. Tomita, H. Shibata, M. Seki, and T. Yasuda, *J. Clin. Microbiol.,* **26,** 804 (1988).

1388. F. Legros, P. Schietecat, C. P. Leroy, and J. P. Van Vooren, *J. Immunoassay,* **10,** 359 (1989).

1389. T. Ishizaki, N. Iwase, T. Ueno, and M. Umeda, *Clin. Chem.,* **36,** 1088 (abs. 640) (1990).

1390. Y. Ishimori, T. Yasuda, T. Tsumita, M. Notsuki, M. Koyama, and T. Tadakuma, *J. Immunol. Methods,* **75,** 351 (1984).

1391. M. Umeda, Y. Ishimori, K. Yoshikawa, M. Takada, and T. Yasuda, *J. Immunol. Methods,* **95,** 15 (1986).

1392. Y. Ishimori, M. Koyama, K. Rokugawa, S. Motoda, and H. Matsuda, *Clin. Chem.,* **35,** 1204 (abs. 662) (1989).

1393. Y. Ishimori, M. Hatoh, and M. Koyama, *Clin. Chem.,* **32,** 1067 (abs. 088) (1986).

1394. K. Hosoda and T. Yasuda, *J. Immunol. Methods,* **121,** 121 (1989).

1395. S. Sekine, S. Motoda, Y. Ishimori, K. Rokugawa, Y. Inui, and H. Matsuda, *Clin. Chem.,* **34,** 1164 (abs. 050) (1988).

1396. J. Barbet, P. Machy, and L. D. Leserman, *J. Supramolec. Struct. Cell. Biochem.,* **16,** 243 (1981).

1397. A. M. Butt, H. Rutner, M. Cobianchi, M. Baran, N. Y. Oraivej, and J. Readio, *Clin. Chem.,* **34,** 1255 (abs. 500) (1988).

1398. A. L. Plant, M. V. Brizgys, L. Locasio-Brown, and R. A. Durst, *Anal. Biochem.,* **176,** 420 (1989).

1399. M. A. Gerber, M.F. Randolph, and K. K. DeMeo, *J. Clin. Microbiol.,* **28,** 1463 (1990).

1400. C. J. Halfman and D. W. Jay, *Clin. Chem.,* **32,** 1677 (1986).

1401. I. Hemmilä and T. Lövgren, Eur. Patent Appl. 324,323 (1989).

1402. E. Soini, I. Hemmilä, and T. Lövgren, US Patent No. 4,587,223 (1986).

1403. V. B. Elings, D. F. Nicoli, and J. Briggs, *Methods Enzymol.,* **92,** 458 (1983).

1404. J. Briggs, V. B. Elings, and D. F. Nicoli, *Science,* **212,** 1266 (1981).

1405. J. E. I. Luotola and H. Harjunmaa, Eur. Patent Appl. 169,434 (1985).

1406. H. Harjunmaa, Eur. Patent Appl. 157,197 (1985).

1407. D. B. Wagner and R. A. Baffi, US Patent No. 4,680,275 (1987).

1408. E. Soini, *Trac.-Trend,* **9,** 90 (1990).

1409. E. Soini and T. Lövgren, "Time-Resolved Fluoroimmunoassay," in T. T. Ngo, Ed., *Non-isotopic Immunoassay,* Plenum Press, New York, 1988.

1410. T. Lövgren, I. Hemmilä, K. Pettersson, J. U. Eskola, and E. Bertoft, *Talanta,* **31,** 909 (1984).

1411. T. Lövgren, I. Hemmilä, K. Pettersson, and P. Halonen, "Time-Resolved Fluorometry in Immunoassay," in W. P. Collins, Ed., *Alternative Immunoassays,* Wiley, Chichester, UK, 1985.

1412. G. J. R. Barnard, J. L. Williams, A. C. Paton, and H. P. Shah, "Time-Resolved Fluoroimmunoassay," in W. P. Collins, Ed., *Complementary Immunoassays,* Wiley, Chichester, UK, 1988.

1413. G. Barnard, "The Development of Fluorescence Immunoassays," in B. D. Albertson and F. P. Haseltine, Eds., *Non-Radiometric Assays: Technology and Application in Polypeptide and Steroid Hormone Detection,* Alan R. Liss, Inc., New York, 1988.

1414. I. Hemmilä, E. Soini, and T. Lövgren, *Fresenius Z. Anal. Chem.,* **311,** 357 (1982).

1415. O. H. Meurman, I. A. Hemmilä, T. N. E. Lövgren, and P. Halonen, *J. Clin. Microbiol.,* **16,** 920 (1982).

1416. A. Kallner, G. Kallner, J.-G. Ljunggren, and H. E. Sjöberg, *OPMEAR,* **29,** 98 (1984).

1417. N. Paterson, E. M. Biggart, R. S. Chapman, and G. H. Beastall, *Ann. Clin. Biochem.,* **22,** 606 (1985).

1418. I. Böttger, H. W. Pabst, R. Senekowitsch, and H. Krieger, *Nucl. Med. Commun.,* **6,** 195 (1985).

1419. H.-L. Kaihola, K. Irjala, J. Viikari, and V. Näntö, *Clin. Chem.,* **31,** 1706 (1985).

1420. H. J. H. Kreutzer, J. F. W. Tertoolen, J. H. H. Thijssen, P. J. Der Kinderen, and H. P. F. Koppeschaar, *Clin. Chem.,* **32,** 2085 (1986).

1421. A. N. Savaser, N. Hosten, E. Schulz, L. Jorno, and R. Felix, *Labor. Praxis,* **10,** 998 (1986).

1422. A. M. Savaser, R. Felix, N. Hosten, E. Schulz, H. Huben, and K. Koppenhagen, *Nuc. Compact-Comp. News Nucl. Med.,* **17,** 146 (1986).

1423. S. Bruce, J. G. Ratcliffe, and A. D. Swift, *Commun. Lab. Med.,* **2,** 49 (1986).

1424. D. W. Chan, J. Kinzler, B. Almaraz, and H. Drew, *Clin. Chem.,* **32,** 1065 (abs. 075) (1986).

1425. N. Lawson, N. Mike, R. Wilson, and H. Pandov, *Clin. Chem.,* **32,** 684 (1986).

1426. J. A. Nisbet and S. Bird, *Clin. Chem.,* **32,** 201 (1986).

1427. A. Burlina, M. Blebani, and L. Perobelli, *Clin. Chem.,* **31,** 953 (abs. 262) (1985).

1428. F. Peter, S. T. Wang, and G. Strung, *Clin. Chem.,* **33,** 881 (abs. 007) (1987).

1429. M. Frölich, M. M. DePlanque, B. M. Goslings, and A. E. Meinders, *Clin. Chim. Acta,* **165,** 127 (1987).

1430. B. Lartigue, C. Lartigue, X. Montagutelli, F. Barreau, and A. Michaudet, *Le Biologiste,* **173,** 15 (1988).

1431. A. J. Parnham and I. F. Tarbit, *Clin. Chem.,* **33,** 1421 (1987).

1432. B. Thonnart, O. Messian, N. Colas Linhart, and B. Box, *Clin. Chem.,* **34,** 691 (1988).

1433. J. C. Libeer, L. Simonet, and R. Gillet, *Ann. Biol. Clin.,* **47,** 1 (1989).

1434. D. Sgoutas, E. Barton, M. Hammarstrom, P. Peters, and S. Sgoutas, *Clin. Chem.,* **35,** 1785 (1989).

1435. J. J. Body, F. Seraj, and V. Keymolen, *Clin. Chem.,* **35,** 497 (1989).

1436. E. M. Biggart, N. Paterson, S. Gillespie, F. C. Logue, B. Berry, R. S. Chapman, I. D. Hay, A. Reid, A. C. A. Glen, and G. H. Beastall, *J. Endocrin.,* **104,** Suppl., 125 (1985).

1437. J. C. Libeer, L. Simonet, and R. Gillet, *Ann. Clin. Biochem.,* **47,** 1 (1989).

1438. D. P. Schutte, W. J. H. Vermaak, W. J. Zakolski, and W. J. Kalk, *Med. Lab. Sci.,* **44,** 312 (1987).

1439. T. E. Torresani and R. Scherz, *Clin. Chem.,* **32,** 1013 (1986).

1440. J. Arends and B. Nørgaard-Pedersen, *Clin. Chem.,* **32,** 1856 (1986).

1441. A. N. Savaser, N. Hosten, E. Schulz, L. Jorno, and R. Felix, *Eur. J. Nucl. Med.,* **13,** 397 (1987).

1442. R. Dominici, C. Carducci, and C. Antonozzi, *Science Tools,* **33,** 27 (1986).

1443. H. W. van Hamersvelt, H. J. H. Kreutzer, J. F. W. Tertoolen, J. H. H. Thijssen, and H. P. F. Koppeschaar, *Netherland J. Medicine,* **35,** 192 (1989).

1444. J. Sander and C. Niehaus, *Clin. Chem.,* **32,** 1231 (1986).

1445. Y.-Q. Zhang and Z. Huang, *Chinese Medical Journal,* **102,** 862 (1989).

1446. U.-H. Stenman, H. Alfthan, L. Myllynen, and M. Seppälä, *Lancet,* **2,** 647 (1983).

1447. H. Alfthan and U.-H. Stenman, *J. Chromatography,* **470,** 385 (1989).

1448. H. Alfthan, *J. Immunol. Methods,* **88,** 239 (1986).

1449. U.-H. Stenman, H. Alfthan, T. Ranta, E. Vartiainen, J. Jalkanen, and M. Seppälä, *J. Clin. Endocrin. Metab.,* **64,** 730 (1987).

1450. H. Alfthan, U.-H. Stenman, and M. Seppälä, *Ann. Clin. Biochem.,* **24,** 250 (1987).

1451. T. Ranta, K. Ylinen, U.-H. Stenman, H. Nikula, and I. Huhtaniemi, *Clin. Endocrinol. Oxf.,* **29,** 495 (1988).

1452. D. Reid, A. Maturen, R. Prasad, and N. Biskup, *Clin. Chem.,* **32,** 1072 (1986).

1453. J. Mäkinen, L. Anttila, K. Irjala, T. Salmi, and H.-L. Kaihola, *Eur. J. Obstet. Gynecol. Reprod. Biol.,* **26,** 219 (1987).

1454. G. Banfi, E. Casari, M. Murone, and P. A. Bonini, *Clin. Chem.,* **35,** 1545 (1989).

1455. J. Brotherton, *Andrologia,* **21,** 407 (1989).

1456. J. Brotherton, *Human Reproduction,* **4,** 837 (1989).

1457. B. Lindblom, M. Hahlin, and P. Sjöblom, *Am. J. Obstet. Gynecol.,* **161,** 397 (1989).

1458. S. Peltyszyn, L. Mathez, and B. Nouri, *Clin. Chem.,* **36,** 1086 (abs. 630) (1990).

1459. H. Alfthan, J. Schröder, R. Fraser, A. Koskimies, H. Halila, and U.-H. Stenman, *Clin. Chem.,* **34,** 1758 (1988).

1460. H. Alfthan and U.-H. Stenman, *J. Clin. Endocrinol. Metab.,* **70,** 783 (1990).

1461. C. M. G. Thomas and M. F. G. Segers, *Clin. Chem.,* **35,** 1791 (1989).

1462. D. Apter, B. Cacciatore, H. Alfthan, and U.-H. Stenman, *J. Clin. Endocrinol. Metab.,* **68,** 53 (1989).

1463. L. Dunkel, H. Alfthan, U.-H. Stenman, and J. Perheentupa, *J. Clin. Endocrinol. Metab.,* **70,** 107 (1990).

1464. G. P. Brothea, A. J. Mills, V. M. Prabhakaran, R. Walsh, and V. Whelan, *Clin. Chem.,* **36,** 1204 (abs. 1179) (1990).

1465. F. Jockenhövel, S. A. Khan, and E. Nieschlag, *J. Clin. Chem. Clin. Biochem.,* **27,** 825 (1989).

1466. C. Bieglmayer and F. Fischl, *J. Clin. Chem. Clin. Biochem.,* **25,** 747 (1987).

1467. U. Fingscheidt, G. F. Weinbauer, S. A. Khan, and E. Nieschlag, *Acta Endocrinol.,* **122,** 96 (1990).

1468. U.-H. Stenman, H. Alfthan, A. Koskimies, M. Seppälä, K. Pettersson, and T. Lövgren, *Ann. N.Y. Acad. Sci.,* **422,** 544 (1984).

1469. K. S. I. Pettersson and J. R.-M. Söderholm, *Clin. Chem.,* **36,** 1928 (1990).

1470. U.-H. Stenman, H. Alfthan, and D. Apter, *Ann. Clin. Biochem.*, **24**, 250 (1987).

1471. C. L. Hughes, Jr., W. C. Dobson, D. K. Walmer, and S. B. Dixon, *J. Reprod. Med.*, **35**, 211 (1990).

1472. A.-M. Haavisto, L. Dunkel, K. Pettersson, and I. Huhtaniemi, *Pediatr. Res.*, **27**, 211 (1990).

1473. G. Banfi, M. Martinelli, M. Murone, and P. Bonini, *Clin. Chem.*, **36**, 1689 (1990).

1474. P. Vilja, *Clin. Chem.*, **36**, 1897 (1990).

1475. H. Dechaud, R. Bador, F. Claustrat, and C. Desuzinges, *Clin. Chem.*, **32**, 1323 (1986).

1476. M. U. Suonpää, J. T. Lavi, I. A. Hemmilä, and T. N. E. Lövgren, *Clin. Chim. Acta*, **145**, 341 (1985).

1477. E. J. Coombes, B. J. Moody, H. James, and C. Kelly, *J. Autom. Chem.*, **9**, 129 (1987).

1478. R. Goberna, C. Gonzales, J. M. Guerrero, and C. Marchante, *Clin. Chem.*, **34**, 1160 (abs. 035) (1988).

1479. A. Drobnies, D. McLellan, M. Tkachuk, and J. Toone, *Clin. Chem.*, **36**, 989 (abs. 177) (1990).

1480. C. Gonzales, J. M. Guerrero, C. Marchante, and R. Goberna, *Clin. Chem.*, **34**, 994 (1988).

1481. E. Toivonen, I. Hemmilä, J. Marniemi, P. Jørgensen, J. Zeuthen, and T. Lövgren, *Clin. Chem.*, **32**, 637 (1986).

1482. G. N. Hansen, B. L. Hansen, P. N. Jørgensen and C. K. Vogel, *Cell. Tissue Res.*, **256**, 507 (1989).

1483. S. A. Patkar, P. N. Jørgensen D. Bucher, I. Jensen, and J. Zeuthen, *Ann. Clin. Biochem.*, **24**, 247 (1987).

1484. S. Dobson, A. White, M. Hoadley, T. Lövgren, and J. Ratcliffe, *Clin. Chem.*, **33**, 1747 (1987).

1485. H. Hashida, K. Tanaka, S. Inoue, K. Hayakawa, and E. Ishikawa, *J. Clin. Lab. Anal.*, **5**, 38 (1991).

1486. C. Strasburger, G. Barnard, L. Toldo, B. Zarmi, Z. Zadik, A. Kowarski, and F. Kohen, *Clin. Chem.*, **35**, 913 (1989).

1487. C. J. Strasburger and F. Kohen, *J. Biolum. Chemilum.*, **4**, 112 (1989).

1488. B. Schmidt and G. Steinmetz, *Clin. Chem.*, **33**, 1070 (1987).

1489. U. Arumäe, T. Neuman, R. Sinijärv, and M. Saarma, *J. Immunol. Methods*, **122**, 59 (1989).

1490. K. Pesonen, H. Alfthan, U.-H. Stenman, L. Viinikka, and J. Perheentupa, *Anal. Biochem.*, **157**, 208 (1986).

1491. K. Pesonen, L. Viinikka, G. Myllylä, J. Kiuru, and J. Perheentupa, *J. Clin. Endocrinol. Metab.*, **68**, 486 (1989).

1492. G.-B. van Setten, *Curr. Eye Res.,* **9,** 79 (1990).

1493. S. Antonsen, *Ann. Clin. Biochem.,* **24,** Suppl. 2, 213 (1987).

1494. R. Bützow, H. Alfthan, U.-H. Stenman, H. Bohm, and M. Seppälä, *Clin. Chem.,* **34,** 1591 (1988).

1495. L. Riittinen, U.-H. Stenman, H. Alfthan, A.-M. Suikkari, H. Bohn, and M. Seppälä, *Clin. Chim. Acta,* **183,** 115 (1989).

1496. R. Koistinen, U.-H. Stenman, H. Alfthan, and M. Seppälä, *Clin. Chem.,* **33,** 1126 (1987).

1497. S. Niemi, O. Mäentausta, N. J. Bolton, and G. L. Hammond, *Clin. Chem.,* **34,** 63 (1988).

1498. C. M. G. Thomas, R. J. Van Der Berg, and M. F. G. Segers, *Clin. Chem.,* **33,** 2120 (1987).

1499. M. C. Patricot, B. Mathian, F. Later, and A. Revol, *Ann. Biol. Clin.,* **48,** 17 (1990).

1500. M. K. Gupta, K. Seifarth, G. P. Redmond, G. Gidwani, and W. Bergfeld, *Clin. Chem.,* **35,** 1143 (abs. 366) (1989).

1501. A. Mannila, I. Hemmilä, T. Lövgren, J. Zeuthen, and J. Marniemi, *Abstract of Papers Presented at the Nordic Congress of Clinical Chemistry,* Odense, Denmark, August 1986.

1502. P. Koskinen and K. Irjala, *Clin. Chem.,* **35,** 327 (1989).

1503. J. U. Eskola, T. J. Nevalainen, and T. N. E. Lövgren, *Clin. Chem.,* **29,** 1777 (1983).

1504. T. J. Nevalainen, J. U. Eskola, A. J. Aho, V. T. Havia, T. N. E. Lövgren, and V. Näntö, *Clin. Chem.,* **31,** 1116 (1985).

1505. J. U. Eskola and T. J. Nevalainen, *Mater. Med. Pol.,* **18,** 132 (1986).

1506. J. U. Eskola, T. J. Nevalainen, and P. Kortesuo, *Clin. Chem.,* **34,** 1052 (1988).

1507. T. J. Nevalainen and J. U. Eskola, *Klin. Wochenschr.,* **67,** 103 (1989).

1508. M. Büchler, P. Malfertheiner, H. Schädlich, T. Nevalainen, T. Mavromatis, and H. G. Beger, *Klin. Wochenschr.,* **67,** 186 (1989).

1509. P. Malfertheiner, T. Nevalainen, W. Uhl, H. Schädlich, and M. Büchler, *Klin. Wochenschr.,* **67,** 183 (1989).

1510. O. Itkonen, E. Koivunen, M. Hurme, H. Alfthan, T. Schröder, and U.-H. Stenman, *J. Lab. Clin. Med.,* **115,** 712 (1990).

1511. I. Joronen, V. K. Hopsu-Havu, M. Manninen, A. Rinne, M. Järvinen, and P. Halonen, *J. Immunol. Methods,* **86,** 243 (1986).

1512. V. K. Hopsu-Havu, I. Joronen, A. Rinne, and M. Järvinen, *Arch. Dermatol. Res.,* **277,** 452 (1985).

1513. I. Hemmilä, K. Pulkki, and K. Irjala, *Israel J. Clin. Biochem. & Lab. Sci.,* **4,** 52 (abs.) (1985).

1514. A. Tienhaara, J. U. Eskola, and V. Näntö, *Clin. Chem.,* **36,** 1961 (1990).

1515. M. Suonpää, T. Halonen, and K. Pettersson, *Clin. Chem.*, **45**, 1205 (abs. 670) (1989).

1516. O. M. Koch, G. Demetriades, G. Heidl, G. Wüst, and C. H. Hardenbicker, *J. Tumor Marker Oncology*, **3**, 197 (1988).

1517. E. H. Cooper, J. C. Knowles, D. Parker, and M. Taylor, *Biomed. Pharmacother.*, **42**, 189 (1988).

1518. P. Masson, B. Pålsson, Å. Andren-Sandberg, *Scand. J. Clin. Lab. Invest.*, **48**, 751 (1988).

1519. K. Hara, F. Mitsuhashi, T. Sakawaki, and H. Ohkura, *Jpn. J. Clin. Pathol.*, **37**, 789 (1989).

1520. O. C. Boerman, C. M. G. Thomas, M. F. G. Segers, P. Kenemans, T. Lövgren, V. R. Zurawski, H. J. Haisma, and L. G. Poels, *Clin. Chem.*, **33**, 2191 (1987).

1521. O. C. Boerman, M. F. G. Segers, L. G. Poels, P. Kenemans, and C. M. G. Thomas, *Clin. Chem.*, **36**, 888 (1990).

1522. O. Nilsson, E.-L. Jansson, C. Johansson, and L. Lindholm, *J. Tumor Marker Oncol.*, **3**, 314 (1988).

1523. C. Haglund, J. Lindgren, P. J. Roberts, P. Kuusela, and S. Nordling, *Br. J. Cancer*, **60**, 845 (1989).

1524. P. Vihko, R. Kurkela, J. Ramberg, I. Pelkonen, and R. Vihko, *Clin. Chem.*, **36**, 92 (1990).

1525. P. R. Huber, H. Fritschi, and Y. Schnell, *Clin. Chem.*, **36**, 1096 (abs. 674) (1990).

1526. K. Pettersson, J. Söderholm, E. Uribe, B. Nørgaard-Pedersen, C. Koch, and T. Lövgren, *Abstracts of Papers Presented at the International Screening Symposium of Newborn Errors of Metabolism*, No. 118, Sao Paolo, Brazil, Nov. 1988.

1527. H. Siitari and T. Lövgren, *Abstacts of Papers Presented at the Int. Symp. Monoclonal and DNA Probes in Diagnostic and Preventive Medicine*, Florence, Italy, April 1986.

1528. B. Nopper, F. Kohen, and M. Wilchek, *Anal. Biochem.*, **180**, 66 (1989).

1529. M. K. Viljanen, C. Backman, T. Veromaa, H. J. Frey, M. Reunanen, and G. K. Molnar, *Acta Neur. Scand.*, **69**, 361 (1984).

1530. Q. Vos and R. Benner, *Abstract of Papers Presented at the 7th International Congress of Immunology*, No. 121-67, Berlin, FRG, August 1989.

1531. Q. Vos and R. Benner, *J. Immunol. Methods*, **122**, 43 (1989).

1532. T. Kohno, T. Mitsukawa, S. Matsukura, and E. Ishikawa, *J. Clin. Lab. Anal.*, **4**, 224 (1990).

1533. C. Bonfanti, O. Meurman, and P. Halonen, *J. Virol. Methods*, **11**, 161 (1985).

1534. I. Hemmilä, M. Viljanen, and T. Lövgren, *Fresenius Z. Anal. Chem.*, **317**, 738 (1984).

1535. A. Aceti, F. Titti, P. Verani, S. Butto, A. Pennica, A. Sebastiani, and G. B. Rossi, *J. Virol. Methods,* **16,** 303 (1987).

1536. H. Siitari, P. Turunen, J. Schrimcher, and M. Nunn, *J. Clin. Microbiol.,* **28,** 2022 (1990).

1537. A. Aceti, A. Pennica, D. Celestino, S. B. Paparo, M. Caferro, S. Sanguigni, M. Marangi, and A. Sebastiani, *Trans. Roy. Soc. Tropic. Med. Hyg.,* **82,** 445 (1988).

1538. A. Aceti, A. Pennica, O. Leri, M. Caferro, A. Grilli, D. Celestino, V. Casale, A. Citarda, A. Grassi, and F. Sciarretta, *Lancet,* **2,** 505 (1989).

1539. A. Aceti, A. Pennica, M. Caferro, D. Celestino, B. S. Paparo, and A. Sebastiani, *Trans. Roy. Soc. Tropic. Med. Hyg.,* **81,** 764 (1987).

1540. H. Siitari, I. Hemmilä, E. Soini, T. Lövgren, and V. Koistinen, *Nature,* **301,** 258 (1983).

1541. H. Siitari and P. Laaksonen, *Abstracts of Papers Presented at the 7th Int. Congress of Virology,* Montreal, Canada, February 1987.

1542. G. Scalia, G. Gerna, and P. Halonen, *J. Medical Virol.,* **29,** 164 (1989).

1543. P. Halonen, C. Bonfanti, T. Lövgren, I. Hemmilä, and E. Soini, "Detection of Viral Antigens by Time-Resolved Fluoroimmunoassay," in K.-O. Habermehl, Ed., *Rapid Methods and Automation in Microbiology and Immunology,* Springer Verlag, Heidelberg, 1985.

1544. P. Halonen, O. Meurman, T. Lövgren, I. Hemmilä, and E. Soini, "Detection of Virus Antigens by Time-Resolved Fluoroimmunoassay," in P. A. Bachman, Ed., *Current Topics in Microbiology and Immunology, New Developments in Diagnostic Virology,* **104,** Springer Verlag, Berlin, 1983.

1545. P. Halonen, C. Bonfanti, M. Waris, T. Lövgren, and I. Hemmilä, "New Developments in Diagnostic Virology," in A. Sanna and G. Morage, Eds., *New Horizons in Microbiology,* Elsevier Science Publisher, Amsterdam, 1984.

1546. M.-T. Matikainen, P. Halonen, I. Hemmilä, and T. Lövgren, *Scand. J. Immunol.,* **18,** 77 (1983).

1547. J. C. Hierholzer, K. H. Johansson, L. J. Anderson, C. J. Tsou, and P. E. Halonen, *J. Clin. Microbiol.,* **25,** 1662 (1987).

1548. V. T. Ivanova, I. V. Ponomare, K. L. Shakhani, M. A. Yakhno, A. N. Slepushk, and A. P. Savitsky, *Vopr. Virusol.,* **35,** 115 (1990).

1549. M. L. Khristova, T. L. Busse, N. V. Zagidullin, S. V. Leonov, S. L. Rybalko, A. F. Frolov, and I. G. Kharitonenkov, *Vopr. Virusol.,* **34,** 538 (1989).

1550. I. G. Kharitonenkov, P. Halonen, M. L. Khristova, M. Kivivirta, T. L. Busse, and M. V. Sokolova, *Vopr. Virusol.,* **34,** 533 (1989).

1551. M. Kleemola and R. Räty, *Proceedings of the Sixth International Congress on Rapid Methods and Automation in Microbiology and Immunology,* No. 384, Espoo, Helsinki, Finland, June 1990.

1552. S. Nikkari, P. Halonen, I. Kharitonenkov, M. Kivivirta, M. Khristova, M. Waris, and A. Kendal, *J. Virol. Methods,* **23,** 29 (1989).

1553. H. H. Walls, K. H. Johansson, M. W. Harmon, P. E. Halonen, and A. P. Kendal, *J. Clin. Microbiol.,* **24,** 907 (1986).

1554. M. Waris, S. Nikkari, P. Halonen, I. Kharitonenkov, and A. Kendal, "Europium-Chelate and Horseradish Peroxidase Labelled Monoclonal Antibodies in Detection of Influenza Viruses," in A. Balows, R. C. Tilton, and A. Turano, Eds., *Rapid Methods and Automation in Microbiology and Immunology,* Brixia Academic Press, Brescia, Italy, 1989.

1555. V. T. Ivanova, I. V. Ponomareva, K. L. Shakhanina, M. A. Yakhno, A. N. Slepushkin, and A. P. Savitsky, *Vopr. Virusol.,* **35,** 115 (1990).

1556. M. Waris, P. Halonen, T. Ziegler, S. Nikkari, and G. Obert, *J. Clin. Microbiol.,* **26,** 2581 (1988).

1557. J. C. Hierholzer, P. G. Bingham, R. A. Coombs, K. H. Johansson, L. J. Anderson, and P. E. Halonen, *J. Clin. Microbiol.,* **27,** 1243 (1989).

1558. P. Middleton, C. Bonfanti, P. Halonen, T. Wall, M. Petric, and I. Hemmilä, *Abstract of Papers Presented at the Int. Conf. Canadian Association Clinical Microbiologists,* Cacmid, Canada, November 1984.

1559. N. De Jonge, O. C. Boerman, and A. M. Deelder, *Trans. Roy. Soc. Tropical Med. Hyg.,* **83,** 659 (1989).

1560. R. Sinijärv, L. Järvekülg, E. Andreeva, and M. Saarma, *J. Gen. Virol.,* **69,** 991 (1988).

1561. L. Järvekülg, J. Sõber, R. Sinijäv, and M. Saarma, *Dokl. VASHNIL.,* **12,** P15 (1987).

1562. L. Järvekülg, J. Sõber, R. Sinijärv, J. Toots, and M. Saarma, *Ann. Appl. Biol.,* **114,** 279 (1989).

1563. H. Siitari and A. Kurppa, *J. Gen. Virol.,* **68,** 1423 (1987).

1564. Y. Xu, Y. Wang, and X. Liu, *Yuan Zineng Kexua Jishu,* **21,** 602 (1987), Chemical abstract 109: 3343h.

1565. R. L. Hale and I. Wieder, US Patent No. 4,925,804 (1990).

1566. V. Näntö, K. Suonpää, J. Eskola, and T. Lövgren, *Isr. J. Clin. Biochem. Lab. Sci.,* **4,** 52 (1985).

1567. A.-C. Höglund, K. Blomberg, H. Mikola, and T. Lövgren, "Direct Measurement of T4 in Blood Spots Using a Time-Resolved Fluoroimmunoassay: A Comparison of Different Tracers," in B. J. Schmidt, A. J. Diament, and N. S. Loghin-Gross, Eds., *Current Trends in Infant Screening: Proceedings of the 7th International Screening Symposium,* Elsevier Science Publisher, Amsterdam, 1989.

1568. K. Blomberg, K. Suonpää, and T. Lövgren, *Biochim. Clinica,* **13,** Suppl. 1/8, 165 (abs. A53) (1989).

1569. P. Nuutila, P. Koskinen, K. Irjala, L. Linko, H.-L. Kaihola, J. U. Eskola, R. Erkkola, P. Seppälä, and J. Viikari, *Clin. Chem.,* **36,** 1355 (1990).

1570. P. Sjöblom, M. Wikland, M. Hahlin, L. Nilsson, and B. Lindblom, *Human Reprod.,* **5,** 396 (1990).

1571. R. Maserati, M. Autelli, P. Colombo, P. Pisati, and L. Bacchella, *Biochim. Clinica,* **13,** Suppl. 1/8, 163 (abs. A49) (1989).

1572. H. Dechaud, R. Bador, F. Claustrat, C. Desuzinges, and R. Mallein, *Clin. Chem.,* **34,** 501 (1988).

1573. M. A. Bacigalupo, L. Ferrara, G. Meroni, and A. Ius, *Fresenius Z. Anal. Chem.,* **328,** 263 (1987).

1574. A. Ius, L. Ferrara, G. Meroni, and M. A. Bacigalupo, *J. Steroid Biochem.,* **33,** 101 (1989).

1575. M. A. Bacigalupo, L. Ferrara, G. Meroni, and A. Ius, *J. Steroid. Biochem.,* **36,** 357 (1990).

1576. T. Ahola, K. Blomberg, and T. Lövgren, *Biochim. Clinica,* **13,** Suppl. 1/8, 164 (abs. A52) (1989).

1577. E. Bertoft, J. U. Eskola, V. Näntö, and T. Lövgren, *FEBS Lett.,* **173,** 213 (1984).

1578. E. Bertoft, O. Mäentausta, C. Sundqvist, and A. Lukola, *Anim. Reprod. Sci.,* **12,** 291 (1987).

1579. F. J. Lüke and W. Schlegel, *Fresenius Z. Anal. Chem.,* **337,** 97 (1990).

1580. F. J. Lüke and W. Schlegel, *Clin. Chim. Acta,* **189,** 257 (1990).

1581. J. A. Vilpo, S. Rasi, E. Suvanto, and L. M. Vilpo, *Anal. Biochem.,* **154,** 436 (1986).

1582. R. C. H. M. Oudejans, H. Voshol, T. K. F. Shulz, and A. M. T. Beenakkers, "Time-Resolved Fluorescence Immunoassay," in L. I. Gilbert and T. A. Miller, Eds., *Immunological Techniques in Insect Biology,* Springer Verlag, New York, 1988.

1583. P. Helsingius, I. Hemmilä, and T. Lövgren, *Isr. J. Clin. Biochem. Lab. Sci.,* **4,** 52 (1985).

1584. N. C. Paterson and M. J. Stewart, *Ann. Clin. Biochem.,* **24,** 205 (1987).

1585. S. M. Tadepalli and R. P. Quinn, *J. AIDS,* **3,** 19 (1990).

1586. J. M. Sailstad, K. H. Yedwell, F. R. Nelson, S. Y. Chang, and J. W. A. Findlay, *J. Clin. Immunoassay,* **13,** 53 (abs. 9) (1990).

1587. M.-L. Mäkinen, K. Pettersson, and M. Suonpää, *Clin. Chem.,* **35,** 1205 (abs. 669) (1989).

1588. E. P. Diamandis, R. C. Morton, E. Reichstein, and M. J. Khosravi, *Clin. Chem.,* **34,** 1157 (abs. 021) (1988).

1589. E. Diamandis, R. C. Morton, E. Reichstein, and M. J. Khosravi, *Anal. Chem.,* **61,** 48 (1989).

1590. T. K. Christopoulos, E. S. Lianidou, and E. P. Diamandis, *Clin. Chem.,* **36,** 1497 (1990).

1591. E. Reichstein, R. C. Morton, and E. Diamandis, *Clin. Chem.,* **34,** 1216 (abs. 309) (1988).

1592. E. Reichstein, R. C. Morton, and E. P. Diamandis, *Clin. Biochem.,* **22,** 23 (1989).

1593. E. Reichstein and E. P. Diamandis, *Clin. Chem.,* **35,** 1139 (abs. 345) (1989).
1594. A. Tan, M. J. Khosravi, and E. P. Diamandis, *Clin. Chem.,* **35,** 1139 (abs. 346) (1989).
1595. Y. K. Tan, M. J. Khosravi, and E. P. Diamandis, *J. Immunoassay,* **10,** 413 (1989).
1596. M. J. Khosravi and E. P. Diamandis, *Clin. Chem.,* **35,** 1138 (abs. 344) (1989).
1597. M. J. Khosravi and E. P. Diamandis, *Clin. Chem.,* **35,** 181 (1989).
1598. M. J. Khosravi, R. C. Morton, and E. P. Diamandis, *Clin. Chem.,* **34,** 1640 (1988).
1599. M. J. Khosravi and R. Sudsbury, *Clin. Chem.,* **35,** 2251 (1989).
1600. G. Ellis, F. J. Holland, and S. K. Makela, *Clin. Chem.,* **35,** 1150 (abs. 397) (1989).
1601. M. J. Khosravi and E. P. Diamandis, *Clin. Chem.,* **34,** 1221 (abs. 336) (1988).
1602. M. J. Khosravi and P. Shankaran, *Clin. Chem.,* **36,** 1101 (abs. 699) (1990).
1603. M. J. Khosravi and E. P. Diamandis, *Clin. Chem.,* **33,** 1994 (1987).
1604. M. J. Khosravi, *Clin. Chem.,* **36,** 169 (1990).
1605. I. Kahan, A. Papanastasiou-Diamandi, M. D'Costa, and E. Diamandis, *Clin. Chem.,* **34,** 1226 (abs. 357) (1988).
1606. I. Kahan, A. Papanastasiou-Diamandi, M. D'Costa, and E. P. Diamandis, *Clin. Chem. Enzym. Commun.,* **1,** 293 (1989).
1607. M. A. Chan and E. Diamandis, *Clin. Chem.,* **33,** 919 (abs. 190) (1987).
1608. M. A. Chan, A. Bellem, and E. P. Diamandis, *Clin. Chem.,* **33,** 2000 (1987).
1609. I. Kahan, A. Papanastasiou-Diamandi, G. Ellis, S. K. Makela, J.-A. McLaurin, M. D'Costa, and E. P. Diamandis, *Clin. Chem.,* **36,** 503 (1990).
1610. V. Bhayana and E. P. Diamandis, *Clin. Chem.,* **35,** 1077 (abs. 059) (1989).
1611. V. Bhayana and E. P. Diamandis, *Clin. Biochem.,* **22,** 433 (1989).
1612. M. J. Khosravi, M. A. Chan, A. C. Bellem, and E. P. Diamandis, *Clin. Chem.,* **34,** 1275 (abs. 600) (1988).
1613. M. J. Khosravi, M. A. Chan, A. C. Bellem, and E. P. Diamandis, *Clin. Chim. Acta,* **175,** 267 (1988).
1614. E. S. Lianidou, T. K. Christopoulos, and E. P. Diamandis, *Clin. Chem.,* **36,** 1130 (abs. 829) (1990).
1615. E. S. Lianidou, T. K. Christopoulos, and E. P. Diamandis, *Clin. Chem.,* **36,** 1679 (1990).
1616. E. P. Diamandis, A. Papanastasiou-Diamandi, V. Lustig, M. J. Khosravi, and A. Tan, *Clin. Chem.,* **35,** 1117 (abs. 241) (1989).
1617. E. P. Diamandis, A. Papanastasiou-Diamandi, V. Lustig, M. J. Khosravi, and A. Tan, *Clin. Chem.,* **35,** 1915 (1989).
1618. E. P. Diamandis, A. Papanastasiou-Diamandi, V. Lustig, M. J. Khosravi, and A. Tan, *Clin. Biochem.,* **22,** 413 (1989).

1619. M. Brown, Y. Shami, M. Zymulko, N. Singhnaz, and P. J. Middleton, *J. Clin. Microbiol.,* **28,** 1398 (1990).

1620. P. Shankaran, E. Reichstein, and E. P. Diamandis, *Clin. Chem.,* **35,** 1153 (abs. 413) (1989).

1621. P. Shankaran, E. Reichstein, M. J. Khosravi, and E. P. Diamandis, *J. Clin. Microbiol.,* **28,** 573 (1990).

1622. E. P. Diamandis and R. R. Ogilvie, *Ann. Clin. Biochem.,* **27,** 232 (1990).

1623. A. Papanastasiou-Diamandi, V. Bhayana, and E. P. Diamandis, *Clin. Chem.,* **34,** 1210 (abs. 281) (1988).

1624. A. Papanastasiou-Diamandi, V. Bhayana, and E. P. Diamandis, *Ann. Clin. Biochem.,* **26,** 238 (1989).

1625. V. Bhayana, Y. A. Tan, A. Papanastasiou-Diamandi, and M. J. Khosravi, *Clin. Chem.,* **36,** 1077 (abs. 586) (1990).

1626. Y. K. Tan, V. Bhayana, A. Papanastasiou-Diamandi, and M. J. Khosravi, *Clin. Chem.,* **36,** 1077 (abs. 585) (1990).

1627. Y. K. Tan, V. Bhayana, A. Papanastasiou-Diamandi, and M. J. Khosravi, *J. Immunoassay,* **11,** 123 (1990).

1628. E. Reichstein, Y. Shami, M. Ramjeesingh, and E. P. Diamandis, *Anal. Chem.,* **60,** 1069 (1988).

1629. E. P. Diamandis, V. Bhayana, K. Conway, E. Reichstein, and A. Papanastasiou-Diamandi, *Clin. Chem.,* **34,** 1216 (abs. 312) (1988).

1630. E. P. Diamandis, V. Bhayana, K. Conway, E. Reichstein, and A. Papanastasiou-Diamandi, *Clin. Biochem.,* **21,** 291 (1988).

1631. M. J. Khosravi, R. C. Morton, and E. Reichstein, *Clin. Chem.,* **36,** 1097 (abs. 681) (1990).

1632. T. Wong, J.-A. McLaurin, S. K. Makela, E. P. Diamandis, and G. Ellis, *Clin. Chem.,* **36,** 1150 (abs. 925) (1990).

1633. Y. Shami, E. Reichstein, M. Ramjeesingh, K. VanGulck, and M. Zywulko, *Clin. Chem.,* **32,** 1072 (abs. 114) (1986).

1634. A. Papanastasiou-Diamandi, K. Conway, and E. P. Diamandis, *J. Pharmaceut. Sci.,* **78,** 617 (1989).

1635. P. Matsson, A. Kuusisto, T. Crippen, I. Hemmilä, and E. Soini, *Cytometry,* **Suppl. 2,** 68 (abs. 409C) (1990).

1636. G. Barnard, F. Kohen, H. Mikola, and T. Lövgren, *Clin. Chem.,* **35,** 555 (1989).

1637. G. Barnard, C. O'Reilly, K. Dennis, and W. Collins, *Fertil. Steril.,* **52,** 60 (1989).

1638. J. M. Scherrmann, *Le Biologiste,* **21,** 481 (1987).

1639. J. Marchand, *Abstracts of Papers Presented at the International CIS Symposium,* Paris, France, January 1987.

1640. H. T. Karnes, J. S. O'Neal, and S. G. Schulman, "Luminescence Immunoassay," in S. G. Schulman, Ed., *Molecular Luminescence Spectroscopy,* Wiley-Interscience, New York, 1985.

1641. A. M. Sidki and D. S. Smith, Eur. Patent Appl. 10,926 (1984).

1642. A. M. Sidki and J. Landon, "Fluoroimmunoassays and Phosphoroimmunoassays," in W. P. Collins, Ed., *Alternative Immunoassays,* Wiley, Chichester, UK, 1985.

1643. A. M. Sidki, D. S. Smith, and J. Landon, *Clin. Chem.,* **32,** 53 (1986).

1644. M. R. Glick and J. D. Winefordner, *Anal. Chem.,* **60,** 1982 (1988).

1645. F. V. Bright and L. B. McGown, *Talanta,* **32,** 15 (1985).

1646. K. Nithipatikom and L. B. McGown, *Anal. Chem.,* **59,** 423 (1987).

1647. T. Vo-Dinh, T. Nolan, Y. F. Cheng, M. J. Sepaniak, and J. P. Alarie, *Appl. Spectrosc.,* **44,** 128 (1990).

1648. O. S. Wolfbeis, *Appl. Fluoresc. Technol.,* **1,** 1 (1989).

1649. M. Aizawa, S. Kato, and S. Suzuki, *J. Membr. Sci.,* **2,** 125 (1977).

1650. N. Yamamoto, Y. Nagasawa, M. Sawai, T. Sudo, and H. Tsubomura, *J. Immunol. Methods,* **22,** 309 (1978).

1651. K. Shiba, Y. Umezawa, T. Watanabe, S. Ogawa, and S. Fujiwara, *Anal. Chem.,* **52,** 1610 (1980).

1652. M. Aizawa, A. Morioka, S. Suzuki, and Y. Nagamura, *Anal. Biochem.,* **94,** 22 (1979).

1653. J. Wangsa and M. A. Arnold, *Anal. Chem.,* **60,** 1080 (1988).

1654. J. F. Place, R. M. Sutherland, and C. Dähne, *Biosensors,* **1,** 321 (1985).

1655. W. R. Seitz, *J. Clin. Lab. Anal.,* **1,** 313 (1987).

1656. R. D. Petrea, M. J. Sepaniak, and T. Vo-Dinh, *Talanta,* **35,** 139 (1988).

1657. N. Opitz and D. W. Lübbers, *Talanta,* **35,** 123 (1988).

1658. R. Parry, G. A. Robinson, J. J. Skehel, and G. C. Torrest, "Surface Plasmon Resonance Immunosensors," in A. Balows, R. C. Tilton, and A. Turano, Eds., *Rapid Methods and Automation in Microbiology and Immunology,* Brixia Academic Press, Brescia, Italy, 1989.

1659. S. G. Weber, D. M. Morgan, and J. M. Elbicki, *Clin. Chem.,* **29,** 1665 (1983).

1660. R. M. Sutherland, C. Dähne, A. Bregnard, E. Hybl, and J.-L. Maystre, "Evanescent Wave Immunoassays," in W. P. Collins, Ed., *Complementary Immunoassays,* Wiley, Chichester, UK, 1988.

1661. J. T. Ives, W. M. Reichert, J. N. Lin, V. Hlady, D. Reinecke, P. A. Suci, R. A. VanWagenen, K. Newby, J. Herron, P. Dryden, and J. D. Andrade, "Total Internal Reflection Fluorescence Surface Sensors," in A. N. Chester, S. Martelluci, and A. M. Verga Scheggi, Eds., *Optical Fiber Sensors,* NATO ASI Series E No. 132, Martinus Nijhoff Publishers, Dordrecht, 1987.

1662. D. De Rossi, A. Nannini, and M. Monici, "Immobilized Antibodies—Fiber Optic Sensor for Biomedical Measurement," in A. N. Chester, S. Martelluci, and A. M. Verga Scheggi, Eds., *Optical Fiber Sensors,* NATO ASI Series E No. 132, Martinus Nijhoff Publishers, Dordrecht, 1987.

1663. R. M. Sutherland, C. Dähne, J. F. Place, and A. R. Ringrose, *J. Immunol. Methods,* **74,** 253 (1984).

1664. R. M. Sutherland, C. Dähne, J. F. Place, and A. R. Ringrose, *Clin. Chem.,* **30**, 1533 (1984).

1665. D. E. Yoshida, J. T. Ives, W. M. Reichert, D. A. Christensen, and J. D. Andrade, *SPIE,* **904**, 57 (1988).

1666. R. A. Badley, R. A. L. Drake, I. A. Shanks, A. M. Smith, and P. R. Stephenson, *Phil. Trans. R. Soc. Lond.,* **316**, 143 (1987).

1667. R. P. Parry, C. Love, and G. A. Robinson, *J. Virol. Methods,* **27**, 39 (1990).

1668. B. J. Tromberg, M. J. Sepaniak, T. Vo-Dinh, and G. Griffin, *Anal. Chem.,* **59**, 1226 (1987).

1669. J. D. Andrade, J. Herron, J. N. Lin, H. Yen, J. Kopecek, and P. Kopeckova, *Biomaterials,* **9**, 76 (1988).

1670. D. Medows and J. S. Schultz, *Talanta,* **35**, 145 (1988).

1671. J. D. Andrade and R. A. Van Wagenen, US Patent No. 4,368,047 (1983).

1672. T. Vo-Dinh, B. J. Tromberg, G. D. Griffin, K. R. Ambrose, M. J. Sepaniak, and E. M. Gardenhire, *Appl. Spectrosc.,* **41**, 753 (1987).

1673. B. Reck, K. Himmelspach, N. Opitz, and D. W. Lübbers, *Analyst,* **113**, 1423 (1988).

1674. M. Thompson and E. T. Vandenberg, *Clin. Biochem.,* **19**, 255 (1986).

1675. R. H. Yolken and F. J. Leister, *J. Clin. Microbiol.,* **15**, 757 (1982).

1676. E. Ishikawa and K. Kato, *Scand. J. Immunol.,* **8**, Suppl. 7, 43 (1978).

1677. B. Portmann, T. Portmann, E. Nugel, and U. Evers, *J. Immunol. Methods,* **79**, 27 (1985).

1678. J. P. Gosling, *Clin. Chem.,* **36**, 1408 (1990).

1679. H. Shah, A.-M. Saranko, M. Härkönen, and H. Adlercreutz, *Clin. Chem.,* **30**, 185 (1984).

1680. N. Watanabe, Y. Niitsu, S. Ohtsuka, J.-I. Koseki, Y. Kohgo, I. Urushizaki, K. Kato, and E. Ishikawa, *Clin. Chem.,* **25**, 80 (1979).

1681. M. Imagawa, E. Ishikawa, S. Yoshitake, K. Tanaka, H. Kan, M. Inada, H. Imura, H. Kurosaki, S. Tachibana, M. Takagi, M. Nishiura, N. Nakazawa, H. Ogawa, Y. Tsunetoshi, and K. Nakajima, *Clin. Chim. Acta,* **126**, 227 (1982).

1682. K. Ruan, S. Hashida, S. Yoshitake, E. Ishikawa, O. Wakisaka, Y. Yamamoto, T. Ichioka, and K. Nakajima, *Clin. Chim. Acta,* **147**, 167 (1985).

1683. R. E. Fulton, J. P. Wong, Y. M. Siddiqui, and M. S. Tso, *J. Virol. Methods,* **22**, 149 (1988).

1684. K. Matsuoka, M. Maeda, and A. Tsuji, *Chem. Pharm. Bull.,* **27**, 2345 (1979).

1685. W. D. Hinsberg, K. H. Milby, and R. N. Zare, *Anal. Chem.,* **53**, 1509 (1981).

1686. S. Hashida, E. Ishikawa, Z.-I. Mohri, T. Nakanishi, H. Noguchi, and Y. Murakami, *Endocrinol. Japon.,* **35**, 171 (1988).

1687. M. Imagawa, S. Yoshitake, E. Ishikawa, Y. Niitsu, I. Urushizaki, R. Kanazawa, S. Tachibana, N. Nakazawa, and H. Ogawa, *Anal. Lett.,* **14**, 1679 (1981).

1688. K. Sugimoto, K. Zaitsu, and Y. Ohkura, *Anal. Chim. Acta,* **169**, 133 (1985).

1689. K. Tanaka, E. Ishikawa, Y. Ohmoto, and Y. Hirai, *Clin. Chim. Acta,* **166,** 237 (1987).

1690. K. Kitamura, K. Matsuda, M. Ide, T. Tokunaga, and M. Honda, *J. Immunol. Methods,* **121,** 281 (1989).

1691. Y. Nishida, H. Kawai, and H. Nishino, *Clin. Chim. Acta,* **153,** 93 (1985).

1692. Y. Oka, K. Sakamoto, H. Ikeda, S. Nagoshi, S. Tsukagoshi, M. Aburada, H. Endou, and K. Fujiwara, *Biochem. Intern.,* **16,** 941 (1988).

1693. T. Hayashi, K. Hashimoto, and S. Sakamoto, *J. Pharmacolbio-Dyn.,* **12,** 410 (1989).

1694. A. Klos, V. Ihrig, M. Messner, J. Grabbe, and D. Bitter-Suermann, *J. Immunol. Methods,* **111,** 241 (1988).

1695. J. R. Dave, P. Taylor, J. M. Grange, and H. Gaya, *J. Med. Microbiol.,* **21,** 271 (1986).

1696. M. W. Harmon, L. I. Russo, and S. Z. Wilson, *J. Clin. Microbiol.,* **17,** 305 (1983).

1697. S. W. Hildreth, B. J. Beaty, J. M. Meegan, C. L. Frazier, and R. E. Shope, *J. Clin. Microbiol.,* **15,** 879 (1982).

1698. N. N. Kushner, C. H. Riggin, M. E. Annunziato, and D. J. Marciani, *J. Immunol. Methods,* **114,** 253 (1988).

1699. M. Leinonen, P. Saikku, M. Nurminen, and A. Lassus, *Eur. J. Clin. Microbiol.,* **6,** 659 (1987).

1700. J. A. Aleixo and B. Swaminathan, *J. Immunoassay,* **9,** 83 (1988).

1701. B. S. Leung and J. R. Scott, *J. Clin. Immunoassay,* **12,** 154 (1989).

1702. N. Schmeer, H.-P. Müller, W. Baumgärtner, J. Wieda, and H. Krauss, *J. Clin. Microbiol.,* **26,** 2520 (1988).

1703. N. Tumosa and L. Kahan, *J. Immunol. Methods,* **116,** 59 (1989).

1704. K. C. Wang and B. S. Leung, *J. Immunol. Methods,* **84,** 279 (1985).

1705. A. Ali and R. Ali, *J. Immunol. Methods,* **56,** 341 (1983).

1706. C. E. Jones, J. F. Pike, R. P. Dickinson, and R. J. Rousseau, *Am. J. Clin. Pathol.,* **75,** 509 (1981).

1707. Y.-G. Tsay and G. M. Halpern, *Immunol. Allergy Practice,* **6,** 169 (1984).

1708. H. S. Rock, J. R. Scott, and S. Harri, *Clin. Chem.,* **33,** 918 (abs. 185) (1987).

1709. E. Crimi, V. Brusasco, P. Crimi, M. Brancatisano, and A. Bregante, *Annals Allergy,* **61,** 371 (1988).

1710. J. L. Gueant, D. A. Moneret-Vautrin, G. Dejardin, C. Algalarondo, J. P. Nicolas, and J. P. Grilliat, *Allergy,* **44,** 204 (1989).

1711. M. Sakaguchi and S. Inouye, *Microbiol. Immunol.,* **31,** 711 (1987).

1712. T. Nakazawa, K. Sato, and J. Tsuchiya, *Ann. Allergy,* **61,** 214 (1988).

1713. A. S. Palacios, J. C. M. Escudero, J. S. J. Diez, J. G. Alonso, and M. A. S. Palacios, *Allerg. Immunopathol.,* **16,** 33 (1988).

1714. M. A. Pesce and S. H. Bodourian, *Clin. Chem.,* **26** 971 (abs. 057) (1980).

1715. E. J. Fione, G. M. Banowetz, B. B. Krygier, J. M. Kathrein, and L. Sayavedra-Soto, *Anal. Biochem.,* **162,** 301 (1987).

1716. R. J. Bjercke, G. Cook, and J. J. Langone, *J. Immunol. Methods,* **96,** 239 (1987).

1717. A. O. Turkes, A. Turkes, B. G. Joyce, and D. Riad-Fahmy, *Steroids,* **35,** 89 (1980).

1718. H. Arakawa, M. Maeda, A. Tsuji, H. Naruse, E. Suzuki, and A. Kambegawa, *Chem. Pharm. Bull.,* **31,** 2724 (1983).

1719. H. Arakawa, M. Maeda, and A. Tsuji, *J. Immunoassay,* **6,** 347 (1985).

1720. H. Shah, A. M. Saranko, M. Härkönen, and H. Adlercreutz, *Clin. Chem.,* **30,** 185 (1984).

1721. G. B. Wisdom, *Clin. Chem.,* **22,** 1243 (1976).

1722. K. Miyai, *Adv. Clin. Chem.,* **24,** 61 (1985).

1723. T. T. Ngo and H. M. Lenhof, *Appl. Biochem. Biotechnol.,* **6,** 53 (1981).

1724. M. Cobb and S. Gotcher, *Am. J. Med. Technol.,* **48,** 671 (1982).

1725. B. A. Berman, P. B. Boggs, R. E. Lee, Jr., and J. G. Leonardy, Jr., *Ann. Allergy,* **61,** 300 (1988).

1726. J. M. Seltzer, G. M. Halpern, and Y.-G. Tsay, *Ann. Allergy,* **54,** 25 (1985).

1727. A. Pécoud, R. Peitrequin, J. Fasel, and P. C. Frei, *Allergy,* **41,** 243 (1986).

1728. L. Yman and A. Kober, *Clin. Chem.,* **36,** 1107 (abs.728) (1990).

1729. J. L. Giegel and M. M. Brotherton, US Patent No. 4,786,606 (1988).

1730. J. L. Giegel, M. M. Brotherton, P. Cronin, M. D'Aquino, S. Evans, Z. H. Heller, W. S. Knight, K. Krishnan, and M. Sheiman, *Clin. Chem.,* **28,** 1894 (1982).

1731. H. T. Wong and S. Hutchins, *Clin. Chem.,* **34,** 1178 (abs. 124) (1988).

1732. D. Sacks, M. Lim, R. Valdes Jr., and G. Kessler, *Clin. Chem.,* **34,** 1211 (abs. 287) (1988).

1733. D. B. Sacks, M. M. Lim, C. A. Parvin, and G. Kessler, *Clin. Chem.,* **36,** 1343 (1990).

1734. P. Bush and J. Rudy, *Clin. Chem.,* **35,** 111 (abs. 215) (1989).

1735. L. C. Rogers, S. E. Kahn, T. H. Oeser, and E. W. Bermes, Jr., *Clin. Chem.,* **32,** 1402 (1986).

1736. J. A. Rugg, K. Leung, P. Singh, S. L. Lamar, R. Tokarski, C. W. Flaa, M. M. Brotherton, and S. A. Evans, *Clin. Chem.,* **32,** 1167 (abs. 584) (1986).

1737. L. C. Rogers, S. E. Kahn, E. W. Holmes, T. H. Oeser, and E. W. Bermes, Jr., *Clin. Chem.,* **32,** 1117 (abs. 334) (1986).

1738. C. J. Beinlich and R. H. Carpenter, *Clin. Chem.,* **33,** 167 (1987).

1739. F. J. Ryan and C. McKenzie, *Clin. Chem.,* **32,** 1168 (abs. 585) (1986).

1740. R. J. van der Berg, M. F. G. Segers, and C. M. G. Thomas, *Clin. Chem.,* **36,** 697 (1990).

1741. K. Leung, S. R. Dawson, and J. A. Rugg, *Clin. Chem.,* **34,** 1221 (abs. 334) (1988).

1742. C. Flaa, L. Rodriguez, K. Leung, S. Dawson, and J. Rugg, *Clin. Chem.,* **34,** 1221 (abs. 333) (1988).

1743. N. Mahmood, S. Srebro, M. McCarthy, M. Brotherton, T. Hunter, and C. DeMarco, *Clin. Chem.,* **35,** 1095 (abs. 141) (1989).

1744. R. Rosecrans, D. Buttita, A. Olley, and F. Serna, *Clin. Chem.,* **35,** 1090 (abs. 115) (1989).

1745. M. Vernet, M.-C. Revenant, A. Ried, C. Naudin, M. Jauneau, T. Olivier, and J.-C. Ruiz, *Clin. Chem.,* **35,** 672 (1989).

1746. J. Singh, E. Pang, L. Lucco, A. W. Dudley, Jr., S. R. Diaz, C. Mayfield, L. Dimanina, K. Kulig, and L. I. Carreras, *Clin. Chem.,* **34,** 1276 (abs. 602) (1988).

1747. D. J. Jirinzu, R. Scarbrough, and J. Williams, *Clin. Chem.,* **34,** 1153 (abs. 001) (1988).

1748. H. T. Wong and A. I. Lipsey, *Clin. Chem.,* **34,** 1165 (abs. 061) (1988).

1749. G. DeSchrijver, R. J. Wieme, and L. Pittoors, *Anal. Chim. Acta,* **170,** 139 (1985).

1750. G. E. Stahlschmidt, C. H. Smith, R. E. Miller, and M. Landt, *Clin. Chem.,* **34,** 433 (1988).

1751. R. Sapin, F. Gassler, and J. L. Schlienger, *Clin. Chem.,* **34,** 2159 (1988).

1752. C. B. Morejon, A. Soto, R. Timmons, J. Delgado, P. Singh, W. C. Ni, and T. Hunter, *Clin. Chem.,* **34,** 1213 (1988).

1753. J. E. Monticello, D. Smith, T. Hunter, P. Singh, M. Manes, and A. Soto, *Clin. Chem.,* **34,** 1257 (1988).

1754. M. Sheiman, S. Srebro, M. McCarthy, P. Singh, and W. Knight, *Clin. Chem.,* **32,** 1083 (abs. 165) (1986).

1755. M. Sheiman, N. Mahmood, S. Srebro, M. McCarthy, P. Singh, and W. Knight, *Clin. Chem.,* **32,** 1084 (abs. 172) (1986).

1756. R. B. Richerson, D. M. Babik, M. E. Venetucci, and E. A. Ogunro, *Clin. Chem.,* **34,** 1219 (abs. 324) (1988).

1757. R. J. M. van Oers, B. Leerkes, and I. Bertschi, *J. Clin. Chem. Clin. Biochem.,* **28,** 59 (1990).

1758. D. S. Trundle, P. P. Chou, and A. Raymond, *Clin. Chem.,* **36,** 554 (1990).

1759. C. H. Keller, P. Fries, E. Kline, R. Kucera, S. Hsu, A. Isaksson, and K. Neider, *Clin. Chem.,* **35,** 1142 (abs. 362) (1989).

1760. C. H. Keller, P. Fries, E. Kline, K. Neider, P. Doles, and E. A. Ogunro, *Clin. Chem.,* **36,** 697 (1990).

1761. D. A. Armbruster and L. C. Hawes, *J. Clin. Lab. Anal.,* **4,** 170 (1990).

1762. K. A. Ford, H. N. Baker, J. G. Baar, D. Balay, D. Marlewski, M. Venetucci, and E. A. Ogunro, *Clin. Chem.,* **35,** 2333 (1989).

1763. J. B. Bodner, L. Klein, J. G. Baar, J. Bogacz, J. Strarup-Brygnes, E. Necklaws, and R. B. Richerson, *Clin. Chem.*, **36**, 1100 (abs. 692) (1990).

1764. B. Dowell, K. Bryg, K. Wikstrom, K. Beykirch, J. Rapp, and M. Shaw, *Clin. Chem.*, **34**, 1161 (abs. 043) (1988).

1765. B. Dowell, K. Borden, and N. Shaw, *Clin. Chem.*, **35**, 1192 (abs. 598) (1989).

1766. G. Barnes, A. Danna, C. Miceli, D. Massie, V. Loos, and N. Shaw, *Clin. Chem.*, **33**, 919 (abs. 192) (1987).

1767. G. Osikwoicz, P. Fries, J. Bogacz, C. Forsythe, K. Chacko, and A. S. Vanderbilt, *Clin. Chem.*, **34**, 1155 (abs. 011) (1988).

1768. P. P. Chou, R. A. Toms, B. King, A. Chang, and S. Longhurst, *Clin. Chem.*, **35**, 1099 (abs. 158) (1989).

1769. E. Mizuochi, H. Yamanashi, K. Obata, M. Takai, K. Iinuma, and K. Kurata, *Clin. Chem.*, **35**, 1192 (abs. 599) (1989).

1770. D. Giacherio and R. Pyzik-Shuler, *Clin. Chem.*, **36**, 1132 (abs. 839) (1990).

1771. D. Delfert, S. George, M. Rojewski, J. McCray, A. Crary, S. Wang, J. Grams, and W. King, *Clin. Chem.*, **36**, 1095 (abs. 671) (1990).

1772. A. Smith, R. Carsters, S. O'Morchoe, B. Prine, E. Tanghal, K. Wikstrom, R. Wilhoite, and M. Hass, *Clin. Chem.*, **36**, 1096 (abs. 675) (1990).

1773. C. Schlesinger, K. Bryg, T. Danna, L. Lauren, C. Miceli, D. Walsh, and N. Shaw, *Clin. Chem.*, **36**, 1096 (abs. 677) (1990).

1774. J. M. Clemens, W. W. Schmidt, and K. W. Wicklund, *Clin. Chem.*, **34**, 1154 (abs. 008) (1988).

1775. W. Schmidt, J. Clemens, L. Rogers, H. P. Covault, and S. Hojvat, *Clin. Chem.*, **35**, 1152 (abs. 406) (1989).

1776. J. Clemens, W. Black, E. W. Holmes, and S. Hojvat, *Clin. Chem.*, **35**, 1095 (abs. 142) (1989).

1777. K. S. Eble, M. Rynning, P. Hutten, and L. Nelson, *Clin. Chem.*, **35**, 1193 (abs. 602) (1989).

1778. K. S. Eble, L. Ducharme, and J. Stojak, *Clin. Chem.*, **35**, 1193 (abs. 603) (1989).

1779. A. M. Spronk, L. Pavlis-Jenkins, L. S. Schmidt, S. Taskar, and J. A. Brady, *Clin. Chem.*, **35**, 1193 (abs. 605) (1989).

1780. R. M. Pennington, L. J. Filar, J. M. Staller, C. K. Hillebrand, and L. S. Paul, *Clin. Chem.*, **34**, 1154 (abs. 007) (1988).

1781. L. E. Schaefer, J. W. Dyke, F. D. Meglio, P. R. Murray, W. Crafts, and A. C. Niles, *J. Clin. Microbiol.*, **27**, 2410 (1989).

1782. A. Raymond, H. Bradley, F. Simpkins, and D. Trundle, *Clin. Chem.*, **35**, 1105 (abs. 189) (1989).

1783. S. Longhurst, P. P. Chou, R. A. Toms, B. King, and A. Chang, *Clin. Chem.*, **35**, 1099 (abs. 159) (1989).

1784. D. R. Brandt, C. M. Forsythe, D. M. Babik, R. C. Gates, K. K. Eng, S. D. Figard, R. J. Kucera, B. J. Green, and R. B. Richerson, *Clin. Chem.,* **36,** 1079 (abs. 593) (1990).

1785. K. Ford, D. E. Caplan, D. D. Tobias, J. E. Turn, and E. Osikowicz, *Clin. Chem.,* **36,** 1099 (abs. 687) (1990).

1786. S. G. Kummerle, G. L. Boltinghouse, S. M. Delby, T. L. Lane, and R. P. Simondsen, *Clin. Chem.,* **36,** 969 (abs. 084) (1990).

1787. P. Freeley, P. Wong, G. Whiteley, K. Conte, K. Dray-Lyons, K. Desplaines, and E. Metzmann, *Clin. Chem.,* **36,** 1091 (abs. 653) (1990).

1788. J. Havelick, M. Fure, P. Gorham, E. Doenges, R. Baker, R. Saul, and E. Metzmann, *Clin. Chem.,* **36,** 1086 (abs. 627) (1990).

1789. S. Pothier, W. Gentzer, J. Bessette, J. Bowser, J. Natale, T. Rigl, R. Saul, and E. Metzmann, *Clin. Chem.,* **36,** 1095 (abs. 672) (1990).

1790. J. Bahar, U. Vaupel, A. Case, K. Farrell, S. Inbar, and E. Metzmann, *Clin. Chem.,* **36,** 1028 (abs. 359) (1990).

1791. T. Yamada, A. Matsui, and M. Yakata, *Clin. Chem.,* **36,** 1050 (abs. 459) (1990).

1792. M. Kanas, C. Wong, T. Saito-Wiedemann, and P. Sohmer, *Clin. Chem.,* **36,** 1208 (abs. 1196) (1990).

1793. B. Jeffery, T. Saito-Wiedemann, J. Pane, C. Wong, and P. Sohmer, *Clin. Chem.,* **36,** 1208 (abs. 1195) (1990).

1794. N. Y. Oraivej, C. Tsalta, and M. McCarthy, *Clin. Chem.,* **36,** 1159 (abs. 966) (1990).

1795. K. Kapsner, M. St. Cyr, and D. Smith, *Clin. Chem.,* **36,** 1162 (abs. 982) (1990).

1796. D. Fitzgerald, S. Hemker, G. Strand, D. Richter, D. Twumasi, and P. Wegfahrt, *Clin. Chem.,* **36,** 1148 (abs. 916) (1990).

1797. B. Simat, T. Peterson, M. Li, J. Dahl, and J. Prit, *Clin. Chem.,* **36,** 1029 (abs. 362) (1990).

1798. B. Simat, J. Dahl, M. Li, T. Peterson, G. Strand, P. Wegfahrt, L. Michels, P. Werness, M. St. Cyr, and D. Enfield, *Clin. Chem.,* **36,** 1039 (abs. 409) (1990).

1799. H. G. Noller, *Clin. Chem.,* **35,** 1209 (abs. 685) (1989).

1800. D. K. Vickery, C. J. Carlson, I. S. Masulli, Y. Tsang, P. M. Tuhy, and E. K. Yang, *Clin. Chem.,* **34,** 1200 (abs. 283) (1988).

1801. D. K. Vickery, C. J. Carlson, I. S. Masulli, S. Y. Tseng, and P. M. Tuhy, *Clin. Chem.,* **34,** 1219 (abs. 325) (1988).

1802. C. W. Benner and D. K. Vickery, *Clin. Chem.,* **34,** 1222 (abs. 337) (1988).

1803. E. G. Gorman, A. R. Briggs, C. C. Lee, I. S. Masulli, B. L. Strasser, and D. K. Vickery, *Clin. Chem.,* **34,** 1156 (abs. 019) (1988).

1804. E. G. Gorman, A. R. Briggs, C. J. Janes, C. C. Leflar, I. S. Masulli, and B. L. Strasser, *Clin. Chem.,* **34,** 1165 (abs. 059) (1988).

1805. T. J. Pankratz, C. C. Leflar, and W. F. Lorelll, *Clin. Chem.,* **34,** 1278 (abs. 616) (1988).

1806. D. J. Newman, E. Medcalf, E. G. Gorman, and C. P. Price, *Clin. Chem.,* **35,** 1205 (abs. 668) (1989).

1807. C.-C. Wang, M. Adamich, R. W. Bussian, R. Chairez, C. J. Lattomus, and G. J. Sam, *Clin. Chem.,* **34,** 1314 (abs. 790) (1988).

1808. G. J. Sam, *Clin. Chem.,* **34,** 1165 (abs. 060) (1988).

1809. M. Adamich, T. Hatfield, and D. Minn, *Clin. Chem.,* **34,** 1315 (abs. 792) (1988).

1810. R. W. Bussian and C. J. Lattomus, *Clin. Chem.,* **34,** 1315 (abs. 793) (1988).

1811. R. Diaco and W. J. Moran, *Clin. Chem.,* **34,** 1315 (abs. 794) (1988).

1812. N. V. Neelkantan, E. J. Friedlander, K. J. Friel, S. A. Hoover, H. P. Lau, I. S. Masulli, and B. L. Strasser, *Clin. Chem.,* **34,** 1211 (1988).

1813. S. J. Zoha, N. V. Neelkantan, H. P. Lau, I. S. Masulli, F. F. Spaven, and P. M. Tuhy, *Clin. Chem.,* **35,** 1202 (abs. 655) (1989).

1814. N. V. Neelkantan, S. Weston, and H. P. Lau, *Clin. Chem.,* **35,** 1202 (abs. 654) (1989).

1815. R. R. Chariton, C. J. Janes, A. A. Jarvis, C. C. Lee, I. S. Masulli, J. H. Nowland, M. C. Reider, D. M. Severino, D. M. Simons, and F. F. Spaven, *Clin. Chem.,* **34,** 1216 (abs. 311) (1988).

1816. B. R. Smith and R. Hall, *Methods Enzymol.,* **74,** 405 (1981).

1817. S. Jacobs and P. Cuatrecasas, *Methods Enzymol.,* **74,** 471 (1981).

1818. R. G. Drake and H. G. Friesen, *Methods Enzymol.,* **74,** 380 (1981).

1819. A. Floridi, *Methods Enzymol.,* **74,** 420 (1981).

1820. E. V. Jensen, S. Smith, and E. R. DeSombre, *J. Steroid. Biochem.,* **7,** 911 (1976).

1821. D. P. Edwards, G. C. Chamness, and W. L. McGuire, *Biochim. Biophys. Acta,* **560,** 457 (1979).

1822. D. P. Byar, M. E. Sears, and W. L. McGuire, *Eur. J. Cancer,* **15,** 299 (1979).

1823. K. Pettersson, R. Vanharanta, J. Söderholm, R. Punnonen, and T. Lövgren, *J. Steroid. Biochem.,* **16,** 372 (1982).

1824. W. P. Dandliker, A. N. Hicks, S. A. Levison, and R. J. Brawn, *Biochem. Biophys. Res. Commun.,* **74,** 538 (1977).

1825. S. A. Levison, W. P. Dandliker, R. J. Brawn, and W. P. Vanderlaan, *Endocrinol.,* **99,** 1129 (1976).

1826. B. G. Joyce, R. I. Nicholson, M. S. Morton, and K. Griffiths, *Eur. J. Cancer Clin. Oncol.,* **18,** 1147 (1982).

1827. G. H. Barrows, S. B. Stroupe, and J. D. Riehm, *Am. J. Clin. Pathol.,* **73,** 330 (1980).

1828. B. R. Rao, C. G. Fry, S. Hunt, R. Kuhmel, and W. P. Dandliker, *Cancer,* **46,** 2902 (1980).

1829. Y. J. Lee, A. C. Notides, Y.-G. Tsay, and A. S. Kende, *Biochemistry,* **16,** 2896 (1977).

1830. K. T. Brunner, J. Mauel, M. C. Cerottini, and B. Chapuis, *Immunology,* **14,** 181 (1968).

1831. H. S. Goodman, *Nature,* **190,** 269 (1961).

1832. G. Holm and P. Perlmann, *Immunology,* **12,** 525 (1967).

1833. J. Szekeres, A. S. Pacsa, and B. Pejtsik, *J. Immunol. Methods,* **40,** 151 (1981).

1834. C. Korzeniewski and D. M. Callewaert, *J. Immunol. Methods,* **64,** 313 (1983).

1835. S. L. Helfand, J. Werkmeister, and J. C. Roder, *J. Exp. Med.,* **156,** 492 (1982).

1836. J. C. Roder, S. L. Helfland, J. Werkmeister, R. McGarry, T. J. Beaumont, and A. Duwe, *Nature,* **298,** 569 (1982).

1837. K. McGinnes, G. Chapman, R. Marks, and R. Penny, *J. Immunol. Methods,* **86,** 7 (1986).

1838. D. Schols, R. Pauwels, F. Vanlangendonck, J. Balzarini, and E. De-Clercq, *J. Immunol. Methods,* **114,** 27 (1988).

1839. M. Brenan and C. R. Parish, *J. Immunol. Methods,* **112,** 121 (1988).

1840. S. E. Slezak and P. K. Horan, *J. Immunol. Methods,* **117,** 205 (1989).

1841. W. G. Wierda, D. S. Mehr, and Y. B. Kim, *J. Immunol. Methods,* **122,** 15 (1989).

1842. R. J. Brawn, C. R. Barker, A. D. Oesterle, R. J. Kelly, and W. B. Dandliker, *J. Immunol. Methods,* **9,** 7 (1975).

1843. K. Blomberg, C. Granberg, I. Hemmilä, and T. Lövgren, *J. Immunol. Methods,* **92,** 117 (1986).

1844. C. Granberg, K. Blomberg, I. Hemmilä, and T. Lövgren, *J. Immunol. Methods,* **114,** 191 (1988).

1845. T. Volgmann, A. Klein-Struckmeier, and H. Mohr, *J. Immunol. Methods,* **119,** 45 (1989).

1846. M. Ranki, A. Palva, A. Virtanen, and H. Söderlund, *Gene,* **21,** 77 (1983).

1847. A.-C. Syvänen, L. Laaksonen, and H. Söderlund, *Nucleic Acids Res.,* **14,** 5037 (1986).

1848. H. G. Pereira, *BioEssays,* **4,** 110 (1985).

1849. J. A. Matthews, A. Batki, C. Hynds, and L. J. Kricka, *Anal. Biochem.,* **151,** 205 (1985).

1850. L. J. Arnold, Jr., P. W. Hammond, W. A. Wiese, and N. C. Nelson, *Clin. Chem.,* **35,** 1588 (1989).

1851. D. Singh, V. Kumar, and K. N. Ganesh, *Nucleic Acids Res.,* **18,** 3339 (1990).

1852. M. S. Urdea, B. D. Warner, J. A. Running, M. Stempien, J. Clyne, and T. Horn, *Nucleic Acids Res.,* **16,** 4937 (1988).

1853. R. K. Saiki, S. J. Scharf, F. Faloona, K. B. Mullis, G. T. Horn, H. A. Erlich, and N. Arnheim, *Science,* **230,** 1350 (1985).

1854. P. O. Dahlén, P. J. Hurskainen, and T. N.-E. Lövgren, "Alternative Labels in DNA Hybridization," in A. Balows, R. C. Tilton, and A. Turano, Eds., *Rapid Methods and Automation in Microbiology and Immunology,* Brixia Academic Press, Brescia, 1989.

1855. P. R. Langer, A. A. Waldrop, and D. C. Ward, *Proc. Natl. Acad. Sci. USA,* **78,** 6633 (1981).

1856. A. C. Forster, J. L. McInnes, D. C. Skingle, and R. M. Symons, *Nucleic Acids Res.,* **13,** 745 (1985).

1857. G. H. Keller, D.-P. Huang, and M. M. Manak, *Anal. Biochem.,* **177,** 392 (1989).

1858. J. P. Ford, B. F. Erlanger, and C. W. Blewett, PCT Int. Patent Appl. WO 88/04,289 (1988).

1859. H. Arakawa, M. Maeda, A. Tsuji, and T. Takahashi, *Chem. Pharm. Bull.,* **37,** 1831 (1989).

1860. A. Giaid, Q. Hamid, C. Adams, D. R. Springall, G. Terenghi, and J. M. Polak, *Histochemistry,* **93,** 191 (1989).

1861. R. Shapiro and J. M. Weisgras, *Biochem. Biophys. Res. Commun.,* **40,** 839 (1970).

1862. B. A. Connolly and P. Rider, *Nucleic Acids Res.,* **13,** 4485 (1985).

1863. P. M. Nederlof, S. van der Flier, J. Wiegant, A. K. Raap, H. J. Tanke, J. S. Ploem, and M. van der Ploeg, *Cytometry,* **11,** 126 (1990).

1864. J. G. J. Bauman, J. Wiegant, P. van Duijn, *Histochem.,* **73,** 181 (1981).

1865. C. P. H. Vary, F. J. McMahon, F. P. Barbone, and S. E. Diamond, *Clin. Chem.,* **32,** 1696 (1986).

1866. G. L. Trainor and M. A. Jensen, *Nucleic Acids Res.,* **16,** 11864 (1988).

1867. I. C. Kilham, *Trends in Biotechnol.,* **5,** 332 (1987).

1868. L. M. Smith, S. Fung, M. W. Hunkapiller, T. J. Hunkapiller, and L. E. Hood, *Nucleic Acids Res.,* **13,** 2399 (1985).

1869. F. Schubert, K. Ahlert, D. Cech, and A. Rosenthal, *Nucleic Acids Res.,* **18,** 3427 (1990).

1870. A. J. Cocuzza, *Tetrahedron Lett.,* **30,** 6287 (1989).

1871. P. Dahlén, A. Iitiä, and M. Nunn, *Abstract of Papers Presented at the Sixth International Congress on Rapid Methods and Automation in Microbiology and Immunology,* No. 286, Espoo, Helsinki, Finland, June 1990.

1872. J. G. J. Bauman, J. Wiegant, and P. Van Duijn, *J. Histochem. Cytochem.,* **29,** 227 (1981).

1873. N. Harris and R. R. D. Croy, *Protoplasma,* **130,** 57 (1986).

1874. M. H. C. Bakkus, K. M. J. Brakel van Peer, H. J. Adriaanjen, A. F. Wierenga-Wolf, T. W. van den Akker, M. J. Dicke-Evinger, and R. Benner, *Oncogene,* **4,** 1255 (1989).

1875. P. M. Nederlof, D. Robinson, R. Abuknesha, J. Wiegant, A. H. N. Hopman, H. J. Tanke, and A. K. Raap, *Cytometry,* **10,** 20 (1989).

1876. M. S. Urdea, B. D. Warner, J. A. Running, M. Stempien, J. Clyde, and T. Horn, *Nucleic Acids Res.*, **16**, 4937 (1988).

1877. F. Coutlée, L. Bobo, K. Mayur, R. H. Yolken, and R. P. Viscidi, *Anal. Biochem.*, **181**, 96 (1989).

1878. F. Coutlée, R. H. Yolken, and R. P. Viscidi, *Anal. Biochem.*, **181**, 159 (1989).

1879. Y. Nagata, H. Yokota, O. Kosuda, K. Yokoo, K. Takemura, and T. Kikuchi, *FEBS Lett.*, **183**, 379 (1985).

1880. P. Pollard-Knight, A. C. Simmonds, A. P. Schaap, H. Akhavan, and M. A. W. Brady, *Anal. Biochem.*, **185**, 353 (1990).

1881. A. Murakami, J. Tada, K. Yamagata, and J. Takano, *Nucleic Acids Res.*, **17**, 5587 (1989).

1882. A.-C. Syvänen, P. Tchen, M. Ranki, and H. Söderlund, *Nucleic Acids Res.*, **14**, 1017 (1986).

1883. P. Dahlén, *Anal. Biochem.*, **164**, 78 (1987).

1884. P. Dahlén, A.-C. Syvänen, P. Hurskainen, M. Kwiatkowski, C. Sund, J. Ylikoski, H. Söderlund, and T. Lövgren, *Molec. Cellular Probes*, **1**, 159 (1987).

1885. P. Hurskainen, M. Tasanne, and H. Siitari, *Abstracts of Papers Presented at the Sixth International Symposium on Rapid Methods and Automation in Microbiology and Immunology,* No. 125, Espoo, Helsinki, Finland, July 1990.

1886. P. Dahlén, P. Hurskainen, T. Lövgren, and T. Hyypiä, *J. Clin. Microbiol.*, **26**, 2434 (1988).

1887. P. Buchert, P. Hurskainen, and H. Söderlund, *Abstracts of Papers Presented at the IIIrd International Symposium on Quantitative Luminescence Spectroscopy in Biomedical Sciences,* Ghent, Belgium, 1989.

1888. L. Huhtamäki, P. Hurskainen, H. Söderlund, C. Syvänen, P. Buchert, T. Lövgren, and H. Siitari, *Abstracts of Papers Presented at the Sixth International Symposium on Rapid Methods and Automation in Microbiology and Immunology,* No. 290, Espoo, Helsinki, Finland, July 1990.

1889. A. Iitiä, P. Dahlén, and M. Nunn, *Abstracts of Papers Presented at the Sixth International Symposium on Rapid Methods and Automation in Microbiology and Immunology,* No. 380, Espoo, Helsinki, Finland, July 1990.

1890. O. Prat, E. Lopez, G. Mathis, and E. J. P. Jolu, *Abstracts of Papers Presented at the Sixth International Symposium on Rapid Methods and Automation in Microbiology and Immunology,* No. 294, Espoo, Helsinki, Finland, July 1990.

1891. M. J. Heller, E. Hennessy, J. L. Ruth, and E. Jablonski, *Fed. Proc.*, **46**, 1968 (1987).

1892. R. P. Ekins, *J. Pharmaceut. Biomed. Anal.*, **7**, 155 (1989).

1893. R. Ekins, F. Chu, and E. Biggart, *Anal. Chim. Acta*, **227**, 73 (1989).

1894. R. Ekins, *Fresenius J. Anal. Chem.*, **337**, 20 (1990).

1895. C. E. Denning, L. A. Schick, and R. C. Boguslaski, *Clin. Chim. Acta*, **98**, 5 (1979).

1896. M. K. Bluett, E. O. Reiter, G. E. Duckett, and A. W. Root, *Clin. Chem.*, **23**, 1644 (1977).

1897. C. J. Beinlich, J. A. Piper, J. C. O'Neal, and O. D. White, *Clin. Chem.*, **31**, 2014 (1984).

1898. T. S. Baker, R. J. Holdsworth, and W. F. Coulson, "The Dual Analyte Assay for the Detection of the Fertile Period in Woman," in J. Bonner and V. Thompson, Eds., *Research in Family Planning,* MTP Press, Lancaster, 1984.

1899. E. A. Lenton, H. King, J. Johnson, and S. Amos, *Human Reprod.*, **4**, 378 (1989).

1900. S. P. Haynes and D. J. Goldie, *Ann. Clin. Biochem.*, **14**, 12 (1977).

1901. R. K. Desal, W. M. Deppe, R. J. Norman, T. Govender, and S. M. Joubert, *Clin. Chem.*, **34**, 1488 (1988).

1902. C. Blake, M. N. Al-Bassam, B. J. Gould, V. Marks, J. W. Bridges, and C. Riley, *Clin. Chem.*, **28**, 1469 (1982).

1903. D. A. Weerasekera, J. B. Kim, G. J. Barnard, and W. P. Collins, *J. Steroid. Biochem.*, **18**, 465 (1983).

1904. T. P. Gillis and J. J. Thompson, *J. Clin. Microbiol.*, **8**, 351 (1978).

1905. K. Pachmann and D. Killander, *Immunol. Lett.*, **13**, 301 (1986).

1906. K. Mossberg and M. Ericsson, *J. Microscopy,* **158**, 215 (1990).

1907. Y. Harabuchi, S. Koixumi, T. Osato, N. Yamanaka, and A. Kataura, *Virology,* **165**, 278 (1988).

1908. G. Pizzolo and M. Chilosi, *Am. J. Clin. Pathol.*, **82**, 44 (1984).

1909. M. R. Chapple, G. D. Johnson, and R. J. Davidson, *J. Immunol. Methods,* **111**, 209 (1988).

1910. J.-P. Aubry, I. Durand, P. De Paoli, and J. Banchereau, *J. Immunol. Methods,* **128**, 39 (1990).

1911. R. Festin, A. Björklund, and T. H. Tötterman, *J. Immunol. Methods,* **126**, 69 (1990).

1912. R. R. Hardy, K. Hayakawa, D. R. Parks, and L. A. Herzenberg, *Nature,* **306**, 270 (1983).

1913. D. R. Parks, R. R. Hardy, and L. A. Herzenberg, *Cytometry,* **5**, 159 (1984).

1914. E. F. Srour, T. Leemhuis, L. Jenski, R. Redmond, and J. Jansen, *Cytometry,* **11**, 442 (1990).

1915. R. K. Sinijärv, L. V. Järvekülg, and M. J. Saarma, *Dokl. VASHNIL,* **8**, 16 (1988).

1916. X. Zhao, H. Fei, K. Tian, and T. Li, *J. Luminescence,* **40 & 41**, 286 (1988).

1917. E. Soini, I. Hemmilä, and P. Dahlén, *Ann. Biol. Clin.*, **48**, 567 (1990).

1918. R. Vihko and L. Koskinen, *Clin. Chem.*, **27**, 1744 (1981).

1919. T. K. Dhar, E. Voss, and M. Schöneshöfer, *J. Steroid Biochem.*, **25**, 423 (1986).

INDEX